The Psychology and Physiology of Breathing

In Behavioral Medicine,
Clinical Psychology, and
Psychiatry

THE PLENUM SERIES IN BEHAVIORAL PSYCHOPHYSIOLOGY AND MEDICINE

Series Editor:
William J. Ray, *Pennsylvania State University, University Park, Pennsylvania*

BIOLOGICAL BARRIERS IN BEHAVIORAL MEDICINE
Edited by Wolfgang Linden

ELECTRODERMAL ACTIVITY
Wolfram Boucsein

HANDBOOK OF RESEARCH METHODS IN CARDIOVASCULAR
BEHAVIORAL MEDICINE
Edited by Neil Schneiderman, Stephen M. Weiss, and Peter G. Kaufmann

INTERNATIONAL PERSPECTIVES ON SELF-REGULATION
AND HEALTH
Edited by John G. Carlson and A. Ronald Seifert

PHYSIOLOGY AND BEHAVIOR THERAPY
Conceptual Guidelines for the Clinician
James G. Hollandsworth, Jr.

THE PHYSIOLOGY OF PSYCHOLOGICAL DISORDERS
Schizophrenia, Depression, Anxiety, and Substance Abuse
James G. Hollandsworth, Jr.

THE PSYCHOLOGY AND PHYSIOLOGY OF BREATHING
In Behavioral Medicine, Clinical Psychology, and Psychiatry
Robert Fried with Joseph Grimaldi

SOCIAL SUPPORT AND CARDIOVASCULAR DISEASE
Edited by Sally A. Shumaker and Susan M. Czajkowski

The Psychology and Physiology of Breathing

In Behavioral Medicine, Clinical Psychology, and Psychiatry

Robert Fried

Hunter College
City University of New York
and
Institute for Rational-Emotive Therapy
New York, New York

With

Joseph Grimaldi

University of Massachusetts Medical Center
Worcester, Massachusetts

Plenum Press • *New York and London*

Library of Congress Cataloging-in-Publication Data

Fried, Robert.
    The psychology and physiology of breathing : in behavioral
medicine, clinical psychology, and psychiatry / Robert Fried, with
Joseph Grimaldi.
        p.   cm. -- (The Plenum series in behavioral psychophysiology
and medicine)
    Includes bibliographical references and index.
    ISBN 0-306-44278-7
    1. Breathing.   2. Hyperventilation--Psychosomatic aspects.
3. Asthma--Psychosomatic aspects.   4. Medicine and psychology.
I. Grimaldi, Joseph. II. Title. III. Series.
    [DNLM: 1. Respiration--physiology. 2. Respiratory--physiology.
3. Psychophysiology.   WF 102 F899p 1993]
QP121.F77 1993
612.2--dc20
DNLM/DLC
for Library of Congress   93-512
                                                                CIP

ISBN 0-306-44278-7

© 1993 Plenum Press, New York
A Division of Plenum Publishing Corporation
233 Spring Street, New York, N.Y. 10013

Printed in the United States of America

To Den (Commander S.), who astutely observed that
"people are like clouds, hundreds passing without recognition,"
in a haiku composed in the sixth grade;
to Steve (Bones), who fashioned designer genes—for bacteria;
and to Paul (Kabloona), who explained the Truman Doctrine to me
as we hurtled over precipitous mountain roads in Pozo.

Foreword

This is Robert Fried's third book on the crucial role of breathing and hyperventilation in our emotional and physical health. The first, *The Hyperventilation Syndrome* (1987), was a scholarly monograph, and the second, *The Breath Connection* (1990a), was a popular version for the lay reader. This book combines the best features of both and extends Dr. Fried's seminal work to protocols for clinical psychophysiology and psychiatry. Hoping to avoid misunderstanding, he has taken systematic care to introduce relevant electrical, physiological, and psychological concepts in operational language for the widest possible professional audience.

Any clinician not thoroughly experienced in respiratory psychophysiology and biofeedback will leave these pages with profound new insight and direction into an aspect of our lives which we innocently take for granted as "common sense"—the role of breathing in health and illness. Einstein viewed such common sense as "that set of prejudices we acquired prior to the age of eighteen." I am impressed that Dr. Fried mirrors Einstein's uncanny genius in not accepting the obvious—breathing is not "common sense" but, rather, is a pivotal psychophysiological mechanism underlying all aspects of life.

The "common sense" that Dr. Fried explores has deceptive roots in history. Hippocrates anticipated Dr. Fried's focal interest some 2,500 years ago in observing that "breathing is the basic rhythm of life." Actually, this observation *was* common sense since the Greeks accepted the intertwined relationship of psyche and soma in a common etymological structure of two expressions: *phren* was used to denote the diaphragm as well as the mind, and *pneuma* represented the vital essence of life as well as breath or air. Any imbalance was used as a basis to explain disease.

Virtually every philosophical system seeking to comprehend human nature since earliest recorded history views breathing as a crucial central link between mind and body. The Old Testament makes the link in describing mankind's creation, where body precedes sustaining breath:

> And God formed man of the dust of the ground and breathed into his nostrils the breath of life, and man became a living soul.
>
> Genesis 2:7

Most yogic systems, which superficially vary in theory and technique, incorporate a common underlying structural assumption that life (mind-body) is a regenerative "given" that may be altered for health or illness through proper or improper breathing.

Ancient wisdom about the importance of "proper breathing" is largely ignored in modern medical practice. We are enthralled by the technological marvels of scientific diagnosis, medication, and surgery. We treat respiratory problems with medication or mechanical assistance such as intermittent positive pressure breathing (IPPB) delivered by a machine. We are taught to treat globus hystericus and its many variants that occur along a continuum from anxiety to panic disorders with medications and/or paper bag rebreathing to increase retention of carbon dioxide without instructing patients in the self-regulation of respiratory dynamics. Ironically, we use hyperventilation to activate and detect brain-wave abnormalities such as epilepsy. Yet normal breathing apparently has been overlooked as a serious subject for modern medical diagnosis and therapeutics. Astute physicians, however, recognize that shallow breathing or hyperventilation is an epiphenomenon, if not an etiologic factor, in 50% to 70% of medical complaints.

Proper breathing is taught in anticipation of natural childbirth and is an important foundation in training vocalists and wind instrument players. Various modalities of biofeedback, sometimes referred to as "scientific yoga of the West," when properly applied, probably exert their most significant nonspecific effect in normalizing breathing patterns. Dr. James Lynch, in *The Language of the Heart*, identified the disruption in breathing accompanying human dialogue as an incipient factor in the 90% of high blood pressure cases previously identified as idiopathic, or "cause unknown."

Dr. Fried ingeniously ties all of these leads together with scientific rigor. He couples a scholarly and rational overview with an operational treatment procedure that satisfies patients, their physicians, and other health-care professionals. For the first time, he validates "faulty breathing" as the etiologic "common pathway" that may be corrected by yoga, meditation, exercise, relaxation, biofeedback, and a variety of other nonmedical techniques used to normalize health. He accomplishes this by using a perspicacious multivariate experimental design that incorporates physiological measurements (respiration rate, respiration mode and pattern, endtidal carbon dioxide, blood oxygen concentration, cardiorespiratory synchrony, electromyography, electroencephalography, and a thermal index of peripheral vascular tone) to establish his case for the crucial role of the hyperventilation syndrome in many medical conditions. He takes heed of the following critical issues raised by Darrow (1943):

> To attain significance a test of autonomic functions must circumvent the mutually antagonistic action of the two branches of the autonomic nervous system so that it may be clear whether an observed peripheral event is due to increase of activity in one branch of the autonomic system or to decrease of activity in the other. There must be no question for example whether an observed pupillary dilation is due to sympathetic excitation or to inhibition of the parasympathetically determined irido-constrictor tone. The problem is literally to determine the weight on either side of a "balance" when neither side is known. The mere knowledge that the balance has been upset by a given condition as afforded by many so-called tests of autonomic function, may be physiologically or clinically of little value except as indication that something has been disturbed. It does not necessarily define the foregoing events in the neural and neurohumoral systems, and in consequence may even be misleading in determining proper corrective procedures. . . . This may explain the sterility which, with few exceptions, has beset attempts to correlate measurements of peripheral autonomic changes with human "behavior." (Quoted from a more detailed explanation in Stroebel, C. F. (1972). Psychophysiological pharmacology. In Greenfield, N. S. & R. A. Sternback (eds.), *Handbook of Psychophysiology*. New York: Holt, Rinehart and Winston.

Before this book, there were many disparate and ornamentally embellished pathways which promised to lead us to the peak of optimal health. But Dr. Fried has identified one direct "final common pathway": *stressed and distressed people hyperventilate*. Like Einstein, he has changed our frame of reference, providing a scientific rationale and treatment protocol for better understanding and for altering the increasingly stressful course of human existence.

CHARLES F. STROEBEL, M.D., Ph.D.

Old Wethersfield, Connecticut

Preface

In 1982, I took a two-year leave from Hunter College, CUNY, to direct the Rehabilitation Research Institute, ICD-International Center for the Disabled, New York. My main objective, supported by a grant from the JM Foundation, was to establish a model program for biobehavioral control of idiopathic epileptic seizures in persons whose disorder was intractable to anticonvulsant medication. What followed was an odyssey through the clinical and research literature on the physiology of respiration because, as I gradually learned, respiration controls blood flow through the brain and therefore its metabolism, neuronal activity, and seizure thresholds. It gradually dawned on me that insufficient tissue oxygen (hypoxia) seemed to underlie other somatic and psychological disorders of concern to behavioral clinicians.

My findings on the effects of breathing, especially hyperventilation, on brain waves, and seizure frequency and severity replicated the data in hundreds of medical physiology studies whose illustrious authors—the Gibbses, Lennoxes, Sargant, Schwab, Penfield, Jasper, Meyer, and many more—are held in awe to this day in traditional neurology circles. I summarized these studies in a scholarly monograph, *The Hyperventilation Syndrome* (Johns Hopkins University Press Series in Contemporary Medicine and Public Health, 1987) which is now out of print. *The Breath Connection* (Plenum Press, 1990) followed. It was intended for the "educated public" (snobbishly said to refer to those who read *The New York Times*).

Now, it is 1993, and I have been at it for over ten years. There is no end in sight. I have become a little less naive about the specificity of physiology in the scheme of things, and I have learned that it is possible to predict reliably some behavioral outcomes despite considerable ambiguity about why things work as they do. This conclusion has led me to expand what I considered important in an extension and update of the previous work.

You will find much in this book that appeared in *The Hyperventilation Syndrome*, but this is by no means only an updated version of that book. For one thing, it is increasingly clear that since many somatic, affective, and psychopathological conditions may stem from hypoxia caused by certain breathing characteristics, we need to know about blood—the medium of respiratory gas transport in the body. So I have added some discussion about that. Because the cardiovascular system moves blood around, and the kidneys keep it viable, I have added something about that also. There have been numerous innovations in computerized assessment of psychophysiological modalities, and it is especially here that my collaboration with Joe Grimaldi has been most productive. Because it is the clinical value of the methodology of objective physiological assessment (Chapter 5), and in the later chapter on assessing the progress of treatment (Chapter 9), on the basis of which the book may ultimately succeed or fail. We are also the first to introduce routine clinical psychophysiological evaluation of alveolar (lung) CO_2 by infrared capnometry, and blood O_2 levels by oximetry, and to integrate CO_2 and O_2 monitoring in therapeutic self-regulation strategies—now made possible by affordable instrumentation.

The discussion of treatment methods has been expanded so that this book may serve virtually everyone in the clinical behavioral sciences. In a few areas the material is very dense and complex, directed toward those with advanced training. In most areas, however, the material is simple, and the methods are detailed step-by-step according to the needs of most clinicians. These practitioners treat clients with complaints running the gamut from "psychosomatic" disorders—such as hypertension, migraine, and colitis—and psychological disorders—including anxiety, panic, and depression—to organic breathing disorders such as asthma.

Finally, after more than ten years of intense study, it is clear that some givens in the psychology and physiology of breathing are fanciful, some are misleading, and some are outright wrong. The many of you who know me will not be astonished when I offer no apology where I say so.

Acknowledgments

Many persons have contributed something to this book. Some contributions were spiritual, others were tangible—and some, thank God, were helpful. For instance, my editor at Plenum, Eliot Werner, bravely overcame his reluctance to accept this manuscript for publication and, for all I know, may yet be hoping at the eleventh hour for a fortuitous reprieve. Thank you, Eliot.

I will be forever indebted to Virginia L. Cutchin, my wife, for the countless hours (actually months) lovingly devoted to the production of this book. Her typing and editorial skills are beyond comparison. I thought I knew something about computerized biofeedback until I met the maven, Joe Grimaldi, Ph.D. It is really a marvel to watch Joe at work: First, he sits contemplating at the keyboard—like Paderewski—then he frowns and devours several hundred eucalyptus drops. When the camphor reaches a critical mass, there is a flurry of keypresses, and a new configuration emerges on the screen. You did it again, Joe! Thank you. This book would not have been written were it not for his contribution.

I thank my mentors, friends, and colleagues at the Institute for Rational Emotive Therapy, New York—Albert Ellis, Ph.D.; Janet Wolfe, Ph.D.; Ray DiGiuseppe, Ph.D.; Dom Dimatia, Ph.D.; Gina Vega; and the directors of the Institute—for their help, their patience with me, and the financial support in the form of grants to purchase equipment for the Biofeedback and Stress Clinic.

It would have been extremely difficult for me to carry out this project without the help and support of Jan Hoover of J & J Instruments in Poulsbo, Washington. When the idea of revising *The Hyperventilation Syndrome* came up, I realized that the instrumentation I had described was antediluvian. To produce a practical guideline, I needed to experiment with every component of a standard and commonly used physiological monitoring interface unit. The obvious choice was the J & J I-330 Physiological Monitoring System. When I proposed this idea to Jan, he unhesitatingly volunteered to contribute a complete set of interface modality units and other hardware, and the appropriate computer software (Physiodata). Thank you, Jan.

My enthusiasm for the use of the OxiCap 4700 to measure end-tidal CO_2 and arterial O_2 saturation must have overwhelmed Judy Stechert and Scott Vierke of Ohmeda in Louisville, Colorado. Ohmeda generously donated a unit to the project.

Once again, I thank Chuck Stroebel, M.D., Ph.D., for reviewing the manuscript and expressing his unabashed support of my work in the Foreword. A number of others also reviewed the manuscript, or segments of it, and made valuable suggestions that are incorporated into it. Among them, in alphabetical order, are K. Naras Baht, M.D. (Fairfield, California); Paul M. Lehrer, Ph.D. (Robert Wood Johnson Medical School); Peter G. F. Nixon, M.D. (Charring Cross Hospital, London); and Erik Peper, Ph.D. (San Francisco State University).

I wish also to express my gratitude for permission to reproduce charts, graphs, figures, or text from the following publishers or other sources:

American College of Physicians, Philadelphia, Pennsylvania
American Medical Association, Chicago, Illinois
American Physiology Society, Bethesda, Maryland
Appleton Lange, East Norwalk, Connecticut
Aspen Publishers, Gaithersburg, Maryland
Blackwell Scientific Publications, Oxford, United Kingdom
The BOC Group, Louisville, Colorado
British Medical Association, London, United Kingdom
Cambridge University Press, Cambridge, United Kingdom
CRC Press, Boca Raton, Florida
European Respiratory Journal, Sheffield, United Kingdom
Federation of American Societies for Experimental Biology, Bethesda, Maryland
Hans Huber Publishers, Bern, Switzerland
Harper & Row, New York, New York
HarperCollins, New York, New York
J. B. Lippincott, Philadelphia, Pennsylvania
Mosby Year Book Medical Publications, St. Louis, Missouri
Pergamon Press, Elmsford, New York
Prentice Hall, Englewood Cliffs, New Jersey

Rockefeller University Press, New York, New York
W. B. Saunders, Philadelphia, Pennsylvania
Uitgeverij Eisma B. V., The Netherlands

Finally, I am indebted to Lynn Krasner Morgan, Director of the Levy
Library, Mount Sinai Medical Center, New York, for permitting me and my
research assistants to use the library.

A note of caution to the reader

Persons with seemingly functional breathing disorders may be referred to nonmedical psychotherapists for treatment. You are cautioned that these conditions may not be functional. Hyperventilation, for instance, may compensate serious metabolic disorders of the acid–base balance—possibly caused by heart disease, diabetes, or kidney failure. Alternately, there may be blood disorders, lung disease, lesions, or other disorders of brain regulation centers. Consequently, you should not undertake to treat anyone until a medical examination has determined that behavioral alteration of breathing is not contraindicated. Organic breathing disorders should be treated only with the approval of a competent medical specialist.

This book does not claim to teach medical diagnoses or treatments. Guidelines and treatment strategies are meant to acquaint you with procedures currently available and the manner in which they may be executed. There are numerous individual differences and unknown conditions in persons with breathing disorders, and there are regional variations in the rules which govern the practice of therapy. Therefore, I cannot endorse, or take responsibility for, any diagnosis or treatment you may make on the basis of the guidelines in this book.

Contents

Chapter 1

Introduction

An Essay Concerning Human Misunderstanding

It is ambition enough to be employed as an under-laborer in clearing the ground a little, and removing some of the rubbish that lies in the way of knowledge.
—JOHN LOCKE

In the foreword to *The Hyperventilation Syndrome* (1987a), Charles F. Stroebel first compared my work to that of Hippocrates and Einstein—favorably, thank God! Some say that was too much for me and that my head is still swollen. With due modesty I would, of course, argue otherwise. But, I might add, to balance the picture, that there is still no consensus regarding either his welcome compliment or the book.

Typically, criticisms of the book centered on a number of issues, not the least of which was that I proposed idiosyncratic hypotheses—*panic* was a case in point: One reviewer thought the theory I endorsed bizarre because it leaned on reports that panic was associated with the constriction of brain arteries, and reduced brain blood flow, observed in most persons when hyperventilating. And though most agree that panic sufferers hyperventilate, they may not agree that this is etiological in panic.

I pulled my punches then. Panic has also been likened to at least one other condition in which the etiology is believed to be related to hyperventilation (HV) and reduced brain blood flow—idiopathic epileptic seizures; Tucker et al. (1986) reported panic in 70% of patients with temporal lobe disorder. Edlund et al. (1987) and Volkow et al. (1986) also found seizure activity in panic sufferers with temporal lobe EEG abnormalities; and Weilburg et al. (1987) suggested a "common neural mechanism" underly-

1

ing seizures and panic attacks. Reiman et al. (1984) appear to be the first investigators to show definitively that panic sufferers have significantly reduced blood flow (oligemia) in a specific region of the brain, the parahippocampus.

Other critics of the book called my persistent suggestion that EEG fundamental frequency may primarily represent brain arterial vasomotor activity rather than that of brain neurons a "fringe" theory. Why? Berger (1929) thought it to be the mechanism underlying the EEG; Wilder Penfield (1933) thought it responsible for seizures: "The vasomotor spasms and changes seen so characteristically in the cerebral cortex of epileptics are due to vasomotor reflexes" he asserted (p. 310). Bremer (1938) thought otherwise—the former were overruled!

When it comes to the psychology, physiology, and related phenomena of breathing, we are sometimes remarkably naive, some launching head-first in support of popular hypotheses as though these were proven by science. This is understandable considering that many of us do not have the means to verify them. We have little alternative but to rely on the conclusions of researchers in the field. This point is nowhere better illustrated than in the controversy over the role of hyperventilation versus lactate in panic disorder discussed in Chapter 7. But paradoxically, some hold that research on hyperventilation, for instance, "is being stifled, limited, narrowed by the overdominance of the researcher" (Fensterheim, 1989). Would that it were so! It is hard work and often frustrating to sort out fact from nonsense about the physiology and psychology of breathing. More systematic effort by researchers would be most welcome, certainly not less!

Then again, well-documented effects of various forms of breathing are still so poorly understood that, in many quarters, they are still considered controversial, though they have been reported in medical publications since the 1920s. The following item appeared in the "Correspondence" section of *JAMA* (vol. 147, p. 182), in 1951:

ALKALOSIS AND HYPERVENTILATION
To the Editor:—In the July 21, 1951, edition of The Journal of the American Medical Association, page 1125, in the article on "Alkalosis Due to Hyperventilation" the authors, Sattler, Marquardt, and Cummins, state, "A review of the literature reveals no clinical reports of hyperventilation alkalosis." In the April 22, 1922 (p. 1193) edition of The Journal, I described several cases of hyperventilation alkalosis in an article entitled "Clinical Tetany by Forced Respiration." In the June 1920, edition of the *American Journal of Physiology*, Grant and I first described the production of tetany by voluntary hyperventilation.

It was penned by Alfred Goldman, a pioneer in this field.

Here are five articles published in English before 1951, located quickly and easily, each with a title that readily identifies a concern with alkalosis:

Carryer, H.M. (1943). Syndrome of hyperventilation with tetany: Report of a case. *Proceedings of the Staff Meetings of the Mayo Clinic*, 18:522.

Fowweather, F.S., Davidson, C.L., & Ellis, L. (1940). Spontaneous hyperventilation tetany. *British Medical Journal*, 11:373–376.

The classic:

Kerr, W.J., Dalton, J.W., & Gliebe, P.A. (1937). Some physical phenomena associated with the anxiety states and the relationship to hyperventilation. *Annals of Internal Medicine*, 11:961–992.

and

McCance, R.A. (1932). Spontaneous overbreathing tetany. *Quarterly Journal of Medicine*, 1:247–255.

Schultzer, P. & Lebel, H. (1939). Spontaneous hyperventilation tetany. *Acta Medica Scandinavica*, 101:303–314.

Five articles from many dozens, all readily accessible in major journals. Where were Sattler and colleagues looking?

In 1983, Dent, Yates, and Hignbottam asked, "Does the hyperventilation syndrome exist?" in the *Proceedings of the British Thoracic Society*. They argued that 70% of HV cases referred to them for treatment were misdiagnosed. Among alternate diagnoses were allergic reactions (atopic), thyrotoxicosis, asthma, and hypothyroidism. As for the remaining, "30% of this group were nonatopic and had no evidence of asthma or hypothyroidism; *the cause of their breathlessness remains unclear*" (italics added).

One would suppose that, being pulmonary physicians, the first thing they did to disprove HV was to cite alveolar or blood carbon dioxide (CO_2) concentration, but there is no such reference. Yet, in their references they cite Evans and Lum (1977), and Pincus (1978), where blood and alveolar carbon dioxide (CO_2) levels in HV are clearly mentioned. What should we make of this? Fortunately, some, like Gardner et al. (1992), propose that arterial blood gas should be taken routinely.

Another example: Just the other day, a news program informed us that epilepsy is "an electrical disease of the brain"; that massive electrical discharges during seizures "cause" epilepsy. This is akin to saying that a fever causes malaria. Where is the logic? Can massive electrical discharge of the brain be anything but the end-product of metabolic disorder?

Clinical neurologists early on noted that disordered breathing was reliably associated with epilepsy and abnormal EEG; that is why HV is still used routinely to evoke abnormal brain waves in neurological and EEG examination. So, is it really unusual to suggest that seizures might be *due to* brain arteries constricting in response to low CO_2 when it has been reportedly observed to do so in HV (Darrow & Graf, 1945; Penfield & Jasper, 1954)?

Some years ago (Fried, Rubin, Carlton, & Fox, 1984a,b; Fried, Fox, & Carlton, 1990), I reported that *percentage of end-tidal CO$_2$* (PETCO$_2$) biofeedback seems to make a major dent on idiopathic seizure frequency and severity, an outcome predicted by previous *metabolic* theories of idiopathic seizures (Meyer & Gotoh, 1960). Since PETCO$_2$ biofeedback is simple and relatively inexpensive, I figured that other investigators would try it, at least to protect *electrogenic* theory. To my astonishment, the study sank out of sight without making a ripple.

The few in the neurophysiology community who bothered to criticize the study expressed doubt about the connection between hypocapnia (low blood CO$_2$), brain blood flow, abnormal EEG, and seizures. The funny thing about this is that no one seemed aware that Schwab et al. (1941) reported on "regulation of the treatment of epilepsy by synchronized recording of respiration and brain waves," a direct though distant antecedent of my CO$_2$ biofeedback study.

One of the conclusions of that study was that the minute respiratory volume and the *delta* index show clearly the effect of change in breathing on the brain wave pattern preceding the seizure (p. 1033). The *delta* index is what we now call *theta*, the occurrence of any frequency lower than 7 Hz—usually associated with a seizure. (The authors of this study were affiliated with Harvard Medical School, Massachusetts General Hospital, and The Maudsley Hospital, London. One of them was a Fellow of the Rockefeller Foundation. The article appeared in *Archives of Neurology and Psychiatry*.)

Recent technical leaps in computerized EEG topography make it possible to see the power spectrum composition of various brain regions. Since *theta* has been consistently shown to correlate with local blood flow, it would seem logical to use the EEG to infer local metabolism. I have never been able to get a single article about *theta* as an inference about brain blood flow past a journal editor. They simply don't believe it. Yet, it has been right there in their literature for years. How is this to be explained?

The ever so aptly named Lord Brain (1964), one of the world's most respected neurologists, pronounced epilepsy to be an electrical problem:

There seems no doubt, however, that whatever its immediate or remote cause, an epileptic attack is the manifestation of a paroxysmal discharge of abnormal electrical rhythms in some parts of the brain. (p. 129)

"A paroxysmal discharge of abnormal electrical rhythms?" That's the disease? Doesn't it matter how they got to be abnormal? Is " . . . whatever its immediate or remote cause?" a satisfactory etiology? Why not mention the connection to disordered breathing and its sequelae: hypocapnia, alkalosis, reduced cerebral blood flow and metabolism, paroxysmal vaso-spasm, *theta*, etc.

Electricity is not what makes the brain work or flounder. It is its *detritus*. And if you want to study brain function, you also need to study breathing and blood.

Blood is a tissue. It may look to you to be just a fluid coursing through veins and arteries, but blood, in the truest sense of the word, is a tissue—albeit a liquid one. It is a differentiated part of the body adapted for a special function. Unfortunately, behavioral physiologists typically don't study blood. Even when they read about homeostasis, they seldom see any reference to the most immediately critical of these "dynamic balances," blood acid-base balance (pH homeostasis).

In order to learn about breathing and its effect on the body and the mind, I propose that it is vitally important to also learn about the function of blood and the red blood cell, and the hemoglobin (Hb) molecule which transports oxygen (O_2) and CO_2 to and from body tissues. It is time that we knew as much about that cell, and the pH of its fluid environment, as we know about the neuron, because that information is much more useful: Whatever mishap befalls that red blood cell may well cause neurons to erupt in a "paroxysmal discharge of abnormal electrical rhythms," frantically lashing out, as it were, as they slowly asphyxiate. Breathing is the key to their regulation.

About This Book

In a recent "clinical supervision," part of my fellowship in Rational Emotive Therapy (RET), my supervisor said to another trainee, "Tell your client to 'take a deep breath now,' that will reduce his tension and anxiety." This is a very simple example, but it occurred to me, at that moment, that this was a good blend of the cognitive and behavioral, and I have found it extremely helpful to integrate psychophysiology with psychotherapeutic methods.

This book is about the connection between breathing and psychological, emotional, and stress-related disorders, with emphasis on their psychophysiological assessment and treatment. In other words, *the breath connection*! And so the title of Lowry's now classic text, *Hyperventilation and Hysteria* (1967), instantly comes to mind. Its subtitle, *The Physiology and Psychology of Overbreathing and Its Relationship to the Mind-Body Problem*, would have been the perfect title for this book.

I should point out that I have long recommended training in psychotherapy for biofeedback practitioners, and training in relaxation methods and biofeedback for psychotherapists. So with that in mind, I chose the title *The Psychology and Physiology of Breathing in Behavioral Medicine, Clinical Psychology, and Psychiatry*. This book is about breathing *and* psychophysiology in clinical psychology and psychiatry practice. Its primary objective is to detail techniques to evaluate breathing using common physiological monitoring methods and the reasons why you should do so if you are concerned with treating clinical syndromes.

Another objective of this book is to show you how you may integrate physiological monitoring methods into treatment strategies by self-regulation, some of which fall more or less within the general framework of biofeedback. Sometimes, in asthma for instance, breathing is the primary target of monitoring and treatment. In most cases, however, the primary concern may be your client's anxiety, blood pressure, migraine, or tension. Then, the focus may be on autonomic nervous system (ANS) arousal; breathing may be a secondary concern. Yet, as you will see, breathing cannot be separated from other physiological events.

I should also advise you that this book is *not* intended to be exhaustively comprehensive; nor does it aim at an uncritical presentation of what does and does not work in clinical practice. Rather, it transmits my experience with the most up-to-date and practical physiological evaluation and treatment skills. It is targeted at clinicians who are, like myself, concerned with the treatment of emotional, stress-related, and psychosomatic disorders. Perhaps it would be helpful to think of this book as the workshop I would present, given enough time to do so. I have chosen that "voice" to address you here.

Many of you have, in the past, commented favorably on *The Hyperventilation Syndrome* (1987a), but some also reported wincing at its density, and the limits to its translation into clinical practice. I try to correct this here by giving you more of my personal point of view and my reasons for approaching evaluation and treatment "philosophy" as I do. Unlike the previous book, intended to be a scholarly monograph, this book is more nearly didactic: a guide to applications—how to and why.

To achieve this end, it takes material from *The Hyperventilation Syndrome*, updates it, and integrates it—with a systematic look at state-of-the-art evaluation and treatment methods, standardized on the J & J Instruments I-330 System, for physiological monitoring (see Chapter 5). I am betting that the success of this approach will be greatly facilitated by the illustration of recording and biofeedback methods using an advanced system popular among researchers and practitioners because of its versatility, comparatively moderate cost, and ease of operation.

Clearly this book still weaves breathing through its fabric because this process underlies all other physiological modalities. For clinicians who apply psychophysiological methods in clinical practice, no physiological modality can make any sense if breathing is not simultaneously considered. Any segment of the ECG, for example, may be in phase with breath.

Respiration and Psychophysiology

The term "respiratory psychophysiology" is a misnomer: breathing is integral to all forms of physiological monitoring: hand temperature (Bacon & Poppen, 1985; Hertzman, 1959; Hertzman & Roth, 1942), the cardiovascular system (Cacioppo & Petty, 1982), the EEG (Rampil, 1984), and reaction time (Beh & Nix-James, 1974) are some examples. Therefore, the plan of this book is to provide a functional description of what relates to breathing and to integrate that knowledge with psychophysiological observations.

Clinical Psychophysiology

Behavioral physiology addresses physiological and mental factors operating when we adapt to each other and to the world we live in. Psychophysiology is one of its major tools. "Clinical" means the treatment of disorders in a client population. "Psychophysiology" is another matter. Perhaps *psychophysiometrics* might be a more accurate word because psychophysiologists are principally concerned with quantitative measures of physiology thought to be related to behavior.

Modern psychophysiological methods and techniques have some illustrious historical antecedents. Among them are such landmark events as the description by Fere (1888) and Tarchanoff (1890) of electrical characteristics of the skin. Einthoven perfected the string-galvanometer for the electrocardiograph in 1903; and Berger described the *alpha* rhythm in brain waves in 1929. What these pioneers have in common with us is a fascination with bioelectrical phenomena, i.e., the apparently electrical nature of living matter. It was a firmly held belief that the study of bioelectrical potentials held the key to understanding behavior and life, until modern advances in biochemistry cast doubt on it. This myth is most clearly recognizable in the popularity of the monster created electrically by Dr. Frankenstein . . . or, according to Gene Wilder, who portrayed him in a recent movie, "Frawnkensteen!"

Although few remember, John B. Dods (1852) was invited by the U.S. Congress to lecture on "The Philosophy of Electrical Psychology." That was heady stuff in its day, seeming to bridge the gap between science and magic. And in a way, psychophysiology attests to the fact that we haven't lost our fascination with the electrical nature of life. Though we have learned empirical applications of its many and varied forms, we are no closer to grasping its meaning. History is less precise about the origin of the thermometer, which also features prominently in the scheme of things. It is attributed to a colleague of Galileo, circa early 1600s.

Rapid advances in electronics technology, especially in the past ten years, have streamlined the observation of minute quantities of bioelectrical energy. This new precision in measurement has shown that variables which we held to be *discrete* may in fact be *continuous*, and that the sheer amount of data out there exceeds anything that can reasonably be analyzed by human senses. Computer technology has coupled high speed data time-sampling with high speed analysis in a way that would have seemed fanciful a mere 25 years ago. This is a remarkably rapid development when you consider that it took 70 years from the time of its invention before the zipper appeared on a pair of trousers.

Clinical psychophysiology is multivariate and alinear. It "sees" some of the characteristic muscle changes, and central and autonomic nervous system changes associated with varying degrees of arousal in normal persons, and in those with psychological, psychiatric, and somatic disorders. It usually, but not invariably, treats these disorders with biofeedback self-regulation of some physiological indications of homeostasis.

Electrical Psychology

Ancient Egyptians discovered electricity when they immersed two strips of metal in a clay jar containing vinegar. With the tip of the tongue in contact with the two strips, they experienced that well-known tingle. They had invented the battery! However, history does not record this as the occasion for the invention of the light bulb. Consequently, science remained in the dark!

It is not until the 18th century that Galvani rediscovered electricity (this is erroneously attributed to Volta). Galvani also discovered that living tissue has electrical properties, and he held that it coursed through the body in nerves, with the brain as its principal source. Thus, clinical psychophysiology evolved from no humble beginnings! In most cases, we now employ noninvasive measures of electrical activity to assess organ or tissue system function. These methods are indirect and deductive, and require a working knowledge of norms and expected values. For instance, the electromyograph (EMG) records electrical activity in muscle from which we infer muscle tension. But there are spontaneous electrical events in resting muscle fibers, quite independent of those produced by the compression of voluntary or reflex contraction. How do you tell them apart, and what do they tell us about tension (i.e., pressure)?

The electrocardiograph (ECG or EKG) records electrical activity of the heart. Some components are associated with the initiation of contraction cycles, while others result from those contractions. What do these electrical events tell us about what the heart is doing, or why?

The electroencephalograph (EEG) records electrical activity of the brain. Why do its components fall into coherent frequency "bands"? What are the characteristics of brain waves from which we may derive useful inferences about physiological or behavioral events? It is helpful to know something about the characteristics of bioelectricity and how it arises from living tissue, and how it is measured and recorded.

In other instances, electrical signals are used as analogs of physiological states. This is typically done by transducers.

Transducers

A transducer interfaces two systems. It converts energy from its original form in one system, to a form manageable by another. It is a functional connection between them. For instance, a capnometer determines concentration of alveolar CO_2 (see Chapter 5). Because CO_2 is not visible, we use a transducer which can "see" it, and translate its concentration to an electrical voltage analog displayed on a meter. We generally compile such direct and indirect measures of biological activity to help us evaluate the "psychology"—the other state of the client. We have also learned that such information may be an integral part of treatment strategies.

Some Rudiments of Electrobiopotentials

The minute electrical currents observed in resting and changing metabolic tissue activity are often the best means available to study them. You may find it useful to know some of the common terms and basic concepts in electrical phenomena, as well as the devices typically encountered in connection with psychophysiology and biofeedback technology. A rudimentary knowledge will usually do.

"Elektron" is the ancient Greek word for *amber*. It has been known for a long time that rubbing this material gives it the ability to attract small, lightweight particles. That attraction is due to *static* electricity, a flow of electrons. Any medium which allows the flow of electrons is called a conductor. Materials such as copper are good conductors while others, such as water, which do not conduct electricity, are called insulators. Water may become a conductor when an *electrolyte*, such as salt, is dissolved in it. An example of this is the gel squeezed on electrodes before applying them to a body surface. This "electrode-paste" is usually a neutral, hypoallergenic substance containing an electrolyte.

We generally believe that an atom is composed of a nucleus made up of protons and neutrons. Neutrons have no electrical charge. Protons have a positive charge. Electrons, which have a negative charge, orbit the nucleus. Protons and electrons are the basic particles that we understand to make up electric energy. Each element has an equal number of protons and electrons. By attracting each other, they tend to hold electrons in "orbit."

Any form of energy such as a magnetic field, or more commonly heat, may free electrons from their orbit around an atom. These "free electrons" then flow as a current if there is a suitable conductor. Current flow may also result from the application of pressure to the apex of a crystal (*piezoelectric*; piezo, for pressure). This is why we use crystals in phonograph cartridges. (It is also one of the sources of current from contracting muscles, including those of the heart.)

Direct Current (dc)

Chemical reactions such as those in the dry-cell battery can cause electrons to flow. The "metal-strip-in-the-vinegar-jar," cited above, is an example of a wet-cell battery, like that found in your car—the vinegar replaced by dilute sulfuric acid.

In the dry-cell, electrons may flow from a *cathode* (+) to an *anode* (−). The potential difference between them is expressed in *volts*, but is not realized until a conductor forms a pathway, or *circuit*, between them. The volt represents the *electromotive force* (emf), with which electrons are made to flow in a circuit. The number of electrons flowing is measured in *amperes*. Biologically generated electricity ranges from micro- to millivolts, and the current is typically measured in microamperes (micro is millionths, milli- is thousandths).

Materials vary in their ability to conduct electrical current. Superconducting materials are those that offer minimal *resistance* to electron flow when they are supercooled. Resistance to electron flow may be used to limit that flow, thereby converting some potential energy to heat. Resistance in a circuit is described by *Ohms law: emf = current × resistance*. It applies only to direct current circuits. The total opposition to current flow in an alternating current circuit is called *impedance*, also measured in ohms.

The Galvanometer

In the ECG, EMG, and EEG, for instance, organ electrical activity may be recorded, perhaps as an ink trace on a moving paper strip; or it might be recorded on magnetic tape for subsequent analysis. The essential integrity of the volt/time relationship is paramount. A transducer might yield an electrical output which is recorded because it captures an indirect volt/time measure of physiological functioning.

Every standard measure of electrobiopotentials is a direct descendant of galvanometer technology. The galvanometer consists of a coil of wire wound around an axis which may rotate on pivots. The axis is perpendicular to a magnetic field provided by a *permanent magnet*. An electric current causes the coil to rotate on its axis in the magnetic field, exerting a force against a "restoring" spring. The degree of deflection of the coil is proportional to the current flowing through it and is sufficiently linear for most applications. It may be calibrated with a pointer, or "needle," moving along a scale.

The pen movement in the polygraph is derived from this arrangement. A resistor "in series" with the coil converts the galvanometer from an ammeter to a voltmeter. A fixed voltage source can be used to calibrate the scale for the voltage decreases that occur with different resistances *in series* with the coil. This application converts the galvanometer to an ohmmeter.

Capacitance

A capacitor stores electrons, and therefore opposes voltage change. It consists, typically, of two conductor surfaces separated by a very narrow gap. It can function in several different ways: (a) If one conductor is charged, the other will charge by induction, like a car battery, but unlike the car battery when it reaches a certain threshold, it will discharge like a cloud in a lightning storm. Or (b) if both conductors are respectively connected to the cathode and anode of a dc source such as a battery, so as to maintain a potential difference between the conductor plates, one will acquire a determinable net positive charge, while the other will have an equal negative charge.

Nerve or muscle cell membranes mimic the capacitor: Ions passing through them can accumulate faster inside than they can leak out. Potassium and sodium are cations (+-charged), passing in and out of the cell through so-called *channels*, accumulating in different concentrations inside and outside the membrane.

Proteins in the cell are negatively charged. The cell membrane, being relatively impermeable to proteins, allows leakage of potassium and sodium and becomes negative inside, relative to outside, until a sort of equilibrium—the resting potential—is established at about −70 uv. You can readily see that this process must be crucially sensitive to the acid-base balance of the cellular and extracellular fluid since the pH is a measure of hydrogen ion (H+) concentration in those fluids.

One *farad*, the unit of *capacitance*, is equivalent to a potential difference of 1.0 v between the plates of the capacitor, at 1.0 amperes per second. Values of capacitance in practical electronic circuits and in biological systems are measured in microfarads.

Alternating Current (ac)

The direction of alternating current (ac) flow reverses periodically. Alternating current has practical and commercial advantages over dc: It can be "stepped up" to facilitate transmission over long power lines and then "stepped down" for local usage, resulting in far less *power* loss than would be the case in dc transmission. Power is determined by multiplying volts by amperes. Power is expressed in *watts*: $P = volts \times amps$.

The *frequency* of the current is the number of direction changes per second. The standard house-current frequency in the United States is 60 cycles per second, or 60 Hz. An oscilloscope permits visualization of the pattern of voltage change during a preset time period—voltage over time. For instance, household current is 115 vac, 60 Hz. With 1.0 second as a time base, 60 reversals, or cycles (Hz), will be displayed on the screen. With the time base at 0.1 second, there is enough space on the average oscilloscope screen for the pattern to reflect the form of one complete reversal cycle; that pattern is a *sine wave*.

Unlike dc, ac voltage is represented by one or more of four values. If the current is 12 vac, 60 Hz:
   (a) *peak* voltage: maximum point on a sine wave, 6 volts.
   (b) *peak-to-peak*: the voltage from maximum (+6 volts) to minimum on a sine wave (−6 volts), 12 vac.
   (c) *root-mean-square* (rms): for practical purposes, rms = 0.7071 × peak voltage; or 6 volts × 0.7071 = 4.24 vac.
   (d) *average*: for practical purposes, average voltage is 0.637 × peak voltage; or 0.637 × 6 volts = 3.82 vac.
Root-mean-square voltage helps to determine the heating value of ac equal in voltage to dc—dc has a greater heat potential, and it has other applications in electronics as well.

Rectifiers and Filters

Many circuits require *either* ac or dc voltage. One may change ac to dc with a *rectifier* which permits current to flow in only one direction. In a *half-wave* rectifier, one half of the alternation cycle is permitted to flow through the device. Consequently, ac is converted to pulsating dc. A *full-wave* rectifier usually employs four diodes so that current flows in the same direction during each half of the alternation cycle.

The rectification of ac results in pulsating dc which introduces a "ripple" effect not suitable to the operation of some circuits. Filters are designed to eliminate this "ripple" effect. *Band-pass* filters eliminate portions of the frequency spectrum present in a complex electric current. Depending on their quality and technical sophistication, band pass filters may be adjusted to eliminate components above or below a designated frequency range. Filtering is common in physiological monitoring because most organs emit complex signals which vary in frequency as well as in voltage.

It is not typically possible, when measuring biopotentials from any site on the body, to restrict the observation to a target organ, since virtually all organ signals can be picked up all over the surface of the body. For example, it is not uncommon to observe a cardiac pattern in the EEG, or in the EMG, though the signal amplitude may vary with electrode placement. Filtering is typically used to eliminate these unwanted signals, inexplicably called "artifacts," as well as 60 Hz radiation emanating from nearby appliances and lights.

Amplifiers

Monitoring biopotentials that may range from a few millionths to several thousandths of a volt requires something more sensitive than a galvanometer. An advantage of ac voltage is that it can easily be stepped-up to a higher value, but technical problems interfere with the use of a transformer when frequency is low. Effective increase in amplitude of these biopotentials is best accomplished with amplifiers.

Fluctuating biopotentials with a finite mean voltage, like those in the ECG, often have two components: a constant-amplitude, dc-component, equal to the mean of the signal, and fluctuations around a mean of zero. *Direct coupled amplifiers* reproduce both components, while *transformer coupled amplifiers* do not transmit dc.

In *linear amplifiers*, the output is directly proportional to the magnitude of the incoming bioelectric current. That means that a *gain* of 1000 multiplies the incoming voltage by 1000.

In a standard electrocardiograph, *lead-I* electrodes attached to each arm and one leg conduct biopotentials to an amplifier. The voltage is amplified so that it can deflect a pen movement. A built-in filter limits the frequency range of the biopotentials to those known to be from the heart proper. The pen movement translates the changing magnitude of the electrical activity of the heart to an ink-trace on a paper-strip chart which moves past the pen at a constant speed of 25 millimeters (mm) per second. The strip-chart is calibrated so that 1 centimeter of vertical pen excursion (10 mm) represent a voltage, at the source (the heart) of 100 millivolts. Horizontally, 1 mm represents 0.04 second (1 second/25mm) (Goldman, 1967) (see Chapter 5). The strip chart is overprinted in millimeters so that measuring excursions of the pen permit both time and voltage measurements of cardiac electrical activity. The height of a waveform represents its voltage, while its width represents its duration, or frequency.

The galvanometer and its descendant, the electromagnetic pen, are also mechanical amplifiers. The excursion of the pen attached to the coil rotating through an arc is proportional to its length: The longer the pen, the larger the excursion of its point for a given degree of rotation of the coil. Naturally, there are limits to mechanical amplifiers imposed by inertia and friction, but the conversion of the galvanometer to the pen was the first functional amplification of biopotentials making it also a transducer. It translates changes in an electric current to perceptible mechanical movement.

There are two common types of amplifiers used in electrophysiology: the *operational amplifier* (op-amp), and the *differential amplifier* (diff-amp). The op-amp is a high gain, linear *integrated circuit* operating in a wide range of frequencies, from dc. Its most common application was in analog computers (Fried, 1972, 1973), but it now largely replaces the transistor as a basic building block in electronic circuits. The differential amplifier, also a high gain linear amplifier, has two separate amplifiers with a common input (one inverting the signal) and a common output. Identical input signals, common to both recording sites, are not amplified due to *common mode rejection*, a characteristic of this system. The ratio of common mode gain (ideally zero) to common mode rejection (CMRR) may be as high as one million to one. Diff-amps are frequently encountered in psychophysiological monitoring and biofeedback. In a *nonlinear amplifier*, a constant signal is emitted by the unit whenever the incoming current reaches a preset threshold value. Such a device is sometimes called a "trigger."

Integration, Time-Series, and Sequential Dependency

Plotting change in voltage of a signal, over time, relative to a baseline, yields the *integral*. Its unit is volts per second (vsec). This is a common technique first implemented with a simple, though not very reliable, *rc* circuit—a resistor and capacitor coupled parallel to a fixed dc source. By selecting the proper combination of capacitor and resistor, a *time constant*—the rate at which the capacitor charges to its maximum value—could be calculated.

Biopotentials may contain fluctuating dc as well as higher frequency components, sometimes centering on a primary fundamental frequency which appears to have the greatest magnitude. For instance, the EEG may be observed to have a fundamental frequency, but, in fact, its dc component is usually overlooked. That is unfortunate because the dc component has been shown to correlate with differences in metabolism and CO_2 production (Cowen, 1967, 1974, 1976; Goldensohn, Schoenfeld, & Hoefer, 1951; Lechner, Geyer, Lugaresi, Martin, Lifshitz, & Markovich, 1967; Lugaresi & Coccagna, 1970).

Rhythm

Rhythm is an attribute of certain kinds of frequency distributions. It is related to an expectation that one or more events will repeat at more or less predictable time intervals. In the preface to *The Hyperventilation Syndrome* (Fried, 1987), C.F. Stroebel reminds us of the Hippocratic aphorism, "Breath is the rhythm of life." Breath was not the only rhythm which concerned the ancient Greeks. They also scrutinized the skies observing the cyclical seasonal changes in the pattern of the stars.

Rhythm is the more or less regular reappearance of events, or the recurrence of the alternating strong and weak elements in any phenomenon. Rhythm is intrinsic to everything that we know in the universe. It should, therefore, come as no surprise that it plays a significant role in physiology. It may take many forms. Frequently, it is embedded in "time-domain" data distributions—data which vary continuously with time, but whose value at any point in time is not independent of its immediate prior value. Our human electrobiopotentials typically constitute a continuous variable in the time-domain. In the immortal words of Shakespeare, "What's in the brain that ink may character which hath not figured to thee my true spirit?" (Sonnet CVIII). Berger (1929) observed that phenomenon in the form of *alpha* waves of the brain.

We tend to forget the limitations of the typical electromagnetic polygraph. For one thing, it doesn't "see" much above 40 Hz. Conclusion: There is nothing there. But as Fischer (1965) has so amply shown, you couldn't be more mistaken:

> Probably because of the history of research on neural electrical activity, especially the fact that the first recordings were made at frequencies of 30 c.p.s. and less, modern clinical EEG's are not adapted to reading much above that figure. Rather, the EEG . . . depends on changes in amplitude of a voltage rather than on frequency changes.

Hence, if voltages are low (10 to 30 microvolts) and frequencies are high (above 40 c.p.s.) there is a question as to how accurately the EEG can measure the brain's electrical activity. (col. 3)

Fischer recorded frequencies up to 120 Hz over the right posterior temporal area of the brain.

Doesn't it strike you as unusually fortuitous that EEG frequencies fall exclusively and conveniently into exactly those "bands" that electromagnetic pen movements can readily "see"? As it typically turns out, tradition dictates accepted practice: Modern EEG instruments are so designed that *despite* advanced electronics, they employ filters that "character" only those frequency components with which experts trained on electromagnetic pen movements are familiar. You can get past those filters, and if you do, you are in for a surprise. But that is by no means the whole story of biological rhythm. There is a definite revival of interest in this area, with the further development of a branch of mathematics, known as "nonlinear dynamics," first developed by Poincare in the 1880s. Nonlinear dynamics integrates mathematics and physiology, and is beyond the capability of most physiologists. However, basic concepts and conclusions are comprehensible to behavioral physiologists and merit consideration for their potential clinical insights.

Most life-variables are distributed in the time-domain (i.e., physiological observations are patterned over time). We note that these time-domain distributions may take the form of "steady states," "oscillations," "noise," and, more recently, "chaos" (Glass & Mackey, 1988). Physiological steady states are those that come to mind when we consider *homeostasis* (Cannon, 1932). Within limits, variations in the parts of a system are such that they result, functionally, in essentially the same ultimate outcome. In respiration, an example is the constant interaction between breathing rate, tidal volume, and resting basal metabolism in a normal person. Other factors being equal, small variations in any one of these occur almost continuously, yet any combination of the others will compensate the system. And, in fact, blood pH, critically dependent on this interaction, will show little variation even if there is a relatively significant momentary departure from the "typical" by any one component. Such a system can be described as a "multiple negative feedback" system.

Oscillations are regular, highly predictable repetitions. The EEG *alpha* rhythm is sometimes described as "8/second oscillations" because, to the naked eye, which cannot discriminate between similar frequencies traced on a polygraph strip chart, it appears almost as though it were a sine-wave compressed by an arbitrarily rapid chart speed.

Figure 1 shows 8 Hz sine-waves recorded on a polygraph paper stripchart running at four different speeds. The density of the waves varies inversely with speed. Figure 2 shows an EEG tracing recorded on the

8 HZ at 1 cm/sec

8 HZ at 2.5 cm/sec

8 HZ at 5 cm/sec

8 HZ at 10 cm/sec

Figure 1. 8-Hz trace at four different chart speeds.

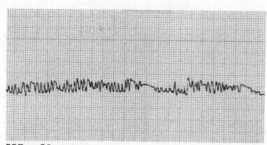

EEG at 25 mm/sec

EEG at 50mm/sec

Figure 2. EEG trace at two different chart speeds.

polygraph strip-chart at two different speeds. At the slower speed, the waves appear to be more nearly sinusoidal because compression causes information loss.

Unpredictable fluctuations are considered "noise" which, before its present definition, was equated with chaos. But now, "chaos" has a special meaning. The term refers to the unpredictability that ultimately occurs in some predictable, determined, systems. For instance, even when all parameters are known at a certain point in time, it has not proven possible to predict weather reliably for much more than five days. The reason for this is that, though any event may be dependent on initial conditions, it may be critically sensitive to small aperiodic disturbances (perturbations).

Consider, for example, a ball rolling down an inclined plane. Other factors being equal, its path will be a straight line from the starting point, *a*, to some end point, *b*. Were the inclined plane suddenly to tilt ever so slightly as the ball is rolling down, its new path would deviate from the path to *b*; and the magnitude of that deviation would increase with the distance traversed. A series of such small, random disturbances renders the path of the rolling ball unpredictable even though at any point, it is a straight line. Thus, chaos arises from highly specifiable initial conditions which may be affected by otherwise virtually insignificant aperiodic variations. This is very different from *random* events comprising noise.

There is an apocryphal story about Marconi, who invented the radio. It is said that when he assembled the first one, and turned on the power, he heard that hiss which we now call "static." When asked what the noise might be, he is alleged to have answered, "Oh, it is *nothing*, just the stars talking."

Rhythmogenesis

Glass and Mackey (1988) describe the major models which present-day mathematicians believe account for the origin of rhythm and oscillation in biological systems. Among them is the "integrate and fire model":

> . . . a quantity called *activity* rises to a threshold leading to an event. The activity then instantaneously relaxes back to a second lower threshold. . . . If the function determining the rise and fall of the activity between the two thresholds is fixed, and if the thresholds are fixed, then the periodic sequence of events will be generated at a readily determined frequency. (p. 8)

There are physiological systems that seem to behave in accordance with this model. The authors cite bladder filling and micturition cycle as an example. It is a linear model with relatively precisely determined frequency, but is not especially typical of physiological systems.

Nonlinear models such as the "limit cycle oscillations" model are more appropriate for such common physiological rhythms as the cardiac cycles. Cardiac oscillations are quite regular when the heart is isolated from sympathetic autonomic innervation. Thus, autonomic stimulation briefly disturbs it, but the pattern reemerges in most cases, when built-in corrections prevent chaos.

The cardiac pattern illustrates the fact that physiological rhythms are typically contextual, that is, they are subject to internal and external disturbance, including interaction with other rhythmic activity—with which they may or may not be in phase. Some rhythms can be terminated by a stimulus of critical magnitude occurring at a critical phase of the cycle. It is hypothesized that infant crib death may be due to this occurrence.

Extrinsic as well as intrinsic factors affect the determination of the point or points in the cycle that are critical. Two cycles interacting out of phase are likely to annihilate each other because two waves traveling in opposite directions cannot pass through each other. There are certain biological cell units which singly, or in combination, are rhythmogenic. We call them "pacemakers." They respond periodically in the face of constant stimulation. The heart and the spontaneous activity of neurons are clearly illustrative of this type of pacemaker.

Negative Feedback Systems

Negative feedback systems are those in which variations from the steady-state are minimized by "feedback." This means *self-limiting*. Some forms of biofeedback incorporate this technology. For instance, one may learn to reduce tension in the frontalis muscle. Relaxation may be learned by trial and error when a tone indicates that the tension in the muscle is above a predetermined threshold value. In this situation, the person is part of the negative feedback "loop." Or alternatively, she or he may learn to increase finger temperature by using a thermometer showing increasing temperature. This is positive feedback, in which deviations from a steady state are increased.

Glass and Mackey (1988) illustrate negative feedback in connection with the control of breathing by blood CO_2 levels: CO_2 is produced by metabolism at a more or less constant rate, given constant conditions, and it is eliminated from the body at a constant rate by breathing. Thus, ventilation is a monotonic increasing function of arterial CO_2 levels of some time in the past. Delay in the feedback system is due to the time required for blood to flow from the brain centers where ventilation is determined, to the lungs where ventilation takes place. Increase in arterial blood CO_2 levels increases breathing rate . . . which decreases arterial blood CO_2 levels, etc.

Hypo- and hyperventilation may be explained by this model if one considers that a more or less constant CO_2 level may become destabilized if (a) there is a change in the CO_2 control function, time delay, or metabolic CO_2 production; or (b) steady state ventilation is otherwise changed. Such a destabilization is noted in Cheyne-Stokes respiration, in which there is alternating (oscillating) increasing and decreasing ventilation. This transition from a steady state to oscillation is called a *Hopf bifurcation*. Cheyne-Stokes respiration is pathological and characteristic of congestive heart disease and renal failure.

Sequential Disinhibition

Szekely (1965) and Kling and Szekely (1968) proposed a different model of rhythmogenesis—sequential disinhibition—in which there is a combination of cell units which have a mutually inhibiting property together with a mechanism for sequential inhibition. A hypothetical set of neural units, when stimulated, inhibits a second set of neurons, which, in turn, when active, inhibits yet a third such set of neurons. When the second set of neurons ceases to fire, the third set is *dis*inhibited and may become active. The proper interaction sequence may result in stable rhythms.

The site and complexity of rhythm generators also varies in physiological systems. For instance, in the heart, intrinsic rhythm is generated by specific cardiac regions (nodes) within the myocardial tissue. But there may be superimposed rhythms such as "respiratory sinus arrhythmia" (RSA) (see Chapter 5), resulting from interaction with respiratory rhythm. Respiratory rhythm depends on generators in the brain and is modified by chemoreceptor and other neural-mediated events. Respiratory rhythmogenesis in the brain is detailed in Chapter 2.

Chapter 2

Elements of the Anatomy
and Physiology of
the Respiratory System

Introduction

The principal function of the respiratory system is to extract oxygen (O_2) from atmospheric air in the lungs, transport it to body tissues, and evacuate excess carbon dioxide (CO_2) and water vapor (H_2O) by expelling them from the lungs back into the atmosphere. In so doing, this system also controls the body's acid-base balance, on which the O_2 transport system and metabolism depend.

This process depends on various components, ranging from the airway passages (mouth, nose, trachea, bronchi, and bronchioles) by which air enters and exits the lungs, to the structures in the lungs (alveoli) where gas exchange takes place, to the medium (blood and hemoglobin) that transports O_2 to body tissues and removes waste and CO_2, and to the individual cell structures that participate in cellular respiration and the production of energy (mitochondria) (Bell, Davidson, & Scarborough, 1968; Brobeck, 1979; Comroe, 1974; Ruch & Fulton, 1961).

This chapter focuses selectively on those aspects of the functional anatomy and physiology of the respiratory system, which, in my opinion, make the basic elements of clinical respiratory psychophysiology understandable.

The Airway Passages

The airway passages—the mouth and nose, trachea, bronchi, and bronchioles—conduct air in and out of the lungs. The nose participates actively in preparing air for the lungs. The mouth is an adjustable aperture, and the rest of the air passages are more or less flexible tubes and tubules that act as conduits for air entering and exiting the lungs.

The Nose

Air may enter the body through the nose which, unlike the mouth, is not simply an airway. Catlin (1869), in a remarkable little book entitled *Shut Your Mouth*, published some rather astute observations:

> The mouth of man, as well as that of brutes, was made for the reception and mastication of food for the stomach, and other purposes; but the nostrils, with their delicate and fibrous linings purifying and warming the air passage, have been mysteriously constructed and designed to stand guard over the lungs—to measure the air and equalize its draughts, during hours of repose.
>
> The atmosphere is nowhere pure enough for man's breathing until it has passed this mysterious refining process; and therefore the imprudence and danger of admitting it in an unnatural way, in double quantities, upon the lungs, and charged with the surrounding epidemic or contagious infections of the moment. (p. 27)

Catlin's observations have since been scientifically verified: Systematic studies have reported the role of the nose in respiration and physiology (Holmes et al., 1950). Breathing, as you can see, can be an "unnatural" act.

The nose consists of two cavities, each with a roof, a floor, and medial and lateral walls, separated by the septum. The right and left nasal cavities communicate with the outside by means of the nares (nostrils), and with the pharynx. Paranasal sinuses and nasolacrymal ducts communicate with the nasal cavities on each side. When air is drawn through the nose, it is separated by the septum and swirls past the turbinates, forming vortices. Due to this vortex action in the nasal passages, coarser particles in the air are removed by the filtering action of nasal hairs. Smaller particles are subsequently removed by the mucous blanket, to which they adhere. In addition to filtering the air, the nose warms and moisturizes it, creates a mucous blanket, provides drainage for the sinuses, and accommodates the sense of smell.

The nasal passages are lined with a densely vascularized mucous membrane populated with ciliated epithelial cells. Air swirling through them, entering the nose at 6°C (43°F), for instance, will be warmed to 30°C (86°F) by the time it reaches the back of the nose, and to body temperature as it passes the trachea (Greisheimer, 1963). The nose also protects the lungs against invading bacteria by the action of lymphocytes and macrophages in the vascular network of the mucous membrane. Likewise, the epithelium participates in its protection. During overventilation, the epithelium near the exterior of the nose changes toward a more "sturdy, stratified, squamous form" (Holmes et al., 1950).

The Nasal Mucous Blanket. There is a layer of tissue that secretes mucus in the inner lining of the nose which forms a sort of "blanket" that also lines the trachea, and reaches all the way down into the bronchi of the lungs. This mucous blanket is in continuous motion, created by the cilia—hairlike cells that move the blanket against gravity, toward the throat. The mucous blanket traps bacteria and debris, and removes it from the respiratory tract by transporting it to the stomach (where it is disposed of by the digestive process). Three-fourths of the bacteria entering the nose are deposited on the mucous blanket and eliminated. The mucus also has an antibacterial agent, the enzyme lysozyme (Ballentine, 1979; Holmes et al., 1950). It is erroneous to think of mucus as excretion; it is, in fact, secretion.

The Turbinates. The turbinates provide water for moisturizing air entering the body. In 20,000 or so daily excursions of air through the nose, the turbinates provide about two quarts of water, coming from the serous (serum-producing) glands abundant in the nasal mucosal lining and in the turbinates (Holmes et al., 1950).

The Nasal Cycle. During quiet breathing, there is alternating cyclical activity of the nasal fossae (channels). The turbinates on one side fill with fluid, narrowing the breathing space; and those on the opposite side shrink as they give up fluid. This "infradian" cycle may last from less than one hour to as long as four hours. Ballentine (1979) reported it to average about once every three-quarter hour. It is not the only change occurring in the nasal mucosa. Others are due to the vasodilation in the mucosal erectile tissues.

The Response of the Nose in Migraine. Holmes et al. (1950) reported their observations of the nasal fossae in persons suffering from migraine. The color of the mucosa, swelling of the turbinates, and amount of mucosal secretion were noted for a period of three days preceding the onset of the attack. Four hours after onset, they noted a marked increase in the color of both the right and left nasal mucosa, with swelling of the turbinates resulting from obstruction, and increase in nasal watery secretion. On the next day, the nasal symptoms subsided.

The Mouth, Pharynx, and Trachea

Air entering the body through the mouth is drawn directly into the lungs through the pharynx and trachea without benefit of filtration, moisturization, and warming. The pharynx extends from the base of the skull to the esophagus. It is a tubular structure made mostly of skeletal muscle lined with mucous membrane. One segment is common to both the respiratory and digestive systems—both food and air pass through it. A mass of lymphatic tissues—the palatine tonsils—line the right and left dorsal wall of a segment of the pharynx (the oropharynx), forming lymphocytes (see Chapter 3).

The larynx, or voice box, connects the pharynx to the trachea, preventing all but air from entering the lungs by the action of the epiglottis (Brobeck, 1979; Greisheimer, 1963). Air enters the lungs via the trachea, a cartilaginous tube about 15 mm wide and 10 to 12 cm long. It is flexible, increasing somewhat in length and diameter during sleep. The trachea divides into bronchi and, in turn, into bronchioles. The latter are elastic tubular structures lined with epithelium. In rare cases, they open directly into alveoli, but generally, they terminate in alveolar ducts.

The Lungs

The lungs are relatively light and porous tissues that lie more or less freely in the thoracic cavity (chest), above the diaphragm. The thoracic cavity varies in size with respiration, since the rib cage and associated muscles are quite flexible. They are separated from the membranes, pleura, which surround them, by serous fluid (surfactant) which lubricates the outer lung surface so that breathing-related expansion and movement may occur with minimum friction. The inferior surface of the lobes of the lungs rests on the diaphragm.

The structure at the end of the alveolar duct is a small, approximately spherical sac called the primary alveolar lobule. It is the physiological unit of the lung. Small vents connect adjacent alveoli within each primary lobule where gas exchange takes place. Atmospheric air and blood are separated in the alveoli by two thin membranes: the endothelium of the pulmonary capillary and the epithelium of the alveolus. There are about 300×10^6 alveoli in the lungs; their total surface available for gas exchange is estimated to be about 75 square meters in an adult male (Bell et al., 1968; Brobeck, 1979; Comroe, 1974; Greisheimer, 1963; Ruch & Fulton, 1961; Shapiro, Harrison, & Walton, 1982; Youmans, 1975).

The secondary lobules are aggregates of primary lobules and form a set of small lungs within the lobes of the lungs. Each secondary lobule has a bronchial tree and circulation. Arterial blood enters the lobule through the bronchial arteries, which branch out through the lobule, close to the bronchioles. After gas exchange (oxygenation and discharge of excess CO_2), blood passes into the pulmonary veins for return to the heart.

Figure 1 is a schematic of the upper respiratory tract showing the trachea and bronchi, and the lungs. The insert enlarges alveoli, the functional units of the lungs.

The alveoli contain an extensive network of capillaries held together by the alveolar endothelium, surrounded almost entirely by alveolar air. O_2 has only to diffuse through the pulmonary and capillary membrane to be absorbed into the blood. The exchange of gases is rapid: venous blood with oxygen pressure (PO_2) below that of alveolar air, and carbon dioxide pressure (PCO_2) exceeding PO_2 of alveolar air, equilibrate within about 0.7 seconds. Numerous physiological variables (including gas tension in the alveoli, state of membrane permeability, etc.) may affect the rate of equilibration.

Differential pressure gradients account for much of the transfer mechanism. Gases diffuse through the membrane until pressure equalization is reached and the arterial blood, leaving the proximity of the alveolar surface, has a gas composition in equilibrium with that in alveolar air. The equilibrium is never exact, since the composition of both blood and alveolar air is continually changing. Dripps and Comroe (1944) reported alveolar air from normal men to have a PO_2 of 97.4 mm Hg, while arterial O_2 pressure (PaO_2) was 97.1 mm Hg.

Inspiration and Expiration

Under ordinary circumstances, air enters the body and lungs by the creation of negative pressure (partial vacuum) in the thoracic cavity (chest). The partial vacuum is created by the action of the diaphragm and/or the intercostal (ribcage) muscles, which create a different pattern of ventilation from that of the action of the diaphragm. This difference is crucial for persons with hyperventilation syndrome (HVS).

Breathing by Contracting the Intercostal Muscles

When the intercostal muscles contract, they lift the rib cage upward and outward, causing a negative pressure which is equalized by the air coming into the lungs, inflating them in the inspiration phase of breathing— the I-phase. In expiration (E-phase), the intercostal muscles are permitted to relax by the release of air from the lungs, and the rib cage falls back to its original configuration with some assistance from intercostal muscle

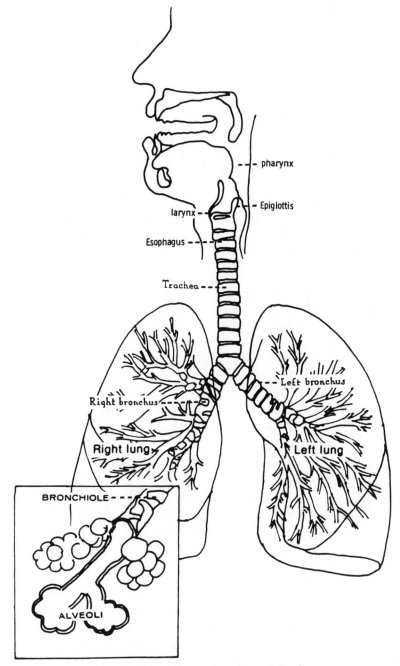

Figure 1. Airways, lungs, bronchi, and alveoli.

contraction. When this breathing mode is at rest, or during moderate activity, the body does a great deal of work—more so than when diaphragmatic breathing prevails—and ventilation of the lungs is incomplete.

Hughes (1979) showed that abdominal (diaphragmatic) breathing is physiologically superior to breathing by using the intercostal muscles. In comparing both breathing methods, he concluded that chest breathing impedes regional pulmonary ventilation; segments of lower lobes of the lungs may remain relatively unventilated. Thoracic, or chest breathing, is variously called "shallow" or "high" breathing.

Breathing by Contracting the Diaphragm

The diaphragm is a dome-shaped muscle. It separates the thorax, containing the heart and the lungs, from the abdominal/visceral region of the body. When the diaphragm is relaxed, it is vaulted upward into the space filled by the lungs in the expiration phase of the breathing cycle. When the diaphragm is contracted, in the inspiration phase, the vault, and thus the upward arching, is reduced. This reduction creates the negative pressure that causes the lungs to expand. It has also been shown that this negative pressure aids venous return of the blood to the heart, thus reducing the amount of work required of the heart in blood circulation (Ballentine, 1979; Melcher, 1976).

When the diaphragm contracts, the abdominal region below it is pushed downward and outward, exerting pressure on the rectus abdominis muscle. The abdomen yields and moves outward. The diaphragm relaxes in the expiration phase of the breathing cycle, and the rectus abdominis returns to its original configuration.

It has been suggested that arterial carbon dioxide pressure ($PaCO_2$) is monitored somehow by the diaphragm through "feedback loops": According to Juan et al. (1984), "diaphragmatic fatigue" may be related to the effects of CO_2 pressure on diaphragmatic contractility. These investigators reported that hypercapnia (increased PCO_2) contributed to reduced contractility of the diaphragm, while hypocapnia (lowered PCO_2) did not. This means essentially that, as CO_2 builds up in the blood, the diaphragm develops a tendency to fatigue and, by reduced contractility, slows down the breathing process. This mechanism is part of the acid-base homeostasis. It would discourage CO_2 build-up (respiratory acidosis). It also explains reduced diaphragm involvement in tachypnea (rapid breathing), in which uneven pulmonary ventilation with CO_2 build-up in pulmonary "dead space" invariably results in prominent thoracic breathing. Please note that gas pressure is frequently called "tension" in pulmonary physiology.

Normal Breathing

The modern study of breathing had its roots in the work of physiologists Pavlov (1928) and Sherrington (1906), who studied the reflex character of this complex behavior and traced neural pathways involved in its apparently automatic execution. Yet, despite that apparent automaticity, breathing is clearly affected by thinking and by emotion. Conversely, abnormalities in breathing may also cause such problems.

There was a time when scientists were also literate, and articulated their thoughts through metaphors. Many of us, unaware of this style, were drawn to finding scientific support for these abstractions, for example, Cannon's "wisdom of the body." This is a *canard*; the body has no wisdom. In fact, it often limits us to repeat what we did in the past. While this may in some cases be helpful, it hardly qualifies as wisdom. The future may be different from the past, but the body seldom modifies its instincts even when they doom it to extinction. Due to conditioning, it responds blindly to the future or to its anticipation.

On the other hand, if there is wisdom of the mind, it may prevent the folly of the body. In biofeedback, we teach the body not to distort the mind. For instance, we teach deep-diaphragmatic breathing to persons suffering from panic attacks so that the folly of the body stops translating into the folly of the mind.

Breathing is under the control of systemic pulmonary reflexes, chemoreceptor-mediated reflexes responding to blood gas composition at different anatomical sites, and brain mechanisms. All of these mechanisms also seem to respond to modulation by the action of the sympathetic and parasympathetic branches of the autonomic nervous system (ANS). But remarkably, these regulatory processes are readily bypassed, up to a point, when breathing is brought under voluntary control.

It affects tissue ventilation, metabolism, heart rate and function (Cacioppo & Petty, 1982), and the maintenance of the body's acid-base balance at an optimum pH of 7.4 (slightly basic) (Brown, 1953; Lum, 1976). In some organisms, notably, the dog, breathing also affects the control of body temperature. All of these processes interact in a complex way, since waste disposal, metabolism, and oxygen delivery to body tissue affect pH (Bell, Davidson, & Scarborough, 1969; Lowry, 1967; Swanson, Stavney, & Plum, 1958; Woodson, 1979).

The exchange of blood gases with the atmosphere takes place in exacting proportions dictated by metabolic rate (usually due to activity level). An increase or decrease in the proportion of gases exchanged in the lungs results in an alteration of the body's acid-base balance, which depends on the amount of CO_2 present in circulating blood. When the body's acid-base balance is disturbed, homeostatic buffer mechanisms restore it. If the balance cannot be restored, life is in jeopardy (see Chapter 4).

The Composition of Atmospheric and Alveolar Air. At sea level, on an average day, atmospheric air has the following composition:

O_2: 20.95 % by volume [P = 158 mm Hg]

CO_2: 0.03 % by volume [P = 0.23 mm Hg]

N_2: 78.09 % by volume [P = 5 mm Hg]

H_2O: 0.66 % by volume as vapor [P = 5 mm Hg]

Inert gases: 0.93 % by volume [P = 7 mm Hg]

At sea level, in a resting person, alveolar air may consist of:

O_2: 13% by volume [P = 97.8 mm Hg]

CO_2: 5% by volume [P = 40.9 mm Hg]

H_2O: 6% vapor by volume

70 percent N_2, and inert gases.

Excess O_2 is toxic and damaging to the body, but homeostatic mechanisms prevent an O_2 overload. Insufficient O_2 (hypoxia) threatens life. Excess CO_2 is also toxic and may cause anesthesia, narcosis, and death. Insufficient CO_2 may cause pH to rise toward alkalosis, inhibiting brain respiratory centers, constricting brain and peripheral arteries and arterioles, reducing brain blood flow, and altering the capacity of hemoglobin to bind and to release O_2 (Darrow & Graf, 1945; Himwich, 1951; Tower, 1960; Woodson, 1979).

The Partial Pressure of Gases. When a gas under pressure is in contact with a liquid like water, it dissolves in the liquid until the pressure in the liquid equals the pressure of the gas outside the liquid. The quantity of gas dissolved in the liquid determines its pressure and is called its tension. Gas tension may vary with ambient temperature and barometric pressure.

When a mixture of gases, such as air, is dissolved in a liquid, the tension of one of the constituent components is called its *partial pressure.* Pressure or partial pressure is commonly expressed by the symbol P. Barometric pressure is air pressure, exerted uniformly on all objects. The common reference point is air pressure at sea level, and is measured in millimeters of mercury (mm Hg). Each unit of mm Hg is called a torr— after Torricelli, who demonstrated its existence in 1643. At sea level, it is approximately 760 mm Hg, or 760 torr, and it decreases with altitude. Common household barometers give air pressures in inches of mercury (in Hg). Air pressure varies slightly with weather conditions, decreasing somewhat (below 30 in Hg) before a storm and increasing somewhat during fair weather "highs."

One may convert from torr to in Hg in this way:

$$1 \text{ meter} = 39.3701 \text{ in}$$

$$\frac{1 \text{ meter}}{1000} = 1 \text{ millimeter (mm)}$$

$$\frac{39.3701}{1000} = 0.03937 \text{ in}$$

Thus, 1 mm equals 0.03937 in and 0.03937 in (760) = 29.92 in. And 29.92 in Hg is the barometric pressure at sea level on an average dry day.

Change in barometric pressure is equivalent to change in altitude. For instance, if barometric pressure decreases, it is equivalent to an increase in altitude, and, other factors being constant, a decrease in oxygen pressure. When barometric pressure dropped from a prestorm level of 30.1 in Hg to 29.2 in Hg as it recently did before a rain storm, it is as though I rose from sea level to an altitude of about 800 feet. Interpolating in Table 5, *U.S. Standard Atmosphere* (Altman & Dittmer, 1971, p. 12), other factors being equal, PO_2 decreased by about 0.1%. For most persons, this represents a negligible change; for some, perhaps not.

Few of us understand why barometric pressure affects physiology. If barometric pressure at sea level is normal, it is 760 torr, and O_2 partial pressure will be 159.1 mm Hg. But at 5000 feet, the average "altitude" to which an aircraft passenger cabin is "pressurized" on a typical interconti-nental flight, air pressure will be about 405 mm Hg, and PO_2, 84.8 mm Hg—a little over half of that at sea level (Altman & Dittmer, 1971). It would not be surprising, in such circumstances, that persons with chronic borderline hypoxia, or a lowered threshold to the effects of hypoxia, would hyperventilate even more and experience symptoms such as headache, panic attacks, migraine, and even angina.

The Normal Respiration Rate. Clausen (1951) reports a breathing rate of 12 to 14 breaths per minute (b/min) in normal men, and slightly higher, 14 to 16 b/min, in normal women at rest. On the other hand, Tobin, Chadha, Jenouri, Birch, Hacik, Gazeroglu, and Sackner (1983) found that in youn-ger persons (mean age = 28.6 years; SD = 5.3), breathing rate was 16.7 (± 2.7) b/min. In older persons (mean age = 68.9 ± 6.5 years), breathing rate was 16.6 (± 2.8) b/min. These subjects were unaware that breathing rate was being observed because, as the researchers point out, the mouthpiece of monitoring equipment results in a lower breathing rate, proportional to the observed increase in expiratory tidal volume. Many other investigators have also cautioned us that we cannot expect to observe normal breathing when using a mouthpiece or noseclips (Chadha, Schneider, Birch, Jenouri,

& Sackner, 1984; Gilbert, Auchincloss, Brodsky, & Boden, 1972; Hormbrey, Jacobi, Patil, & Saunders, 1988; Maxwell, Cover, & Hughes, 1985; Weissman, Askanazi, Milic-Emili, & Kinney, 1984). Respiration rate is smaller in men than it is in women, and it is lower in those in their early 20s than it is in older persons (Jammes, Auran, Gouvernet, Delpierre, & Grimaud, 1979).

Respiratory Rate in Diseased Persons. Tobin et al. (1983) also reported breathing rate in persons with pulmonary and nonpulmonary disorders. In comparison to normal subjects, asymptomatic smokers (who had abstained from smoking for 3 hours before the test) showed significant increase in breathing rate—18.3 ($\pm$ 3.0) b/min; asymptomatic and symptomatic asthmatics showed virtually no difference: 16.6 ($\pm$ 3.4) and 16.0 ($\pm$ 4.1) b/min, respectively. Those with chronic obstructive pulmonary disease (COPD), with or without elevated end-tidal CO_2 (hypercapnia), showed statistically significant breathing rate differences: 20.4 ($\pm$ 4.1) and 23.3 ($\pm$ 3.3) b/min, respectively.

Persons with breathing difficulty (dyspnea) at rest and on mild exertion, and with reduced lung capacity, showed significantly elevated breathing rate: 27.9 ($\pm$ 7.9) b/min. Tidal volume, Vt (see next section), was normal, though minute volume (Vmin) was elevated. Unfortunately, these authors do not report end-tidal CO_2 because in persons with elevated minute volume (Vt) at rest, one would expect significantly decreased end-tidal CO_2 (hypocapnia)—a clinical indication of HV.

Finally, persons with a "chronic anxiety state" showed the following breathing patterns: frequent sighing to a volume three times greater than mean tidal volume (Vt), occurring from 4 to 15 times during a 15-minute observation period; 8- to 15-second suspension in breathing (apnea) at the end-inspiratory position (breath-holding); occasional erratic breathing with rapid shallow breathing alternating with apnea and intermittent large sighs. Breathing rate was 18.3 ($\pm$ 2.8) b/min in these subjects. Unfortunately, no alveolar CO_2 values were obtained. Persons with pulmonary hypertension showed significantly elevated breathing rate (21.1 $\pm$ 6.4 b/min).

It has been my experience with persons showing these breathing patterns and exhibiting elevated anxiety levels that, though tidal (Vt) and minute volume (Vmin) may be normal, they tend to have low end-tidal CO_2 and are, by definition, hyperventilating.

The Normal Respiration Volume. Ventilation of the lungs is usually specified in liters per minute (l/min), or 1/1000th (milliliters per minute— ml/min), and is called minute volume (Vmin). It is the product of respiration rate, or frequency (f), and the tidal volume (Vt): Vmin − f(Vt). Tobin et al. (1983) report tidal volume (Vt) in their younger and older subjects to be 383 (± 85) and 382 (± 108) ml/min, respectively. This difference is not statistically significant. Minute volume is reported in liters: 6.02 (± 1.32) and 5.92 (± 1.59). Here also, the difference is not statistically significant. In general, tidal volume (Vt) divided by *inspiratory time* can be used as an index of *respiratory center drive* under normal breathing conditions (Macklem & Mead, 1967).

The average normal adult with a minute volume of 6 l/min, or 6000 ml/min, and a breathing rate of about 14/min has a tidal volume of about 430 ml. Vt increases linearly with body weight or height, and is greater in men than in women (Jammes, Auran, Gouvernet, Delpierre, & Grimaud, 1979).

Alveolar ventilation is not the same as minute ventilation because of the "dead airspace" in the lungs—air not ordinarily evacuated with breathing (Vd). The volume of Vd is about 150 ml. Alveolar ventilation is, thus: Valv = f(Vt − Vd) = 15 (430 − 150) = about 4,200 ml/min (Altman & Dittmer, 1971; Comroe, 1974; Fehn & Rahn, 1964; Greischeimer, 1963; Haas et al., 1979; Tobin et al., 1983).

Respiratory Volume in Diseased Persons. According to Tobin et al. (1983), in the study cited above, chronic smokers showed a statistically significant increase in both tidal and minute volume: Vt = 484 (± 187) ml/min, and Vmin = 8.18 (± 2.4) l/min. Asymptomatic asthma sufferers showed no significant differences in either Vt or Vmin: 386 (± 133) ml/min, and 6.07 (± 1.39) l/min. Symptomatic asthmatics, on the other hand, showed significantly elevated Vt and Vmin: 679 (± 275) ml, and 9.45 (± 2.50) l/min (see also Chapter 9).

In COPD sufferers, breathing volume was significantly elevated in both nonhypercapnic and hypercapnic subgroups: Vt was 447 (± 139) ml/min, and 476 (± 158) ml/min; and Vmin was 8.59 (± 2.92) l/min, and 10.14 (± 2.96) l/min. And in both restrictive lung disease and pulmonary hypertension, Vt was not significantly elevated—395 (± 70) ml/min, and 431 (± 106) ml/min—but Vmin was 10.28 (± 1.90) l/min, and 10.14 (± 2.90) l/min, respectively. In these chronic anxiety sufferers, neither Vt (403 ± 133 ml/min) nor Vmin (6.65 ± 1.84 l/min) was significantly different from the normal group. These findings are entirely consistent with most such studies published by pulmonary physiologists, controlling for variations in sampling posture and sampling method.

Ruch and Fulton (1960), for instance, list the following values (p. 375):

These parameters are standard, differing little from textbook to textbook. They are not disputed in the *Handbook of Physiology* (Fehn & Rahn, 1964) or in *Respiration and Circulation* (Altman & Dittmer, 1971). That is why it is surprising that some research efforts which report data and con-

Table 1. Lung Volumes*

Inspiratory capacity	3600 ml
Expiratory reserve volume	1200 ml
Vital capacity	4800 ml
Residual volume (RV)	1200 ml
Functional residual capacity	2400 ml
Total lung capacity (TLC)	6000 ml
100 × (RV/TLC)	20%

*Reprinted with permission from T. C. Ruch and J. F. Fulton (1961): *Medical Physiology*, 18th ed. Philadelphia: W. B. Saunders.

clusions entirely inconsistent with basic respiratory physiology norms and conventions find their way into publication.

For instance, in "Ventilatory physiology of patients with panic disorder," by Gorman, Fyer, Goetz, Askanazi, Liebowitz, Fyer, Kinney, and Klein (*Archives of General Psychiatry*, 1988, 45:31–39), the authors compared 13 normal controls to 31 persons with panic, or panic with agoraphobia (PD), and 12 with "anxiety disorder."

I figured that the anxiety group was included here so that both client-groups might be assumed to contain chronic hyperventilators. As it turned out, I was wrong. It would have been consistent, though, with previous reports (Brodtkorb, Gimse, Antonaci, Ellersten, Sand, Sulg, & Sjaastadt, 1990; Carr & Sheehan, 1984; Fried, 1987, 1990; Fried & Golden, 1989; Ley, 1988; Lowry, 1967; Salkovskis, Warwick, Clark, & Wessels, 1986) that most anxiety sufferers, be they PD sufferers or otherwise, tend to hyperventilate. The issue, I thought, is whether hyperventilation is causal or secondary in such clients, and not whether they hyperventilate.

The authors claim, on the basis of minute volume (Vmin), that experimental and control group subjects were not hyperventilating at the time of

Table 2. Lung Volumes*

Sex	Males	Males	Females
Age	20–30	50–60	20–30
Inspiratory capacity	3600	2600	2400 ml
Expiratory reserve capacity	1200	1000	800 ml
Vital capacity	4800	3600	3200 ml
Residual volume (RV)	1200	2400	1000 ml
Functional residual capacity	2400	3400	1800 ml
Total lung capacity (TLC)	6000	6000	4200 ml
100 (RV/TLC)	20%	40%	24%

*Reprinted with permission from J. H. Comroe (1974): *Physiology of Respiration*, 2nd ed. Chicago: Year Book Medical Publishers.

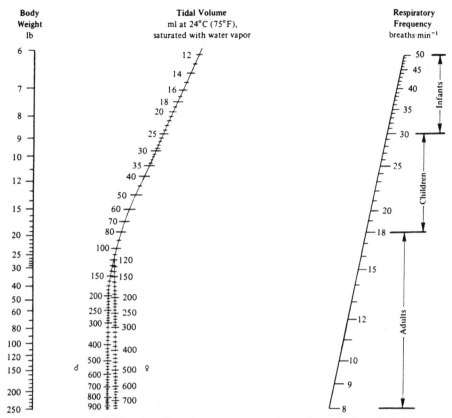

| Body Weight lb | Tidal Volume ml at 24°C (75°F), saturated with water vapor | Respiratory Frequency breaths·min⁻¹ |

Figure 2. Radford nomograph. Reproduced with permission from the *Journal of Applied Physiology*. Vol. 7, p. 451.

the baseline recording. But their data contradict that conclusion, and defining hyperventilation by Vmin is unconventional, if not misleading. If alveolar PCO_2 is not the criterion, then a nomograph such as the one by Radford (see Comroe, 1974; Chernick & Raber, 1972) might have been used. Such a nomograph gives tidal volume, versus body weight, for breathing frequency.

The Radford alignment nomograph permits a straight line connecting a point on each of the two outer axes to determine a value on the one in the center, and a point connecting the right or left axis with a point on the middle one can be extended to determine a value on the third (Figure 2).

Assuming men and women in both groups to be of about average body weight, ranging between 120 and 170 pounds, mean respiration rate should be around 15 b/min, with tidal volume at about 450 to 550 milliliters. Yet, their data do not come close to these values. Keep in mind that at ambient temperatures around 75° F, end-tidal CO_2 ($ETCO_2$) should be around 40 torr. In most texts, $ETCO_2$ at less than 38 torr is taken as the *criterion* for hyperventilation. But of course, symptoms don't emerge at that value.

Further, their reported average Vt and average Vmin must be taken as either erroneous, or as paradoxical. In their Table 4, page 35, the mean Vt for "patients" is 243.6 ml/min, and the standard deviation is 137.3 ml/min, reflecting phenomenal variability and raising yet additional questions. In the last paragraph, page 36, we are told that "SD of tidal volume was significantly higher for the patients than the controls, indicating a more chaotic breathing pattern."

Comparing patients and controls: F = 406.45 (squaring SDs). Certainly this F-ratio would be significant at the .05 level, with 25 and 11 df (but nonhomoscedasticity invalidates the t-test which they report). Then, mean tidal volume reported for patients, 243.6 ml/min, is half of the normal value. Were they breathing twice as fast as the normal rate? We are not told. But on page 38, the authors report a minute volume of 5.5 l/min—normal! Now if minute volume is normal, and tidal volume is half of normal, they must be breathing at twice the normal rate. But, with double normal breathing rate, how do they maintain normal mean PCO_2 (39.5 torr)—especially if they show "chaotic breathing?" And, "Of note is the fact that mean Vmin for patients with panic disorder at baseline was 5.5 (SD = 2) l/min . . . indicating that neither group was hyperventilating in the canopy . . ." (pp. 36–37). How can one explain these data in persons with no reported pulmonary or metabolic disorder, with a breathing rate that is chaotic and estimated at 23/min, and with a textbook normal $ETCO_2$ (39.5 torr). Let's look at the controls: Half are anxiety sufferers with an even lower tidal volume: 150 ml (SD = 7) (1/3 of normal). And their minute volume is 4.5 l/min (normal). Their breathing rate must be 31/min, or about one-third faster than the patients and again, paradoxically, their PCO_2 is higher (42.8)! The controls presumably breathe at an accelerated rate the same as that used in the *hyperventilation challenge*, with 1/3 normal tidal volume, and they show normal PCO_2!

The data in their Table 5, for epoch 5, "recovery from room air hyperventilation," are equally unusual: PaO_2 is elevated somewhat at 116.4 torr in the patients, whereas in the controls, it is somewhat decreased. This suggests high oxyhemoglobin (OHb) saturation in the patients and low OHb in the controls. The pH is near normal for the patients, and somewhat lower for the controls. Arterial CO_2 tension is markedly decreased in the patients, while it is near normal in the controls.

Taken together, these data tell us that the patients fit the profile of chronic hyperventilators, while the others do not. High O_2 saturation with low CO_2 tension suggests a right-shifted OHb dissociation curve, with compensated near-normal pH (i.e., alkalosis).

Once again, data are missing. We are not given breathing rate so we do not know what they are doing during recovery. It is possible to guess, but the data are incomplete and cannot be interpreted with any certainty. Then, inexplicably, 14 patients are dropped from the study. It is hard to know what to make of this "ventilatory physiology" report because the data are uniformly inconsistent, paradoxical, and they defy conventional interpretation.

Here is a different example. In "Brief focused cognitive therapy of panic disorder" (Alford, Freeman, Beck, & Wright, 1990), the authors report treating an 18-year-old woman with mild agoraphobia (DSM-III-R 300.21). Remarkably, with the exception of the study they challenge (Sheehan, 1982), they cite no other report that asserts that panic attacks may have a physiological etiology; and from their references, one may also conclude that none have ever been reported. And, though they employ the HV-challenge, not a single citation in their references has the word "hyperventilation" in its title. Yet the most superficial literature search would have turned up many dozens, including "Hyperventilation as a cause of panic attacks" (Hibbert, 1984), "Panic disorder, the ventilatory response to carbon dioxide and respiratory variables" (Pain, Biddle, & Tiller, 1988), and "Respiratory control as a treatment for panic attacks" (Clark, Salkovskis, & Chalkley, 1985). Not to mention Fried (1987a,b)!

The young woman's symptoms include nausea, heart racing, shakiness, muscle tension, difficulty breathing (dyspnea), and the urge to leave the situation—all typical of mild agoraphobia. Physical examination was said to rule out any medical condition which would be adversely affected by the hyperpena, and she was instructed to hyperventilate. But no data are provided. What was her breathing rate? For how long did she do it? What was her pulse rate and blood pressure before and after the maneuver? What was her alveolar PCO_2 before and after? How long did it take to recover? It is as if time stood still when Rosett performed exactly the same experiment in 1924.

Did the medical examination include an ECG? We are cautioned by Wildenthal, Fuller, and Shapiro (1968) that HV can induce paroxysmal atrial arrythmia, and Lum (1976) and Nixon (1989) caution us that HV should never be assumed to be benign in persons with any chest symptoms. Was there a neurological examination? Gottstein, Berghoff, Held, Gabriel, Textor, and Zahn (1970) warn that:

> Based on these findings (cerebral metabolism during hyperventilation and CO_2 inhalation) one might assume that hyperventilation with a $PaCO_2$ less than 20 torr and a jugular venous PO_2 as low as 20 torr will cause an inadequate oxygen supply even in

healthy subjects. This should be considered with regard to therapeutic hyperventilation.

I hope that if this book accomplishes anything, it is to make you more critical of studies that concern breathing so that you will not take their validity for granted; that you will know what the data mean; and that you will know what questions to ask.

Parameters of Lung Ventilation

Pulmonary ventilation consists of the movement of various quantities, or volumes of air, in and out of the lungs. In addition, there is a volume of air which remains in the lungs between breaths. It is helpful to know something about the way in which respiratory specialists classify and measure these ventilation air volumes.

The total ventilation of the lungs is measured by the pulmonary function test. This procedure establishes the parameters of the volume and the rate of flow of gases in and out of the lungs. These parameters are, in the final analysis, the principal ways of establishing that a person is breathing normally, is tachypneic, or is hyperventilating.

The Total Lung Capacity

The total lung capacity (TLC) is the maximum amount of air that the lungs can hold. It is usually thought to comprise four primary volumes:

(a) Tidal volume (Vt): the amount of air moved in and out of the lungs; Vt is usually around 500 ml;
(b) Inspiratory reserve volume (IRV): the quantity of air that can be forcefully inspired above normal Vt inhalation; if TLC is 6.000 ml, then IRV is 5.500 ml (6,000 ml − 500 ml);
(c) Expiratory reserve volume (ERV): the quantity of air that can be forcefully exhaled after normal Vt exhalation (about 1,200 ml);
(d) Residual volume (RV): the amount of air left in the lungs after forced exhalation (about 1,200 ml).

Capacities are combinations of various air volumes in ventilation. The vital capacity is the sum of the inspiratory and expiratory reserve capacities:

(a) Vital capacity (VC): IRV + Vt + ERV, the amount of air that can be forcefully exhaled after maximum inspiration (about 4,500 ml);
(b) Inspiratory capacity (IC): Vt + IRV, the maximum volume that can be taken into the lungs;

Table 3. Typical Values for Pulmonary Function Tests*

These are values for a healthy, resting, recumbent young male (1.7 m² surface area) breathing air at sea level, unless other conditions are specified. They are presented merely to give approximate figures. These values may change with position, age, size, sex, and altitude; there is variability among members of a homogeneous group under standard conditions.

Lung volumes

Inspiratory capacity, ml	3,600
Expiratory reserve volume, ml	1,200
Vital capacity, ml	4,800
Residual volume (RV), ml	1,200
Functional residual capacity, ml	2,400
Thoracic gas volume, ml	2,400
Total lung capacity (TLC), ml	6,000
RV/TLC × 100, %	20

Ventilation

Tidal volume, ml	500
Frequency, respirations/min	12
Minute volume, ml/min	6,000
Respiratory dead space, ml	150
Alveolar ventilation, ml/min	4,200

Distribution of inspired gas

Single-breath test (% increase N_2 for 500 ml expired alveolar gas), % N_2	<1.5
Pulmonary nitrogen emptying rate (7 min test), % N_2	<2.5
Helium closed-circuit (mixing efficiency related to perfect mixing), %	76

Alveolar ventilation/pulmonary capillary blood flow

Alveolar ventilation (L/min)/blood flow (L/min)	0.8
(Physiological shunt/cardiac output) × 100, %	<7
(Physiological dead space/tidal volume) × 100, %	<30

Pulmonary Circulation

Pulmonary capillary blood flow, ml/min	5,400
Pulmonary artery pressure, mm Hg	24/9
Pulmonary capillary blood volume, ml	75–100
Pulmonary "capillary" blood pressure (wedge), mm Hg	8

Alveolar Gas

Oxygen partial pressure, torr	104
CO_2 partial pressure, torr	40

Diffusion and gas exchange

O_2 consumption (STPD), ml/min	240
CO_2 output (STPD), ml/min	192
Respiratory exchange ratio, R (CO_2 output/O_2 uptake)	0.8
Diffusing capacity, O_2 (STPD) resting, ml O_2/min/torr	>15
Diffusing capacity, CO (steady state) (STPD) resting, ml CO/min/torr	17
Diffusing capacity, CO (single-breath) (STPD) resting, ml CO/min/torr	25
Diffusing capacity, CO (rebreathing) (STPD) resting, ml CO/min/torr	25

Arterial blood

O_2 saturation (% saturation of Hb with O_2), %	97.1
O_2 tension, torr	100
CO_2 tension, torr	40
Alveolar-arterial PO_2 difference (100% O_2), torr	33
O_2 saturation (100% O_2), %	100
O_2 tension (100% O_2), torr	640
pH	7.4

Mechanics of breathing

Maximal voluntary ventilation, L/min	125–170
Forced expiratory volume, % in 1 sec	83
% in 3 sec	97
Maximal expiratory flow rate (for 1 L), L/min	400
Maximal inspiratory flow rate (for 1 L), L/min	300
Compliance of lungs and thoracic cage, L/cm H_2O	0.1
Compliance of lungs, L/cm H_2O	0.2
Airway resistance, cm H_2O/L/sec	1.6
Work of quiet breathing, kgM/min	0.5
Maximal work of breathing, kgM/breath	10
Maximal inspiratory and expiratory pressures, mm Hg	60–100

*Reprinted with permission from J. H. Comroe et al. (1962): *The Lung*, 2nd ed. Chicago: Year Book Medical Publishers.

(c) Functional residual capacity (FRC): ERV + RV, the sum of the expiratory reserve volume and the residual volume;

(d) Total lung capacity (TLC): IC + FRC, the sum of inspiratory capacity and functional residual capacity.

The change in volume of the lungs produced by a given unit of pressure is called "compliance." A high degree of compliance indicates that a given pressure change results in moving a large volume of air in the lungs. If the lungs become less elastic, compliance decreases.

Lung capacity is measured by the volume of air that comprises different components of the total ventilation volume. For instance, of the approximately 500 ml of air (Vt) entering the lungs during quiet respiration, only a portion reaches the alveoli of the lungs. The remainder occupies the space in the nose and mouth, trachea, bronchi, and bronchioles. This is the anatomical dead space (Vd), or volume of air in the pulmonary passages and airways. The Vd is usually about 140 milliliters. It may be noted that the volume of these air passages is fairly constant: about 1 milliliter/pound (2.2 Kg) of normal body weight—Vmin = f(Vt).

There are two principal ways of measuring Vt: (a) directly, by spirometry (Latin *spirare*, to breathe + Greek *metron*, to measure); or (b) indirectly, by pneumography or plethysmography (Greek *plethysmos*, increase + *graphein*, to write). A note of caution has been introduced by most of the investigators who use these breathing observation methods. Direct and indirect methods may be used reliably and extensively to measure lung capacities, but their use in connection with psychological and psychiatric clinical populations is relatively unsound because they have been consistently shown to alter breathing patterns in these populations (Askanazi et al., 1980; Gilbert et al., 1972). Breathing pattern, Vt, f (breathing frequency), and ventilation changes have been reported.

Direct Measurement of Volume: Spirometry

The development of adequate air seals permits the use of a dry piston in a cylinder, attached to a kymograph drum or other suitable recording device. The displacement of the piston may be used to indicate the alteration in Vt or any other capacity. Christie (1935) was one of the earliest investigators to address respiration in the "neuroses" using spirometric methods.

Indirect Measurement of Volume: Pneumography and Plethysmography

There are a number of variations on methods of indirect (derived) observations of Vt. Vest and belt pneumographs have been used to observe relationships between chest expansion and Vt. The pneumographic technique employs a flexible, sealed tube, with a known quantity of air inside, allowed to stabilize to body temperature when it is fastened around the thorax. As the chest expands, the air in the tube is compressed and the increase in pressure is calibrated with a spirometer to indicate chest expansion and Vt (Schafmeister et al., 1983; Smith, Jukes, & Timmons, 1983). It appears to be the consensus that pneumographic methods may be reasonably accurate if used with care and properly calibrated, but each method has its own limitations and most effective applications (Timmons, 1982).

Strain gauges (Timmons et al., 1972) and a number of thoracic impedance and inductance plethysmography methods have been tested (Allison, Holmes, & Nyboer, 1964; Allison & Luft, 1964; Bonjer, Van den Berg, & Dirken, 1964; Goldensohn & Zablow, 1959; Hamilton & Shock, 1936; Kubicek, Kinnen, & Edin, 1964).

Hamilton, Beard, and Kory (1965) reported the use of a thoracic impedance measurement of tidal volume and ventilation. Impedance is comparable to dc resistance in that it is measured as a function of the decrease in an ac voltage traversing the thorax. By measuring Vt with a spirometer (direct) and comparing the measurement with their observation of transthoracic resistance, capacitance (the way the thorax will hold an electrical charge), or impedance, they were able to show a linear relationship between lung volume and impedance change for persons in varying body positions and attitudes (standing, sitting, supine, etc.). They were also able to show the respiration mode (abdominal or chest breathing).

Thoracic impedance plethysmography requires placement of the electrodes directly on the chest and the calibration of the instrument against a spirometer. Electrode placement is crucial, as is electrode type. Thus, this method is not practical for typical applications in connection with the observation of HV in psychological and psychiatric populations. Use of inductive plethysmography has also been reported (Chadha et al., 1982; Tobin et al., 1983).

These noninvasive methods consist, essentially, of two Teflon-insulated wire coils sewn into elastic bands, one to encircle the ribs and the other to encircle the abdomen. These coil bands are coupled to an oscillator. Changes in the diameter of the coils alter their inductance (magnetic field generated by an electric current in a coil), and the frequency of the oscillator may be calibrated to reflect a change in Vt.

Hyperventilation

Shapiro, Harrison, and Walton (1982) defined alveolar HV not due to pulmonary or cardiac disease as having the following characteristics when the person is breathing room air: (a) arterial blood pH is above 7.40; (b) arterial PCO_2 is below 38 mm Hg; (c) blood-O_2 saturation is above minimal normal level; and (d) the typical ventilatory pattern is hyperpnea (elevated Vt) and tachypnea (elevated respiration rate). According to Comroe (1974), HV is defined as "Increased alveolar ventilation in relation to metabolic rate" (i.e., decreased alveolar PCO_2 to less than 37 torr). Since normal PCO_2 can be expected to be around 37 to 40 torr, the criteria of Shapiro et al., and of Comroe, are academic. I think that the confusion surrounding the definition of HV given by behavioral clinicians centers, erroneously, on the appearance of symptoms. This can be very confusing.

Brashear (1983), for instance, provides an elaborate description of the manifestations, symptoms, and treatment of HV-syndrome (HVS), specifying the role of hypocapnia (low alveolar PCO_2) and respiratory alkalosis (elevated pH). But he presents only data on the outcome of 30 to 60 seconds of acute HV which can decrease PCO_2 to half of normal (38 torr is normal) after 30 seconds. Howell (1990) defines HV as ". . . a syndrome characterised by a variety of somatic symptoms induced by physiologically inappropriate hyperventilation and usually reproduced in whole or in part by voluntary hyperventilation" (p. 287). In other words, hyperventilation is what hyperventilation does! Tobin (1990), on the other hand, identifies HV as a "unique form of dyspnea" (see Chapter 5) which, he holds, affects between 6 and 11% of the general patient population. He attributes it to (a) organic causes including neurologic disorders, salycilate intoxication, hepatic failure, severe pain, asthma, interstitial lung disease, and pulmonary and vascular disease; and (b) psychogenic factors especially anxiety. He categorically separates hyperventilators from others who have dyspnea citing evidence for a "hypocapnic set-point" first described by Gardner, Meah, and Bass (1986): After breathing CO_2 enriched air, HV patients rapidly return to a particular PCO_2 level when breathing room air.

Respiratory physiologists uniformly define HV as alveolar PCO_2 reduced below the normal value of 37 to 38 torr, irrespective of the presence or absence of symptoms. For the behavioral clinician, this is not a sensible criterion since she or he tends to view HV only as that physiological state in which symptoms emerge. Thus, you would never hear someone say, "The client had a PCO_2 of 32 torr. That is moderate hyperventilation, but no symptoms were noted." I have seen symptoms emerge in some clients when PCO_2 drops below about 30 torr. Rafferty, Saisch, and Gardner (1992) firmly established the emergence of symptoms at a mean PCO_2 of 20 torr ($PETCO_2$ = 2.6%). This is a good signpost.

Hyperventilation is a complex breathing behavior. It may also involve chest (thoracic) breathing, irregular breathing cycles (dysrhythmic inspiration and expiration), sighing, interrupted breathing (apnea), spasmodic gasps, and so forth. The physiological effects of these behaviors may be profoundly disturbing: Just a few minutes of overbreathing (HV-challenge) may cause the average person to experience dizziness, faintness, vertigo, and, if prolonged, tetany or syncope (Rosett, 1924). This should serve as a strong indication that acute or chronic HV is not a condition to which the body is accustomed to react with impunity.

While acute HV is readily observable in most persons, chronic HV may be quite subtle, and its effects may not always be obvious. In clinical practice, it is infrequently the case that a given client may present tachypnea and grossly exaggerated chest movements. More typically, breathing may be rapid and shallow, or there may be much sighing.

One way of establishing that there is HV is to observe the gas composition of alveolar air (end-tidal air is usually the medium for this observation). This can be accomplished by using an infrared gas analyzer, a *capnometer*, that samples air for PCO_2 (Bass & Gardner, 1985a,b; Fried, 1987a,b) (see Chapter 5). If the end-tidal (alveolar) gas composition is such that PCO_2 falls below the commonly accepted criterion (Comroe, 1974; Fried, 1987a,b), the diagnosis of HV is valid. This procedure is, in many ways, superior to sampling arterial blood (which entails some medical risk).

Most studies that purport to examine the effects of HV do so on not much more than supposition that the populations observed are, in fact, hyperventilating. These studies relate symptoms and findings to persons who show many of the clinical signs present in hyperventilators but in whom a positive identification of alveolar gas composition is absent (Grossman & DeSwart, 1984). Although this is not the best way to do it, it is neither unreasonable nor necessarily invalid from a clinical standpoint.

According to my clinical experience, it is much more likely that a person with no overt dyspnea may be hyperventilating than that a person with typical signs is not doing so. This seems to be a common experience for most clinicians, because they typically report that when they encounter these signs, they will employ the HV-challenge, having the person breathe deeply and rapidly (perhaps twenty to thirty breaths per minute) for two to three minutes. I do not recommend this procedure. I consider it hazardous. Among other things, HV has been shown to trigger paroxysmal vasospasms in the brain and the heart. As early as 1924, Rosett showed its ability to induce seizures, and more recently, Lum (1976) cautioned against its use in persons with chest pain and neuromuscular disorders. Other notes of caution are cited throughout this book. But I must add, in fairness to my colleagues, that a number of them use the procedure and have reported no consequent ill effects in their clients.

Since HV-challenge will induce the symptoms from which the client is seeking relief, the procedure is often used to validate their origin. I am not convinced of the usefulness of this technique, though many studies report that the client shows a sense of relief upon discovering that the chest pain is not due to "something more serious." That in itself should raise a red flag. For instance, HV-induced chest pain can be an exacerbation of angina. This sends the wrong message to both the client and therapist. We must always take physical symptoms seriously—never dismiss them as "hysteria." Even panic sufferers may suffer a heart attack or stroke.

I support the practice of diagnosing HV by symptomatology; so do other investigators (Grossman and DeSwart, 1984; Nixon and Freeman, 1988; van Dixhoorn and Duivervoorden, 1985). With a little practice, anyone can learn to recognize the signs. Lum (1976) listed the following:

(a) Breathing is predominantly thoracic;
(b) Little use is made of the diaphragm;
(c) Breathing is punctuated by frequent sighs;
(d) Sighing has a peculiar "effortless" quality, with a marked "forward and upward" movement of the upper sternum but little lateral expansion;
(e) Normal breathers can imitate the breathing chest movements used by hyperventilators only with difficulty.

These observations have been coupled with the additional fact that speech utterances in chronic hyperventilators are often preceded by a deep sigh or a deep breath. I have noted this phenomenon frequently during initial intake interviews, and it has been reported by many other investigators.

There are varying reports of the frequency with which HV is encountered in different populations. Huey and Sechrest (1981) reported a frequency of 10.8% in a sample of 289 students, McKell and Sullivan (1947) reported the incidence to be 5.8% in gastroenterology practice, and Rice (1950) cited 10.7% in about 1,000 consecutive office patients. More recently, Brashear (1983) proposed 6% to 11%, depending on the client population. Lum (1976) reported that the incidence of detection of HV by medical professionals increased with the degree to which an effort was made to alert them to its existence. In 1963, two patients were seen at the Respiratory Physiology Department of Papworth Hospital; one of these was referred with the suggestion of HV. In 1972, the number of patients seen in that treatment unit had increased to 143, about 115 of whom were referred by other physicians with a "hyperventilation" suggestion.

Given these studies and my own clinical experience, I would estimate that the 10% to 16% incidence of HV in the general population proposed by Huey and Sechrest (1981), and Brashear (1983), is on the conservative side. I have rarely seen a client who does not hyperventilate. Fewer than 1 in 100 of my clients show normal PCO_2. For instance, it has been long known that it is rare among persons with seizure disorders, heart disease, asthma, anxiety, stress, panic disorder with or without agoraphobia, other phobias, hyperthyroidism, migraine, chronic inflammatory joint disease with chronic pain, and so on, not to hyperventilate. We're probably looking at more than half the U.S. population. On the other hand, Gardner, Bass, and Moxam (1992) and Rafferty, Saisch, and Gardner (1992) correctly remind us that many persons with hypocapnia (low alveolar PCO_2) are relatively symptom free.

Hypoventilation

You are far more likely to encounter HV than hypoventilation in clinical practice. But, it is important to consider the possibility that there are some persons who may have that condition. Alveolar hypoventilation is CO_2 retention and is observed with a capnometer as PCO_2 elevated above normal ($PETCO_2$ over 5.00, or PCO_2 in excess of 38 torr). The practical question is what constitutes excessive PCO_2? What criterion should one adopt? This is a difficult question to answer and hinges, to all extents and purposes, on the value at which one may expect to see symptoms emerge. Hypoventilation, unlike HV, is not usually accompanied by the expected psychological and psychiatric signs and symptoms.

The client with HV may present somatic and/or psychological symptoms with no discernible organic basis. Alveolar gas values obtained with a capnometer may support the diagnosis of hyperventilation syndrome (HVS) if PCO_2 is below about 30 torr (Bass & Gardner, 1985a). Implementation of the HV-challenge by some investigators might then be initiated to confirm the diagnosis.

I caution repeatedly against this procedure because, though many have reported using it routinely with no adverse effects, there is at least one report that it may prove fatal in hypoventilation, and few clinicians today routinely observe alveolar PCO_2. This case cited by Bates, Adamson, and Pierce, in the *New England Journal of Medicine* (1966:274), leads the authors to conclude that ". . . although prolonged hyperventilation is not regarded as dangerous in normal patients . . . it may be catastrophic in patients with chronic alveolar hypoventilation not caused by airway obstruction" (p. 1372). Both hypoventilation and HV may be routinely observed in persons with the airway obstruction common to the bronchoconstriction of asthma (see Chapter 9).

Medical physiology distinguishes between idiopathic and centrally caused hypoventilation (Erslev & Gabuzda, 1975; Sodeman & Sodeman, 1979; Stein, 1983). Central hypoventilation may result from brain lesions, various organic diseases, or the use of certain drugs and medications. The so-called Ondine's curse is a syndrome in which the individual in apnea, bereft of the usual automatic neural and other breathing controls, seemingly "forgets" to breathe, resuming when commanded to do so. Monge's polycythemia (Winslow & Monge, 1978) is otherwise known as mountain sickness. The idiopathic forms are of greater concern to us.

The symptoms of primary alveolar hypoventilation may be vague fatigue, headache, perhaps cyanosis (bluishness of the lips, commonly), and sleep apnea in the absence of pulmonary disease. It is usually accompanied by secondary polycythemia (elevated red cell count), hypoxemia (chronic low blood and tissue O_2 level), methemoglobinemia (increased ratio of methemoglobin to hemoglobin—methemoglobin does not bind O_2), and in some cases, congestive heart failure. CO_2 retention worsens during sleep, and sleep apnea is the rule rather than the exception. It might seem paradoxical, but there is rarely dyspnea.

One should suspect alveolar hypoventilation in the very obese client, especially when sleep apnea is reported. This condition is known as Pickwickian syndrome. Under no circumstances would I treat a client with this disorder with deep diaphragmatic breathing because, when executed properly, deep diaphragmatic breathing tends to elevate alveolar CO_2. If breathing slows in persons with hypoxemia, blood O_2 may also drop precipitously. Paradoxically the combination of increased alveolar PCO_2 and lowered PaO_2 impairs ventilatory response and may cause apnea. Apnea was blamed for the fatality in the Bates et al. (1966) report.

Respiratory Control Centers of the Brain

The common textbook reference to "pons and medullary respiration centers" suggests a rather simple arrangement, perhaps also involving the vagus and phrenic nerves. For too many of us, this explanation suffices, although it is as unsophisticated an explanation as the "vegetative function of the ANS"—with which many of us are also quite content. This lack of sophistication has led to some really naive and pedestrian work masquerading as breathing research. A serious effort to study respiratory psychophysiology requires a more detailed knowledge of what happens in breathing and how it relates to systemic and cerebral physiology.

There are different categories of stimuli for known respiratory control mechanisms in the brain including (a) afferent respiratory muscle activity; (b) blood or perfusion pressure, and cerebrospinal fluid pressure; (c) $PaCO_2$; (d) pH; and (e) PaO_2. These stimuli modulate the activity of centers in the lower brain stem which stimulate, inhibit, synchronize, or give rhythmicity to inspiration (I-phase) or expiration (E-phase) in respiration.

Inspiration (I-phase) and expiration (E-phase) are separate events. The reason for this dichotomy is that separate mechanisms and centers appear to control each phase and may, in certain circumstances, do so independently of each other. Normal functioning is, of course, the synchronous interplay of these sensors and mechanisms. Efferent impulses set inspiration in motion. For expiration to take place, inspiration must be inhibited. Thus, rhythmic breathing synchronizes sequences of excitatory and inhibitory efferent impulses based on the prevalence of specifiable sets of afferent stimuli, typically part of reflex mechanisms.

The Pneumotaxic and Apneustic Centers of the Pons and Medulla

The principal respiratory rhythm generator is located in the lower brain stem, that is, the pons and the medulla (Cohen, 1979; Fink, Katz, Reinhold, & Schoolman, 1962).

Bilateral lesioning of the nucleus *parabrachialis medialis*, in the rostral dorsolateral pons, results in apneusis (Breckenridge & Hoff, 1950; Gautier & Bertrand, 1975). This nucleus is considered to be the site of the pneumotaxic (to set the lungs into motion) center.

The lower pons facilitates inspiration by the *apneustic* (arrested breathing) center. This system is prevented from promoting apnea by rostral vagal and afferent stimulation (Wang, Ngai, & Frumin, 1957), and by antiapneustic action of the reticular activation system (RAS).

Lesioning or transsection of the apneustic region results in respiratory slowing with increased amplitude (Breckenridge & Hoff, 1950; Tang, 1953; Wang, Ngai, & Frumin, 1957), ultimately stopping at the deep inspiration position, the "inspiratory cramp," or *apneusis*. The apneustic center is located in the middle and caudal pons (Ngai & Wang, 1957). Electrical stimulation of its various regions suggests that there are discharges related to inspiration-expiration and phase-spanning neurons involved in building up inhibition during inspiration, promoting transition to expiration (Cohen & Wang, 1969). This process seems analogous to that of vagal inhibitory discharges, and the function of expiratory-inspiratory phase-spanning neurons seems to be to inhibit expiration and to build up excitability of the inspiratory center, that is, to promote inspiration. After lesioning, apneusis may partially reverse with recovery, suggesting the existence of some degree of redundancy in this system.

Generally, I-phase *duration* is governed by rate of increase, and maximum level of phrenic nerve activity at the end of the I-phase (inspiratory off-switch level). The *rate of rise* of the I-phase varies with body temperature and CO_2. *Termination* is affected by vagal afferents relaying pulmonary stretch receptor discharge, and activity of the nucleus parabrachialis medialis.

Cohen (1979) posits several different types of I- and E-phase "respiration-related units" (RRU) as the basis of brain neural rhythmicity, and suggests two ways of quantifying their activity: (a) the *respiratory modulation ratio*, the degree of deviation from mean discharge frequency in the cycle; and (b) the *respiratory modulation index*, the degree of deviation from minimum frequency in the cycle-triggered histogram.

The picture is even more complex because there is a variety of RRU discharge patterns, most of which seem to maintain a fixed phase relationship to the respiratory cycle despite changes in such variables as CO_2 level. This relatively stable peak firing frequency, relative to phrenic nerve discharge, suggests a "stable functional connection between different neurons of the RRG [respiratory rhythm generator]" (Cohen, 1979).

But anatomical examination reveals that the incidence of different types of respiratory neurons is not the same in the pons and the medulla. The predominant type of discharge in the medulla is *phasic*—alternating bursts and silent periods; in the pons, it is tonic, and/or phase-spanning. Efferent projection ascending from the pons and medulla respiratory rhythmicity generator is evident in the occurrence of respiratory modulation of the EEG recorded from the cortex and elsewhere. It takes the form of "preferential occurrence of low frequency bursts in certain portions of the respiratory cycle" (Cohen [1979], citing a personal communication with A. Hugelin).

In addition to I-phase synchronization, I-neuron discharge originating in the brain-stem synchronizes on a shorter time scale than that of the I-phase. Oscillations in the 60 to 100 Hz range have been recorded (Suthers, Henderson-Smart, & Read, 1977; Wyss, 1956).

Brain Respiratory Neuron Response to Arterial CO_2 Concentration. A significant decrease in $PaCO_2$ causes apnea. Cohen (1968) detailed three types of response of the brain stem respiratory rhythmicity units to high and low CO_2: A Type 1 response, consisting of lowered CO_2, reduces discharge frequency, and firing eventually ceases. This occurs in most I- and E-neurons. Only two thirds of phasic neurons show this response.

In the Type 2 response, hypocapnia increases firing in the low frequency portion of the cycle, with the discharge becoming tonic (not modulated with the respiratory cycle) when CO_2 is sufficiently low. This response is observed in about half the medullary E-neurons—the "silent period" disappears along with phrenic nerve discharge resulting in expiratory apnea. In the Type 3 response, hypocapnia causes reduction of discharge in the high frequency portion, with little change in the low frequency portion of the cycle, in neurons with tonic respiratory modulated activity.

Eventually, these neurons, found mostly in the pons, lose their respiratory modulation and fire tonically. This suggests that the respiratory modulated portion of the discharge comes from respiration-related units (RRU) sensitive to CO_2, while the tonic portion of the discharge comes from outside the respiratory rhythm generator. Table 4 summarizes the different types of respiration-related neurons proposed by Cohen (1979).

Cohen (1979) teaches us that there are basically two kinds of medullary neurons. Dorsal respiratory-group neurons are predominantly I-neurons; the ventral respiratory-group neurons have about one-third E-neurons; and the caudal region, has a larger proportion of E-neurons. Most dorsal-region neurons project into the spinal cord and respond to hypocapnia by augmentation. There is a significant number of direct afferent and efferent connections between the pneumotaxic center and the ventral respiratory group neurons. Vagal afferents and carotid chemoreceptors project extensively to the dorsal respiratory group neurons.

Dorsal respiratory group neurons transmit IXth and Xth afferent nerve input to the respiratory rhythm generator and control phrenic motor neuron activity. Ventral respiratory group neurons control thoracic respiratory motor neurons, and transmit information between pneumotaxic center RRUs and cranial respiratory motor neurons. The rostral ventilatory group neurons seem to play a major role in rhythm generation, whereas the dorsal respiratory group, is involved in switching from the I- to the E-phase. A minimum of respiratory rhythm can be generated by ventral respiratory group neurons, but the addition of the dorsal respiratory group is required for normal rhythm.

Finally, according to Cohen (1979), "the most important tonic input to RRUs are those derived from central and peripheral chemoreceptors." At low CO_2 levels some RRUs cease firing, whereas others exhibit tonic nonrhythmic firing. Its importance to rhythm generation is derived from the fact that I-neurons inhibit E-neurons, thus contributing to phase-switching.

The Respiratory Centers of the Cerebral Cortex

Guz, Mier, and Murphy (1988) reported a study of the ventilatory response to CO_2 inhalation, in which they recorded diaphragm muscle compound action potential amplitude (using esophageal electrodes), in response to magnetic stimulation of the cortex. They concluded that the cortex may play a variable role in the ventilatory response to inhaled CO_2. Ruch and Fulton (1961) reported accelerator and inhibitory areas in the presylvian cortex. Respiratory movement appears to be localized in the cortical representations of the corresponding body musculature. There are also respiratory functions in the limbic area of the cortex. The larger part of the insular orbital area is inhibitory, as is most of the cingulate gyrus. There is a close association between these areas and the olfactory area, as well as to *Broca's Areas*: speech and breathing seem to be integrated in the

Table 4. Anatomical-Functional Types of Respiratory Neurons*

Location	Type	Discharge pattern	Response to hypocapnia	Response to inflation	Major known projections
DRG (NTS)	I_α	↗	1	0	Sp, c; NRA, c, I (?)
	I_β	↗	1	+	Sp, c; NRA (?)
	P	↘	?	+	?
	Early E	↗	?	+	?
	I_γ	↗	1	0	Sp, c; NTS, c (some); NRA, i; NPBM + KF; i
Rostral VRG	I_δ	↗↘	1	—	NRA, c
	I (V)	↗	1	—	V; i
	Early E	↗↘	2	+	V
	Late E	↗	2	—	V (?)
Caudal VRG	Late E	↗	1, 2	0, —, + (?)	Sp, c
Caudal pons, rostral medulla	EI	↗	2, 3	—, 0	?
Rostral pons NPBM	I, E, IE (tonic)	↗	3	—	NRA, i (?); NPBM + KF; c
KF	I	↗	?	?	NRA, i (?); NPBM + KF; c

Abbreviations: c, contralateral; i, ipsilateral; ↗, augmenting; ↘, decrementing; DRG, dorsal respiratory group; E, expiratory; EI, expiratory-inspiratory; I, inspiratory; IE, inspiratory-expiratory; KF, Kölliker-Fuse nucleus; NPBM, nucleus parabrachialis medialis; NRA, nucleus retroambigualis; NTS, nucleus tractus solitarius; P, pump; Sp, spinal; V, vagal; VRG, ventral respiratory group.
*Reprinted with permission from M. I. Cohen (1979): Physiological Review, Vol. 59, p. 1153.

cortex. The orbital and other limbic areas also mediate emotions. Stimulation of these areas results in breathing changes as well as in the expression of emotion, and these areas affect autonomic activity.

Unlike the heart, the lungs do not have intrinsic rhythm mechanisms. Chemoreceptors and stretchreceptors in the lungs and the musculature associated with breathing send afferent impulses through the vagus to sections of the subcortical portions of the brain (the medulla, pons, and reticular formation) and to the cortex.

In summary, the medulla, pons, and reticular formation are part of the brain-stem and are the location of the major automatic respiratory centers. The medullary center can initiate and maintain sequences of inspiration and expiration (albeit irregular sequences). The apneustic center in the middle and lower pons, if uninhibited, produces prolonged uninterrupted inspiratory spasms (apneustic breathing). The pneumotaxic center in the upper pons inhibits the apneustic center with the aid of vagal impulses.

There are also chemoreceptor cells associated with the vascular system of the brain and the cerebrospinal fluid. They alter breathing through their effect on changes in cerebral vasotonus and blood flow to the brain, depending on their response to $PaCO_2$ and pH (Gotoh, Meyer, & Takagi, 1965; Raichle & Plum, 1972).

Centrally Mediated Abnormal Breathing

A number of breathing patterns deviate from normal rhythm. Comroe (1974) listed the following:

(a) Hyperpnea: increased breathing (usually refers to increased tidal volume [Vt] with or without increased metabolism);
(b) Tachypnea: increased breathing frequency (f);
(c) Hyperventilation: increased alveolar ventilation in relation to metabolic rate (e.g., decreased alveolar PCO_2 to less than 37 torr);
(d) Apnea: cessation of respiration in resting expiratory position;
(e) Apneusis: cessation of respiration in the inspiratory position;
(f) Apneustic breathing: apneusis interrupted periodically by expiration; may be rhythmic;
(g) Gasping: spasmodic inspiration effort, usually maximal, brief, and terminating abruptly; may be rhythmic or irregular;
(h) Biot's respiration: irregular respiration with pauses (originally described in patients with meningitis; now refers to sequences of uniformly deep gasps, apnea, then deep gasps);
(i) Cheyne-Stokes respiration: cycles of gradually increased Vt followed by gradually decreased Vt.

Some investigators relate Cheyne-Stokes respiration to heart failure and others (Lum, 1976) to brain damage. Sensitivity to CO_2 seems greatly increased in persons with this type of breathing disorder, and HV is noted frequently. But, since there is no evidence of heart disease in some cases, brain impairment is hypothesized. Guyton, Cromwell, and Moore (1956) induced Cheyne-Stokes respiration in their subjects by increasing lung-brain circulation time from the typical 10 seconds to as long as 300 seconds. These observations support the hypothesis that this breathing pattern may be due to prolonged circulation time between the lungs and the chemoreceptors.

Endorphins and Breathing Control

Research on endogenous opiates in pain control has led some investigators to note their considerable effect on breathing. Hughes (1975) showed that β-endorphin is especially involved in ventilatory control. Opioid receptors have been located in numerous animal species, as well as in humans, and are found in high concentration in the medulla (Chernick, 1981). They have received some attention in connection with prenatal and neonatal asphyxia, as well as apnea, because it has been noted that β-endorphin levels are elevated in babies at birth and are found in highest concentration when the infant is hypoxemic (Chernick, 1981; Davis, 1981). This endogenous opioid is thought to depress ventilation, especially motor response to hypocapnia (Moss & Friedman, 1978; Moss & Scarpelli, 1981), and to do so by inhibition of pontile respiratory neurons (Denavit-Saubie, Champagnat, & Zieglgansberger, 1978).

The endorphin antagonist, naloxone, has been shown to reverse respiratory failure (Williams et al., 1982), and has been successfully used in the treatment of neonatal respiratory dysfunction (Chernick, 1981), and the reversal of anaphylactic shock—acute respiratory failure. Naloxone has also recently been shown to inhibit the effects of alcohol which, apparently, binds to some of the same receptor sites as the opioids (Mackenzie, 1979; Volpicelli, Alterman, Hayashida, & O'Brien, 1992). Although it is not commonly thought that naloxone has agonistic action, it has been reported to block GABA, an inhibitory neurotransmitter, and further research into its action is being conducted (Lawson et al., 1979).

Klee, Ziouchou, and Streaty (1977) isolated *exorphins*—morphine-like substances—from the pepsin digest of wheat gluten. These exorphins, paradoxically, also contain substances which are morphine antagonists. The mixed agonists/antagonists have been shown to produce profound euphoria and have been implicated in schizophrenia. The relevance of this finding to respiration is that breathing patterns in schizophrenia differ from those in anxiety and panic disorder. They tend to be rapid in anxiety and panic, and slow in schizophrenia. Endorphins, like morphine, slow breathing—sometimes fatally.

The Hering-Breuer Reflex

If there were no inhibition of inspiration, one could, in theory, inflate the lungs until the alveoli burst. In fact, this does not happen. Inflation of the lungs results in inhibition of inspiration, followed by expiration (Hering & Breuer, 1868). Conversely, deflation of the lungs is followed by reflexive inspiration. This circuit is disabled by section of the vagus (Bell, Davidson, & Scarborough, 1968; Brobeck, 1979; Wang & Ngai, 1964).

The Biological Role of Air Ions

When I first wrote this chapter, this section was part of the earlier section, *The Composition of Atmospheric and Alveolar Air*. I then decided to expand and isolate it, assuming that in so doing, I would implicitly express my own ambivalence about the validity of some of these findings. Though outside of the mainstream, bioactivity of air ions may turn out to be of considerable clinical significance, and, based on my own experience, I am not prepared to dismiss this. Nevertheless, it has something of a controversial nature.

One would think it reasonable, at first blush, to assume that the electrical charge of air particles might be bioactive. And indeed, considerable effort has been expended in examining the assumption that they probably influence physiology when their density reaches a certain level. But additional controversy centers on their more or less naturally occurring low per-air-volume density of about .000000000001 parts per million (ppm).

The reason for general skepticism centers on the fact that (a) charged air particles occur in such extremely low concentrations that they are thought to be too sparse for bioactivity; (b) they leave no footprint—no scar, as it were; (c) no known receptors have been located; and, (d) they are so unstable that it is virtually impossible to isolate them for study. This is because they interact so readily with other environmental elements that they lose their identity. These attributes do not favor empirical validation, an essential criterion in a research grant-dependent "publish or perish" world.

What are air ions? The smaller ones are clusters of air molecules consisting of a single molecule that may be positively charged, such as H_3O, or negatively charged, such as O_2^-, typically surrounded by fewer than 10 water molecules (Charry & Kavet, 1989). They possess electrical properties and may combine with other molecules or attach to condensation nuclei or airborne particles. Density of these small air ions in urban air ranges from 10^{-12} to 10^{-11} parts per million (ppm), and 10^{-11} to 10^{-10} ppm in clean rural air.

According to Johnson (1982), the human body collects about 0.01 na (nanoamperes, billionths of an ampere) in clean air, but "worse case" current induction in a person standing below a high voltage dc transmission line is only about 3 uA (microamperes, millionths of an ampere).

You may recall, from Chapter 1, that resistance (the opposition to a current) causes heat. The effect of ions flowing through the body result in an estimated heat production 10^{12} times lower than average basal metabolic heat production, and biopotentials in the human nervous system which are 10^6 times weaker than those required to trigger an action potential, and 10^5 times weaker than extracellular EEG signals (Elul, 1962). These and similar facts strongly support the theory that, as far as we know, ions do not constitute "stimuli"—we simply can't perceive them, and we have a historical tendency to equate effectiveness with perception.

That air ions are 10^4 times lower than the minimal dc currents perceptible by human beings (Kruger & Reed, 1976) lends support to the argument that by virtue of their imperceptibility they cannot be bioactive. This argument is neither devastating nor conclusive. On the one hand it is argued that the male silkworm's responsiveness to female attractant pheromone is based on a concentration of only 200 molecules per cm^3 (Kruger & Reed, 1976). But the relatively low density of pheromone required to produce a response—the definition of a stimulus, after all—only indicates that different receptors have different threshold requirements, not that low molecule density defies the traditional definition of a stimulus. If he responds to it, the silkworm clearly perceives it. Another argument is that aldosterone, an antidiuretic hormone in the kidney, affects sodium and water conservation in concentrations of between 2×10^{-10} and 10^{-12} molecules (Guyton, 1981)—an aqueous concentration not very different from that of ions in air. But then again, we don't "perceive" aldosterone either.

Numerous problems plague the study of air ions: They are highly water soluble, they cannot be visualized microscopically or otherwise, they produce no known acute response, and they readily relinquish their charge and leave no trace. But, an aggregate of research studies in which attempts have been made to control their ambient density yields some preliminary conclusions. Kavet (1989) lists them in his Table 2, p. 165. He also cites the references supporting each.

If we omit, for the moment, those studies which showed no effects, we can see that the findings are quite equivocal (see Tables 5a and b), yet they inspire curiosity because they are by no means consistently negative. Kavet's (1989) Table 4, page 167, is more germane to our concerns. It is

Table 5a. Effect of Positive Ions on Human Physiology and Behavior*

	Increase	Decrease
Galvanic skin response	+	+
Reaction time	+	•
Mood	•	+
Vigilance	+	•
EEG alpha frequency	•	+
Relaxation	+	•
Sleepiness	+	•
Dry mucosa	+	•
Critical flicker fusion	•	+

*Reprinted with permission from R. Kavet (1989): Hypothetical neural substrates for biological response to air ions. In J. M. Charry and R. Kavet (eds.): *Air Ions: Physical and Biological Aspects*, p. 165. Boca Raton: CRC Press.

Table 5b. Effect of Negative Ions on Human Physiology and Behavior*

	Increase	Decrease
EEG alpha frequency	•	+
Amplitude	+	•
Synchronization	+	•
Metabolism (bipolar high)	+	•
(bipolar low)	•	+
Anxiety	•	+
Motor performance	+	•
Reaction time	+	+
Vigilance	+	•
Skin resistance	+	•
Blood pressure	•	+
Pulse finger volume	+	•
Relaxation	+	•
Sleepiness	+	•
Dry mucosa	+	•
Mood	+	•

*Reprinted with permission from R. Kavet (1989): Hypothetical neural substrates for biological response to air ions. In J. M. Charry and R. Kavet (eds.): *Air Ions: Physical and Biological Aspects*. Boca Raton: CRC Press.

based on an earlier report by Charry (1984). The variables that showed increase or decrease to positive or negative ions are listed in Table 6.

Taken together, the most salient results of consistent exposure to air ions appear to be related to serotonin changes in brain and blood together with various effects on mood, learning, performance, reaction time, and perception of pain. In general, positive ion exposure is followed by increased peripheral (blood, urine) serotonin and behavioral decrement; while negative ion exposure appears to have the opposite outcome. Research reports give no clear indication of the range of ion concentration and exposure duration in many studies.

The most intriguing effect of ion exposure is on blood and brain levels of serotonin. Systematically, serotonin constricts vascular smooth muscle as well as that of pulmonary airways, and promotes platelet aggregation. Blood platelets have high affinity serotonin takeup mechanisms. But

Table 6. Clinical Symptoms in Humans*

Symptoms	Ions	
	Positive	Negative
Burn pain		decr.
Postoperative discomfort		decr.
Bronchial asthma		decr.
Respiratory spasticity	incr.	decr.
Asthmatic bronchial spasticity	incr.	decr.
Irritation syndrome (5-HT urine)	incr.	
(5-HIAA urine)	incr.	
Exhaustion syndrome (NE, EPI urine)	decr.	
(17KS, 17-OH urine)	decr.	
Hyperthyroidism (5-HT urine)	incr.	
(NE, EPI urine)	incr.	
(17-KS, 17-OH urine)	incr.	
(histamine urine)	incr.	
Migraine—serotonin	incr.	
EEG alpha and synchronization		incr.
5-HT, 5-HIAA (weather-sensitive)		decr.
(nonweather-sensitive)		•••••
Headache	incr.	
Dizziness	incr.	
Sore throat	incr.	
Smarting eyes		incr.
Congested throat		incr

*Reprinted with permission from R. Kavet (1989): Hypothetical neural substrates for biological response to air ions. In J. M. Charry and R. Kavet (eds.): *Air Ions: Physical and Biological Aspects*, p. 167. Boca Raton: CRC Press.

peripherally circulating serotonin is not thought to cross the blood-brain barrier.

Serotonin constricts brain arteries, according to Giannini, Malone, and Piotrowski (1986), who urge us to recognize a *serotonin irritation syndrome* (SIS). Giannini et al. (1983) report that patients with SIS-like symptoms show increased serum serotonin and urinary 5-HIAA is decreased. This suggests that positive ions promote decrease of monoamine oxidase (MAO) activity, but it does so selectively in SIS-sensitive persons. In the nonsensitive, no such reaction was observed. It is suggested that, metabolically, the SIS-sensitive react differently to cation exposure.

Ordinarily, plasma (free-circulating) serotonin is removed from blood by pulmonary endothelial cells, metabolized by monoamine oxidase, and excreted in urine (Kavet, 1989). In the central nervous system (CNS), neurons containing serotonin are concentrated in the raphe nuclei near the midline from the medulla to the mesencephalon (Douglas, 1980). There are projections from these cell nuclei to the limbic system, thalamus, and cortex, laterally along the reticular formation, and caudally, into the lower brain stem and spinal cord.

According to Douglas (1975), it is possible that one function of tryptaminergic raphe neurons is to control, or "dampen," overreactiveness to stimuli affecting social and adaptive behavior. This may include sexual behavior, aggressiveness, motor activity, and, perhaps, temperature regulation, neuroendocrine functions, and extrapyramidal activity. It has been proposed that air ions exert their action through monoamine oxidase (MAO) (an intramitochondrial enzyme), affecting not only serotonin, but also norepinephrine and dopamine. In fact, Krueger and Smith (1960) reported that administration of iproniazid, an MAO inhibitor, mimics exposure to positive ions, while reserpine, which depletes tissue serotonin, simulates exposure to negative ions. Kavet (1989), however, doubts the MAO hypothesis because (a) inhaled ions are not known to have access to the central nervous system; and (b) peripheral effects of MAO, via the autonomic nervous system (ANS), are not observed.

Krueger is the better known of the air ion research pioneers, but Vasiliev (1960) proposed "pulmonary interoceptors" in the mediation of the physiological reaction to ions. These putative mechanisms are pulmonary neuroendocrine cells—chemoreceptors. The hypothesis of such chemoreceptors essentially yields to the pressure of puzzling physiological reactions to varying climate and weather conditions.

Galen (131 to 201 A.D.) suggested the salutary effects of sea air for certain pulmonary diseases. He also suggested breathing exercises (Wehner, 1989).

Chapter 3

The Circulatory System and the Heart

Introduction

I recently read a wonderful story in the newspaper. There was the American Museum of Natural History with proverbial egg on its face—dinosaur egg! *Brontosaurus*, it was forced to admit, apparently with some reluctance, was wearing the wrong head. The mistake was soon corrected by attaching the right head which, it turns out, had for decades been lying in a carton in the basement.

"Look, Johnny! A Brontosaurus."

"Da-a-ad?"

"What?"

"Such a teeny-tiny head?"

"Yea, Johnny. Didn't need much of a head to be a dinosaur. And anyway, whaddaya think . . . they'd put the wrong head on it?"

I am citing this story to illustrate the politics of science. A further explication of this snafu, in *The New Yorker* (May 6, 1991), follows:

> In 1975, two paleontologists working at the Carnegie Museum with a third brontosaurus proved that Marsh's Brontosaurus was wearing the wrong skull, and therefore so was Osborn's. (By then, the Brontosaurus itself had been scientifically discredited, too. The dinosaur that March had named Brontosaurus was actually a larger version of an Apatosaurus, a dinosaur he had described a year or so earlier.) (p. 33)

Not only was it the wrong head, but it wasn't even a Brontosaurus! Now, maybe we should rethink what we claim controls what in *behavior*, especially when it comes to the brain. A brain is, after all, even more abstruse than a skull, and its descriptors are such vague terms as "relay," "activating system," "sensory projection area," and so on.

We still can't tell much more than where a lesion might be when we note a dysfunction; we only have theories about how we remember; we use a "scientific" term, *idiopathic*, for "of unknown origin," to explain most seizures; and we can't predictably prevent them with medication or surgery in much more than about 45% of cases (Yahr, 1951). As Kluver and Bucy (1939) so aptly demonstrated, we can get along without a cortex. But we pay virtually no attention to blood without which we really can't get along. Unlike the brain, blood and the circulatory system have not been accorded the importance they deserve in psychophysiology. The metaphors, cliches, and traditions of science die hard.

According to the great Harvard neurophysiologists, W.G. and M.A. Lennox, and F.A. and E.L. Gibbs (1938), "The brain is master, the blood, servant." What does this aphorism mean? They concluded that the brain controls circulation rather than the other way around by noting increased brain volume with increased mental activity (Carmichael, Doupe, & Williams, 1937), and inferring increased brain blood flow from the response of a thermocouple embedded in the brain (Gerard, 1938; Lennox & Leonhardt, 1931; Schmidt & Hendrix, 1938). Yet, as early as 1927, Schmidt showed that respiration and systemic blood pressure, among other things, control brain blood flow. These findings are not disputed to this day.

Subsequently, the Lennoxes (1960) quoted Luys as having said in the 1880s:

> It is the blood that carries everywhere with its uninterrupted currents the vivifying stimulation which causes the cells to feel, to become erect, and to associate for co-ordinated action.

What a field day psychoanalysts would have with the metaphors in this quote. It was immediately followed by the Lennoxes' assertion that:

> Many look on the brain as at the mercy of the circulation and helpless in the face of failing blood-borne supplies. There is indeed a reciprocal relationship between brain and circulation, but the former is distinctly the ruler. (p. 740)

Metaphors aside, they nevertheless correctly pointed out that the key element controlling brain blood flow and metabolism is CO_2 and not O_2: Small variations in CO_2 content of blood produced significant changes in brain blood flow and metabolism, while moderate variations in O_2 had little effect. Yet, respiration serves, fundamentally, to provide the body with the required quantity of O_2 according to its needs at a particular momentary level of activity (metabolism). Everyone agrees with this assertion. (Lavoisier, who discovered it, thought O_2 might be dangerous. Little did he know.)

For instance, reduction of O_2 to water in living cells results in intermediates including the extremely reactive superoxide radical, O_2^-. Cells contain relatively large amounts of enzymes, superoxide dismutases, that lower their superoxide levels. Extracellular fluids, on the other hand, have extremely low superoxide dismutase levels. Superoxide can be very damaging, as we see in inflamed tissue. The product of superoxide dismutase is hydrogen peroxide, itself a powerful oxidant. And there are other oxidants each requiring protective enzymes such as peroxidases and catalases.

Cell respiration is not simply limited to availability and distribution of O_2. There is little reason to doubt that "there must be an intracellular O_2 pressure at which biological activity is optimal" (Shapiro, Harrison, & Walton, 1982) ("pressure" here means concentration). Thus, familiarity with O_2 homeostasis is fundamental to understanding respiration: What factors in the present biology of the individual dictate breathing rate, minute volume, and gas composition? What are the effects of variation in any of them?

Such questions are underscored in behavioral physiology, with its special interest in the central nervous system (CNS) and autonomic nervous system (ANS), by reports by Blass and Gibson (1979) on the effects of graded hypoxia: Hypoxia is a graded (versus absolute) reduction in O_2 supply. It differs from anoxia in that the latter is a total absence of O_2. According to W.G. Lennox (1960), "The chief symptom of anoxia is death." An unusually abstract definition of "symptom." That's Harvard for you.

Anoxia has rapid and profound effects on synthesis of neurotransmitters when energy metabolism becomes impaired. CO_2, an end-product of local brain metabolism, falls rapidly as O_2 delivery decreases, and acetylcholine synthesis drops proportionately. Decreased catecholamine and serotonin are also reported (Davis & Carlsson, 1973). Yet, behavioral consequences of hypoxia are largely ignored by behavioral physiologists. This oversight has led to the publication of a number of unusual theories about what breathing behavior is all about, what it should consist of, and mind-numbing (pun intended) behavioral interventions.

For the serious student of respiration, it must be clear, in the final analysis, that the *only valid criterion in any behavioral breathing intervention must be blood gases.* Anything short of that misses the mark by the proverbial "country mile." Failure to comprehend this simple proposition is responsible for the chaos that characterizes this discipline and has led to confusing and misleading ideas and techniques. For instance:

A recent issue of *Biofeedback and Self-Regulation* featured an article by Clark and Hirschman (1990) titled, "Effects of paced respiration on anxiety reduction in a clinical population." Everyone knows that breathing is more rapid in anxious persons, so what's wrong with just slowing it down? I could forgive Clark and Hirschman had they simply failed to cite my work on deep-diaphragmatic breathing, appearing in the same journal just two years before (Fried, 1987b). But their report, like many others, perpetuates myths about "slowing down breathing" that conflict with physiology.

It is often the case that anxious or "hysterical" persons are admonished to breathe more slowly. If you stop to think about it, this makes no sense. What the "experts" really mean is breathe more fully and more deeply, thereby increasing tidal volume and reflexively (Hering-Breuer) decreasing breathing rate. Clearly, the end product should be volume, not rate.

The article cites neither pretreatment breathing rate nor tidal volume in the experimental group, which must have been affected by metabolic acidosis typical in their subjects (alcoholics). There are no data on alveolar CO_2 concentration, and none on changes in CO_2, or tidal volume during and after training—in fact, no reference anywhere to volume.

What was the procedure? Subjects followed tone-cues pacing breathing to about 10 breaths/min, and reported feeling better. The psychogalvanic skin response (PGR) (the most unstable and uninterpretable physiological index known) was used to corroborate subjective reports. Inferring from the statistical analysis, there were no significant differences between the treatment and control group "pre-"breathing rates; and breathing rate dropped from approximately 17 to 18 breaths/min to the "paced" 10 breaths/min.

Did minute volume (Vmin) change? Had the researchers taught deep-diaphragmatic breathing, the rate would have dropped to between 3 and 4 breaths/min in their subjects (Fried, 1990b); and were end-tidal CO_2 levels known, volume could have been estimated. Or they could have consulted *Respiration and Circulation* (Altman & Dittmer, 1971) for the nomograph (see Chapter 2). Other factors being equal, if 10 breaths/min is better than 17 breaths/min, 3 breaths/min should be even better, assuming relatively constant minute volume. The idea is to breathe as much air as activity level demands, in fewer breaths, isn't it?

As we begin to understand more about the interaction of breathing and blood gases in behavioral physiology, we can look more critically at the literature which features these parameters. For instance, it is generally accepted that panic attacks are a psychological disorder. DSM-III-R confirms it. So please consider the following which appeared in the *Australian and New Zealand Journal of Psychiatry*:

> Evidence has been found that physiological variables such as $paCO_2$ and pH are involved in the aetiology of panic attacks and panic disorder but the extent and the nature of the involvement of cognitive variables is undetermined. (Kenardy, Oei, & Evans, 1990, p. 261)

Shouldn't somebody send them a copy of the DSM-III-R? Not only does water swirl down the drain in the opposite direction "down under," but isn't this assertion also upside down? It contradicts just about everything that has ever been written about panic attacks and panic disorder. Naturally, I support the view of Kenardy et al. (1990) completely.

Consider also the following:

> Hyper- and hypocapnia have both pronounced effects upon cerebral function. . . . It has been claimed that pronounced hyperventilation can decrease CBF to such an extent that cerebral hypoxia occurs. . . . (Granholm, Lukjanova, & Siesjo, 1968, p. IV:c)

and

> Future studies should take into account the multiple mechanisms through which anxiety may influence CBF, including arousal, the autonomic nervous system, CO_2 and blood viscosity. CO_2 seems to be the most serious source of confusion, because of its profound effect on blood flow, the marked changes during acute anxiety, the nonlinear relationship between CO_2 and CBF . . . (Mathew & Wilson, 1990, p. 846)

Finally, in "Hyperventilation syndrome: Clinical, ventilatory, and personality characteristics as observed in neurological practice," one may read that:

> Compared with controls, the patients had significantly decreased end-tidal pCO_2 even during symptom free periods. After hyperventilation, hypocapnia followed a protracted course. . . . (Brodtkorb, Gimse, Antonaci, Ellersten, Sand, Slug, & Sjaastad, 1990, p. 307)

Each statement links a mental state to blood or its circulation: excessive loss of blood CO_2 (hypocapnia) in exhaled (end-tidal) breath, cerebral blood flow (CBF), change in blood pH, and low oxygen (hypoxia). Many investigators, including Brodtkorb et al. (1990), report inducing abnormal states, even triggering psychosomatic symptoms, abnormal EEGs and seizures, with the HV-challenge—forced overbreathing.

Yet, some persistently deny that HV may be the primary cause, and insist that panic attacks and other symptoms are due to stress, neurosis, or anxiety, in the face of evidence that HV has a rapid and profound effect on tissue oxygenation. Table 1 of the Brodtkorb et al. study (cited above) is labeled "Referral diagnoses in 25 patients who ultimately were shown to suffer from the hyperventilation syndrome." Numbers 1 and 2 on the list were "epilepsy" and "transient ischemic attack" (TIA) with an 11 and 4 out of 25 frequency, respectively.

Ischemia is a spasmodic arterial narrowing usually attributed to local O_2 deficit (hypoxia). TIA has been solidly linked to angina, heart attack, and stroke, and is also implicated in migraine and idiopathic seizures. With no preconceived notions about such disorders, might you not now come to the conclusion that they must somehow be tissue respiration related? Well, why don't you?

There may be historical explanations. In 1933, Wilder Penfield, one of the world's most respected neurosurgeons, read a paper before the American College of Physicians, in Montreal, "The evidence for a cerebral vascular mechanism in epilepsy." He attributed epilepsy, as did Hughlings Jackson, and Gowers, in the 1800s, to vasomotor reflexes. But since it was already known that the autonomic nervous system *does not* control brain vasomotor reflexes, it became necessary to postulate a "local vascular nerve plexus."

Several years later, other researchers "doped out" the vasomotor reflex mechanism: arteries constrict and dilate in response to blood CO_2 concentration (Brody & Dusser de Barenne, 1932; Bronk, 1966; Cobb, Frantz, Penfield, & Riley, 1966; Cobb, Sargant, & Schwab, 1938; Darrow & Graf, 1945; Davis & Wallace, 1942; Forbes & Cobb, 1966; Gibbs, Williams, & Gibbs, 1940; Gibbs, Lennox, & Gibbs, 1940; Gotoh, Meyer, & Takagi, 1965; Lennox, 1928; Lennox, Cobb, & Gibbs, 1936; Lennox, Gibbs, & Gibbs, 1938; Gibbs, Williams, & Gibbs, 1949; Penfield & Jasper, 1954; Schmidt, 1928; Schmidt & Hendrix, 1966; Von Santha & Cipriani, 1966; Weiss, 1966). Yet, belief in the existence of a hypothetical local vascular nerve plexus persists despite the fact that the *real* mechanism is known and there is no such "nerve plexus" (Fried, Fox, & Carlton, 1990). You see, it isn't even a Brontosaurus.

Look up panic disorder in the DSM-III-R: Criteria 1 (dyspnea) and 5 (choking or smothering sensation) are breathing related—two out of 12 criteria. Adding Criteria 2 (palpitation), 3 (chest pain or discomfort), 5 (dizziness, vertigo, or unsteady feeing), and 10 (faintness), we have symptoms of hypoxia; and 6 out of 12 symptoms of panic disorder are also those of HVS. Consider that in the Brodtkorb et al. study, the second most common diagnosis was "transient ischemic attack" (TIA). We may now be much more impressed by earlier findings of Neill and Hattenhauer (1975) of impaired myocardial O_2 supply due to HV.

What is even more impressive is that Brodtkorb et al., who are neurologists, make no reference whatever to the exact same findings reported by Neill and Hattenhauer 15 years earlier in the journal *Circulation*, or to similar findings relating HVS to hypoxia and coronary arterial spasms (Yasue, Nagao, Omote, Takizawa, Miwa, & Tanaka, 1978; Yasue, 1980). Curiously, brain and systemic physiologists don't seem to read each other's work. No model integrates terms such as "hypocapnia," "alkalosis," "pH," and "hypoxia," with mental and somatic disorders. No model integrates the head and the body . . . not only was it the wrong head. . . .

Concerning panic attacks, history does not show that theories about "subconscious conflict" are disposed to crumble in the face of contradictory empirical evidence. I think that these "sacred cows" would make delicious barbecue.

The Model

In simple unicellular organisms, O_2 seeps through the membrane by diffusion, and reaches mitochondria governing energy production. CO_2 seeps out due to difference in concentration (pressure differential gradient) inside and outside the cell wall. In time, cell aggregates form organisms. At first, inside cells are supplied and evacuated by diffusion through the intracellular fluid (i.e., bathing the cells within the aggregate), creating the beginning of the lymphatic system. The lymphatic system is older, phylogenetically, than the vascular system.

Before the appearance of the capillary system, whole blood discharged directly into fluid in the intracellular space. Blood cells and other constituents drained into lymphatic vessels which pumped it back to the heart. Our lymphatic system still performs the function of collecting debris from intracellular (interstitial) fluid (Sodeman & Sodeman, 1979). But as organisms increased in complexity, the lymphatic system became insufficient to meet their need for ventilation, nutrition, and excretion.

As organisms evolved and grew in size and complexity, they would have required enormous amounts of fluid in the vascular system to provide the required O_2 and nutrients, and to remove the wastes, soluble in fluid under normal conditions. The solution (pun intended): "Watson, my good fellow, what is there that could possibly absorb more O_2 than an equal volume of fluid?" "Elementary, my dear Holmes, hemoglobin." Under normal conditions, each molecule of hemoglobin (Hb) can capture one molecule of O_2.

Imagine the red cells crammed with Hb molecules circulating in the body, each one like a miniature baseball glove reaching out and capturing an O_2 molecule in the lungs, for later distribution. One condition affecting the affinity of Hb for O_2 is the concentration of hydrogen ions (H+) in its surroundings. Hydrogen is the "H" in pH, a measure of that concentration. If pH rises, the little glove holds on tightly to the O_2-ball. If it decreases, O_2 is released.

Temperature also affects O_2 retention. Normal temperature favors release; fever favors retention, taking into account that excess O_2 saturation must be avoided at all costs or the organism burns up. But how does Hb know when to hold and when to release O_2? That is the role of pH: A "saturated" Hb molecule arrives at a capillary in the brain, for instance. Concentration of CO_2 due to local metabolism decreases the pH (it is slightly less alkaline) and that favors release of the O_2.

Of course blood is never fully desaturated. But the relatively desaturated blood then goes back to the lungs to pick up more O_2, and so the cycle repeats. Since body temperature varies little in the absence of fever, the critical component in the oxy-hemoglobin (OHb) binding and dissociation is pH. Red cell function is an important factor in breathing. The acid-base homeostasis is quite intolerant of even small deviations.

To know the events in malfunctioning red cells makes it easier to explain the effects of HV on the threshold of psychosomatic and emotional disorders, in terms of "hypoxia" (Katz, 1982).

General Organization of the Cardiovascular System: The Circulatory System and the Heart

The circulatory system comprises the heart, the blood vessels, and the lymphatic system. It might, more appropriately be termed the *re*circulatory system since it "recirculates" blood through the body. It entails more or less specific routes by which blood reaches organs of the body.

Systemic circulation. Oxygenated blood leaves the left ventricle of the heart via the aorta, travels through all the organs of the body and, when deoxygenated, returns via veins to the right atrium. It also has pulmonary, coronary, and hepatic portal routes which supply the lungs, the heart, and the digestive organs and the liver.

Cerebral circulation is controlled at the Circle of Willis, at the base of the brain where the left and right internal carotid arteries converge with the basilar artery. The Circle of Willis provides the brain with alternate circulation routes in case of impaired incoming blood flow. But, it is the capillary "bed" that is the business end of the cardiovascular system because it is from there that O_2 and nutrients diffuse into tissues, and that CO_2 and other "waste products" exit.

Long before psychophysiologists thought of thermal biofeedback, the importance of the peripheral vascular system was underscored by Deutsch, Ehrentheil, and Peirson (1941) and Hauptmann and Myerson (1948). They suggested that anatomical abnormalities of capillaries noted in their clients might account for their Raynaud's, migraine, depression, psychoses and, in some, epileptic seizures. Such studies make us aware of what actually happens at stimulation sites, and what the important exceptions are to the general rules.

For instance, all physiology textbooks point to ANS innervation of

arterial vasculature, and the vasoconstrictive effects of sympathetic stimulation. But they fail to emphasize that low arterial blood CO_2 (low $PaCO_2$)
is as powerful a peripheral vasoconstrictor as sympathetic stimulation.

Arteries, Arterioles, Capillaries, and Veins

Depending on diameter, structure, and function, blood vessels are
designated as arteries, arterioles, capillaries, venules, and veins. Arteries
are composed of three distinct layers. The outermost layer is principally
collagenous fibers; a middle layer, thicker than the other two, is made of
elastic fibers and smooth muscle; an inner layer of endothelial cells is in
contact with circulating blood (endothelium is said to be squamous, or
scalelike). The hollow part of this muscle tubing, the bore, is called the
lumen.

Arteries expand when the heart contracts and blood is forced into
them; then they recoil to their previous diameter between pulses because
they are elastic. This action helps to move the blood along its way. Some
smooth muscle fibers form adjacent rings along the length of the artery.
They are innervated by sympathetic (ANS) fibers which, when stimulated,
constrict reducing the diameter of the lumen. Vasodilation occurs in the
absence, or inhibition, of sympathetic ANS stimulation. Coronary arteries
emerging from the aorta, delivering blood to the heart, are exceptions:
sympathetic impulses cause dilation, while parasympathetic impulses
result in constriction (Schlossbergh & Zuidema, 1986).

Large arteries (such as the aorta and common carotid), which carry
blood from the heart to smaller diameter arteries, are called "elastic," or
conducting, arteries. Medium-sized distributing, or muscular, arteries
distribute blood throughout the body. Their walls are thinner and more
elastic than those of conducting arteries. In many cases, regions of the
body are served by several arteries that may unite to form a common
branch. The point of junction is called an *anastomosis*. "End arteries" do not
anastomose. Stemming blood flow in an end artery is clearly more serious
than occluding one that anastomoses, since anastomosis provides alternate routes or "collateral circulation." The physiology of vascular resistance to blood flow may be found in Bevan, Halpern, and Mulvaney (1991),
Colantuoni, Bertuglia, and Intaglietta (1985), and Slaaf, Huub, Vrielink,
Tangelder, and Reneman (1988).

Arterioles are basically small arteries. But as they become smaller,
they undergo anatomical change which varies with distance from the
artery. Arterioles deliver blood to capillaries and are of singular importance in regulating the blood flow into capillaries. Arteriolar smooth
muscle may constrict or dilate in response to decreased blood concentra-

tion of CO_2 (below about 30 torr) and/or ANS stimulation. It is important to remember that brain arteries and arterioles ordinarily *do not respond to ANS stimulation*, unlike their peripheral counterpart. The only variable known to affect their caliber (diameter of the lumen), and therefore blood flow in the brain, is CO_2 concentration in arterial blood (Heistad, Marcus, & Abboud, 1978). They typically transport oxygenated blood, alternately under systolic (pulse pressure) and under diastolic pressure exerted by their tonic state (constriction).

The aorta is the main artery, exiting just above the heart. It has two main branches, the ascending aorta and the aortic arch. The latter contains blood pressure-regulating "baroceptors." The descending aorta consists of the thoracic and abdominal segments. Two important branches of the ascending aorta, the right and left coronary arteries at the junction of the aorta and the heart proper, just beyond the aortic valve, supply blood to the heart.

Figure 1 is a schematic representation of the circulatory system showing the major arteries (dark) and the veins (light).

The ascending aorta divides into right and left trunks, branching to the neck and right and left arms. Rising further, they form the right and left aortic arch in the neck. Dividing again, one branch goes to the scalp; the other, via the Circle of Willis, forms the basilar and cerebral arteries. The descending portion supplies the thoracic and abdominal regions, including the lungs and diaphragm. The celiac artery has a hepatic (liver), splenic, and gastric segment. The femoral artery, in the groin, descends into the legs and feet.

There are comparable veins for the return trip. The superior vena cava returns blood to the heart from the upper portion of the body, while the inferior vena cava serves blood returning to the heart from its lower parts. In pulmonary circulation, desaturated (deoxygenated) blood flows through the pulmonary trunk exiting from the right ventricle of the heart. It rises upwards from the heart, backwards, and to the left before dividing into the right and left pulmonary arteries. These arteries branch and terminate in capillaries around the alveoli in the lungs.

Pulmonary veins, *the only veins that carry oxygenated blood in an individual after birth*, exit from each lung with oxygenated blood flowing to the left atrium of the heart. Contraction of the left ventricle causes blood to flow into systemic circulation.

Figure 2 shows the heart and lungs as well as the major arteries and veins which make up the pulmonary circulation.

Arteries gradually dwindle in diameter to arterioles, which terminate in capillaries, about 1 millimeter long, distinguished not only by their diameter—about that of a red blood cell, 7 to 8 microns (millionths of a

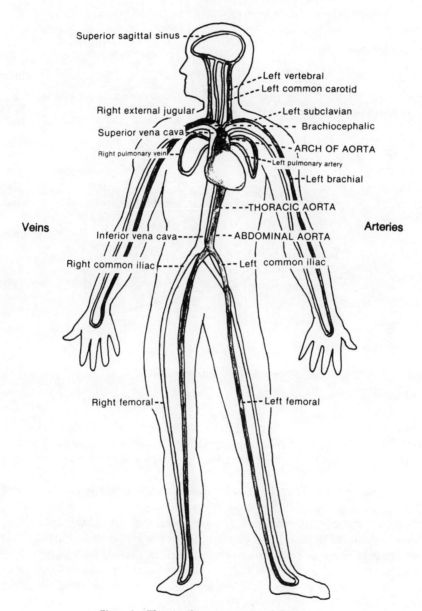

Figure 1. The circulatory system and the heart.

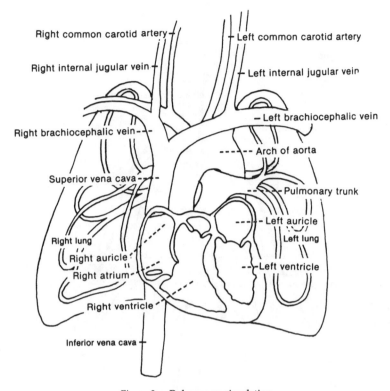

Figure 2. Pulmonary circulation.

meter)—but also by the fact that their wall of endothelial cells is only one cell thick. There is a capillary in proximity to virtually every cell in the body. And it is estimated that no cell lies more than 30 to 50 microns from a capillary.

Exchange at the capillary is by diffusion through the capillary wall into interstitial (intracellular) fluid. It is rapid and pervasive because of the continuous motion of water molecules in and out of the capillaries, mixing the constituents in blood and interstitial fluid as blood flows through the capillaries. There is continuous disequilibrium between contents of the capillary and those in interstitial space because of osmotic (colloid) pressure due to blood proteins inside the capillary, and fluid pressure in the interstitial space.

Ordinarily, interstitial fluid will be at a pressure below that of atmospheric pressure. But increase in interstitial pressure above atmospheric pressure may lead to edema. Pressing the edematous area with a finger will cause the fluid to be forced out of the tissue at the point of contact, leaving a pit. Several factors may contribute to "pitting edema": High capillary pressure, low plasma osmotic pressure, increased capillary permeability, and lymphatic blockage.

Under ordinary circumstances, interstitial space is not filled with fluid, but with gel. Were it otherwise, gravity would cause fluid to flow from the upper body and settle in the lower body and limbs. Gel also retards the spread of bacteria and provides a space that separates cells from each other, facilitating excretion and diffusion. Most blood substances that diffuse through the capillary wall diffuse with almost equal ease through fluid or gel. Ideally, diffusion of fluid from the capillary wall into interstitial space results in an amount equal to that required to form gel.

Blood Circulation through the Brain

Numerous psychophysiological studies report rhythms in the EEG associated with seizures, anxiety, relaxation, meditation, childhood attention-deficit and hyperactivity disorder (ADHD), Tourette's syndrome, and many more. We also have strong evidence that each of these conditions is related to brain neuron function. We are told that the EEG tells us something about how brain neurons function during consciousness and these other mental states. But what do we mean by function?

Cell function depends on metabolism and that means oxidation of glucose. Glucose availability and cell respiration are both directly dependent on brain blood flow. I refer here to "respiration" rather than simply to O_2 delivery since the inter- and intracellular concentration of CO_2 is equally important in determining brain blood flow and metabolism (see also Chapter 4). Countless meditation studies report that breathing alters metabolism, the EEG, and mental states (Badawi, Wallace, Orme-Johnson, & Rouzere, 1984; Beary, Benson, & Klemchuck, 1974; Benson, Beary, & Carol, 1974; Fried, 1987a, 1987b, 1990, 1990a; Kasamatsu & Hirai, 1969; Morse, Martin, Furst, & Dubin, 1977; Wallace, 1970a). Yet few investigators seem to have put two and two together to conclude that breathing must affect the EEG precisely because it affects brain blood flow.

Rapid breathing reduces brain blood flow, while slow, deep breathing enhances it, other factors being equal. Enhanced brain blood flow makes you feel good and is good for you; while reduced brain blood flow makes you feel bad and is bad for you. The idea that one might *condition* brain waves to alter mental states is comparable, in my opinion, to conditioning a gas gauge to fill the fuel tank. Brain waves are epiphenomena of cerebral circulation and metabolism. They are like the sparks that fly when you strike flint. This is not to say that the conditioning doesn't work, just that the variable that you observe changing is not necessarily the one being conditioned. More on this in Chapter 6.

Reading about biofeedback and conditioning of rhythms such as *alpha*, *theta*, and the *sensorimotor rhythm* (SMR)—sometimes known as *mu*—(Chase & Harper, 1971; Finley, 1976; Fried, 1987a,b, 1990; Fried, Carlton, & Fox, 1990; Fried, Rubin, Carlton, & Fox, 1984; Gastaut, 1975; 1975; Harper & Sterman, 1972; Kuhlman, 1979–80; Lubar & Bahler, 1976; Lubar, Shasbin, Natelson, Holder, Whitsett, Pamplin, & Krulikowski, 1981; Qui, Hutt, & Forrest, 1979; Sterman, 1973, 1977a; Sterman & Friar, 1972; Sterman, McDonald, & Bernstein, 1977; Wyrwicka & Sterman, 1968; Upton & Longmire, 1975; Wyrwicka & Sterman, 1968)—leaves one with the distinct, though erroneous, impression that the EEG is a response, a behavior, as it were, like blinking, salivating, leg flexion, or any other reflexive involuntary response. Empirical observations of the brain reveal that EEG invariably changes with metabolism. Here is an example from conditioning of the so-called "seizure suppressing" SMR. According to Chase and Harper (1971), one observes that:

> Onset of each epoch [of SMR] was correlated positively with the inspiration phase. . . . Termination of 12 to 14 c/sec activity tended to occur during expiration in all cats. . . . Short bursts were time-locked to the respiratory pattern described above. (p. 87)

You can see why I opt to begin this section on brain blood flow with the EEG. I plan to press the point that brain blood flow is what the EEG actually "talks about."

Despite a long history dating to Lennox, Gibbs, and Gibbs (1938), incontrovertibly showing EEG fundamental frequency to be related to local arterial vascular caliber, brain blood flow, and metabolic activity, we continue to favor it as evidence of lesion, or rebellious neurons, rather than as an epiphenomenon of blood flow and metabolism. Why? None of the reports cited above include any attempt to correlate cortical rhythms to brain vascular physiology or metabolism, despite the vast literature suggesting that one should do so. Instead, we read such metaphors as "inhibitory rhythm," and so forth.

But a very quiet revolution is taking place. The field of applied neurophysiology must have been keenly aware for some time of the inadequacy of the EEG as a diagnostic tool, for it is ever so quietly phasing it out in favor of new techniques such as the Positron Emission Tomography (PET) scan (Baxter, Phelps, Mazziotta, Schwartz, Gerner, Selin, & Sumida, 1985; Buchsbaum, De Lisi, Holcomb, Cappelletti, King, Johnson, Hazlett, Dowling-Zimmerman, Post, Morihisa, Carpenter, Cohen,

Pickar, Weinberger, Margolin, & Kessler, 1984; Engel, 1984; Stefan, Bauer, Feistel, Schulemann, Neubauer, Wenzel, Wolf, Neundorfer, & Huk, 1990; Wilkinson, Bull, Du Boulay, Marshall, Russell, & Symon, 1969). The most recent study of regional cerebral blood flow (rCBF) by PET scan (Drevets, Videen, Price, Preskorn, Carmichael, & Raichle, 1992) shows with considerable elegance the increased activity in the left prefrontal cortical region and the amygdala, in major depression. And why not discard the EEG? Sixty years of study of this phenomenon have taught us absolutely nothing that was not known within 10 years of Berger's report in 1929.

Although the brain constitutes only about 2% of body weight, it receives about 16% of cardiac output and consumes, at rest, about 20% of the O_2 used by the entire body (Ruch & Fulton, 1961). In steady state conditions, O_2 delivery to brain tissue *must* match metabolic consumption of O_2 (Lubbers & Leniger-Follert, 1978). Oxygen delivery to brain tissues depends on blood flow, in turn depending on the caliber in the arteriolar bed of the brain. We have, therefore, a considerable stake in determining the structures and mechanisms that regulate cerebral blood flow and metabolism.

Brain blood flow has its own set of characteristics that sets it apart from systemic blood circulation. These are important to clinical psychophysiology since the body is more or less elastic, and systemic circulation can undergo some degree of increase in blood volume and pressure. But the brain is confined in bone and increasing blood volume and pressure would damage it by compression. A number of physiological mechanisms ensure that the total volumes of brain tissue, of blood in its circulatory system, and of cerebrospinal fluid remain fairly constant.

Blood is supplied to the brain by two main routes, the internal carotid and vertebral arteries converging at the *Circle of Willis*. Their branches supply the brain with blood. The two vertebral arteries form the basilar artery.

Figure 3 is an unusual schematic representation of the blood supply to the brain. It shows the basilar artery and the *Circle of Willis*, viewed from beneath the brain.

However, there is relatively little division of blood flow taking place between the right and left halves of the Circle of Willis. Thus, restricting blood flow in one carotid artery may seriously affect blood flow to the brain as a whole. On the return side, cerebral veins lead to venous sinuses, relatively large spaces contained between the *dura mater* (one of the meninges) and the bone (cranium). These drain into the internal jugular veins and subsidiary venous channels from which blood exits the brain.

The arteries and veins of the brain are histologically different from those in the body. They have somewhat thinner walls and are more elastic.

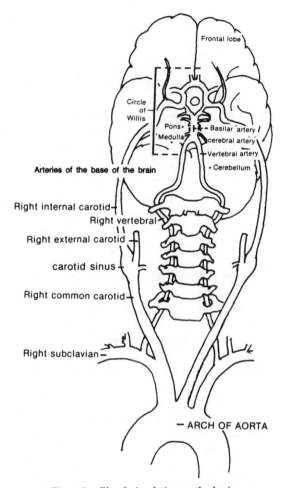

Figure 3. Blood circulation to the brain.

Veins contain more connective tissue. Arteries and veins have numerous vasomotor fibers which, it is generally conceded, do not function in ordinary circumstances. Though they can induce vascular dilation or constriction with strong electrical stimulation, they do not do so under normal conditions:

> . . . [we] support the traditional concept that reflex mechanisms are unimportant in the regulation of cerebral blood flow. (Heistad, Marcus, & Abboud, 1978, p. 100)

and

> Our feeling is that there is now sufficient evidence to conclude that sympathetic

stimulation, under normal conditions, produces little if any reduction in cerebral blood flow. (Heistad, Marcus, & Abboud, 1978, p. 101)

Severe hypertension seems to be an exception.

The density of vascularization of the brain conforms to metabolic demand. Gray matter has a denser supply than white matter, and it also has a higher rate of metabolism. Regional blood flow is regulated by metabolic demand. Local blood flow is distributed among brain structures "in exact proportion to their rate of glucose utilization" and changes together with local glucose consumption in response to altered local functional activity (Sokoloff, 1978).

A number of methods have been used to measure brain blood flow and "local" glucose utilization (i.e., regional metabolism), including *impedance* indices (Jevning, Fernando, & Wilson, 1989) and *rheoencephalography* (Cooper, Moskalenko, & Walter, 1964; Laitinen, Johnasson, & Sipponen, 1966; Tachibana, 1966). Tachibana, Kuramoto, Inanaga, and Ikemi (1967) reported that in the thalamus, for instance, increased blood flow is accompanied by an increase in regional heat production (Gerard, 1938; Schmidt & Hendrix, 1938).

The arterial and arteriolar bed of the brain is autoregulated, that is, it has the intrinsic ability to maintain a relatively constant blood flow despite moderate changes in (perfusion) pressure. This autoregulation serves to ensure that the O_2 and glucose supply to the brain remains more or less constant over wide variations in systemic blood pressure. It is achieved by dilation of arterioles in the vascular bed of the brain in response to decreased perfusion pressure (Edvinsson, Hardebo, & Owman, 1978).

Increased perfusion pressure beyond *maximal*, by a further increase of systemic (peripheral) blood pressure, may result in increased cerebral blood flow. A sudden increase in perfusion pressure above this point can occur and can cause cerebral blood vessel damage and brain edema. Perfusion pressure is the difference between brain arterial and exiting venous blood pressure (A-V).

When metabolism in a part of the brain changes, there is compensatory change in local blood flow (Purves, 1978). Levels of activity in a particular brain structure regulate local energy metabolism, and local blood flow adjusts to the metabolic demand by compensatory flow regulation (Lubbers & Leniger-Follert, 1978). Compensatory flow regulation suggests that local arterioles can adjust capillary microflow in a particular region involving, perhaps, only a few capillaries. The evidence for this mechanism at the capillary level comes from studies of hypoxia which show that decreased O_2 concentration may cause an increase in regional blood flow, despite decreased microflow. Thus, regional flow can remain constant despite change in microflow. Regional compensatory flow regulation suggests that the brain is organized into functional units according to O_2 supply. They regulate O_2 supply by local redistribution without affecting regional and main circulation.

Electrical stimulation of a particular cortical area results in increased local activation with a commensurate increase in O_2 consumption and an outflow of extracellular potassium. As O_2 consumption increases, blood flow to the region rises to meet the demand. Increased flow carries away hydrogen ions (H^+) and pH shifts toward increased alkalinity. Subsequently, the release of H^+ from increased cellular metabolism causes extracellular H^+ to rise despite increased blood flow. When stimulation ceases, the process reverses. The time course of pH change follows that of microflow change (Lubbers & Leniger-Follert, 1978).

The studies by Lubbers and Leniger-Follert have led to the conclusion that one must distinguish between local and regional blood flow in the brain, since it is a fairly unique property of the brain that local capillary blood flow can react differently at different sites without change in regional blood flow. Somehow or other, capillaries must communicate with each other. The idea that capillaries communicate initially suggests involvement of sympathetic and parasympathetic mechanisms, since that is the case in systemic circulation, and such fibers are observed in the brain. It also follows that adrenergic and cholinergic mechanisms must be involved. However, there is evidence for other means by which vascular structures can communicate and these involve various other amines and peptides. Owman and Edvinsson (1978) make reference to "aminergic" and "peptidergic" nerves in the brain.

A system for microregulation makes it possible to explain why brain O_2 consumption may not be significantly different during intellectual activity and during sleep (Mangold, Sokoloff, Conner, Kleinerman, Therman, & Kety, 1955; Sokoloff, Mangold, Wechsler, Kennedy, & Keaty, 1955). Regional flow can remain constant despite considerable change in microflow.

The cerebrovascular system is also the *blood-brain barrier*. Vascular endothelial cells, connected by tight junctions, restrict intracellular diffusion (Rapoport, 1978) so that the vascular endothelium as a whole acts as a barrier. Water soluble substances, proteins, and ions are generally excluded, while lipid-solutes, O_2, and CO_2 traverse readily. This barrier regulates composition of the brain and cerebrospinal fluid ensuring delivery of sufficient glucose to support metabolism. Likewise, essential amino acids diffuse into the brain through various transport mechanisms. But competition among them determines relative quantities passed from the blood to the brain.

For instance, blood concentration of tryptophan, relative to other amino acids, affects tryptophan uptake and serotonin synthesis in the brain (Fernstrom & Wurtman, 1972). Sometimes, lactic acid may accumulate in the brain if production exceeds the rate at which it can diffuse into the bloodstream, given the concentration of competing substances (metabolic substrate) in the blood.

The blood-brain barrier is not a totally rigid filter, according to Rapoport (1978). Hypertonic solutions (having greater osmotic [fluid] pressure) alter its permeability with resultant greater brain uptake. In a normal, recumbent person, that arterial blood pressure will be about 95 mm Hg. Pressure in the internal jugular vein may be only about 10 mm Hg. Thus, venous pressure does not seriously impede blood outflow.

Chemical Control of Cerebral Blood Flow: CO_2

Normal consciousness rapidly disintegrates when cerebral blood flow is impaired; brain cells depend on O_2 for normal metabolic function.

Figure 4 shows the relationship between arterial blood CO_2 concentration ($PaCO_2$) and cerebral blood flow within normal limits. Cerebral blood flow decreases rapidly as $PaCO_2$ decreases.

Schmidt (1927) was one of the first physiologists to report that *cerebral blood flow varies inversely with respiration rate*. This finding has been replicated repeatedly (Gibbs, Lennox, & Gibbs, 1940; Gibbs, Williams, & Gibbs, 1949; Himwich, 1951; Meyer & Waltz, 1961; Penfield & Jasper, 1954; Swanson, Stavney, & Plum, 1958; Tower, 1960; Wolf & Lennox, 1930). The principal factor affecting brain blood flow is concentration of CO_2 in arterial blood ($PaCO_2$) (Gibbs, Maxwell, & Gibbs, 1947; Ingvar & Soderberg, 1956; Kety & Schmidt, 1945; Krueger, Rockoff, Thomas, & Ommaya, 1963; Lambertsen, Semple, Smyth, & Gelfand, 1961; Rockoff, Doppman, Krueger, Thomas, & Ommaya, 1966; Wolff & Lennox, 1930). Figure 4 shows an increasing monotonic relationship between cerebral blood flow and CO_2 concentration in arterial blood.

Figure 5 shows the relationship between concentration of CO_2 in arterial blood in the brain, inferred from blood in the jugular vein, and fundamental frequency of the EEG. As CO_2 concentration decreases, EEG frequency decreases from *alpha* to *theta*.

In 1938, Lennox, Gibbs, and Gibbs demonstrated that the fundamental frequency of the EEG reflects this relationship to $PaCO_2$. This is also an almost linear, increasing monotonic function. Reduction of O_2 does not have nearly so rapid and profound an effect on blood flow and EEG:

As for the effect of oxygen on cortical electrical waves, anoxaemia causes a significant slowing of frequency of the waves only when the anoxaemia is so extreme that unconsciousness impends. The breathing of pure oxygen does not appreciably affect frequency of brain waves. (p. 219)

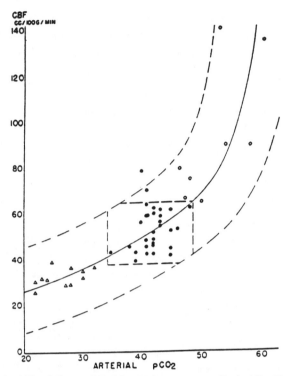

Figure 4. Cerebral blood flow and PaCO₂. With permission: Rockefeller University Press. S.S. Kety, and C.F. Schmidt (1948): The effects of altered arterial tensions of carbon dioxide and oxygen on cerebral blood flow and cerebral oxygen consumption of normal young men. *Journal of Clinical Investigation,* 27:484–492.

Thus, fundamental frequency of the EEG correlates directly with caliber in the cerebrovascular bed, and therefore cerebral blood flow, PaCO₂, and fundamental EEG frequency. They should, in theory, be interchangeable. You may want to keep this in mind as we look at EEG in Chapter 5.

Kety and Schmidt (1948) showed that inhaling 5% to 7% CO₂ produces an increase in cerebral blood flow averaging 75%. Inhalation of 85% to 100% O₂ reduced cerebral blood flow by 13%. Inhaling 10% O₂ increased cerebral blood flow, as we would expect. The effects of reduced brain blood flow are not simply restricted to immediate O₂ unavailability. Kety and Schmidt (1948) showed that HV and hypoxia may show no reduction in O₂ *utilization,* yet be associated with definite mental changes:

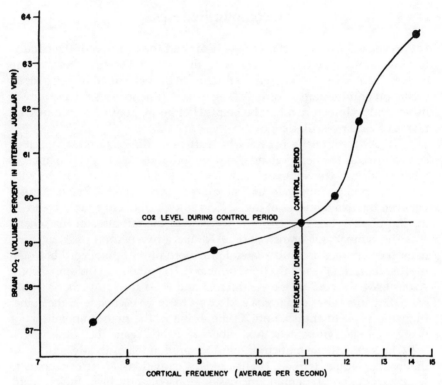

Figure 5. PaCO₂ and EEG. With permission: British Medical Association. W.G. Lennox, E.A. Gibbs, and E.L. Gibbs (1938): The relationship in man of cerebral activity to blood flow and blood constituents. *Journal of Neurology and Psychiatry*, 1:222–225.

> . . . derangements in consciousness may occur when the complex oxidation processes with which consciousness is associated are forced to operate at a lower oxygen tension even though the gross oxygen consumption of the brain as a whole may be within normal limits. (p. 489)

They conclude that "higher psychic functions" are associated with bio-chemical changes so subtle and complex that they cannot be readily described in terms of O_2 utilization. Their conclusions anticipate the work of Blass and Gibson (1979), cited earlier in connection with altered neuro-transmitter synthesis in graded hypoxia. Cerebral blood flow increases with an increase in $PaCO_2$, perfusion pressure, or a decrease in PaO_2 (Lubber & Leniger-Follert, 1978).

Vasomotor Reflexes

In considering the action of the heart and the function of the circulatory system, numerous references to the role of the ANS were made earlier. The ANS is well known to students of the behavioral sciences for its excitation or inhibition of various "vegetative" functions. A brief review of its general architecture might be helpful before we go further into mechanisms of cardiovascular control.

The ANS stimulates organs which are not ordinarily under conscious control such as the heart, glands, and smooth muscles. It has two antagonistic branches, the sympathetic and the parasympathetic, which, with some exceptions, innervate the same organs. A dynamic balance exists between the two branches of the ANS, resulting from either an increase in the impulses of one branch, or a decrease in the impulses of the other.

The sympathetic branch of the ANS has a two-neuron pathway: First neuron cell bodies are in the lateral gray horn of the spinal cord between the first thoracic (T1) and the third lumbar (L3) segments of the spinal cord. Axons leave the cord by the ventral root and enter the sympathetic trunk, consisting of a series of ganglia and axons lying on each side of the spine, from the neck to the sacrum. Epinephrine is the neurotransmitter for postganglionic sympathetic ANS fibers and the organs they innervate.

The sympathetic branch of the ANS predominates in stressful, or as they are sometimes termed, "fight-or-flight" situations: Muscles prepare to work harder and O_2 demand increases. Consequently, bronchioles dilate; the heartbeat is stronger and faster; arteries to the heart and muscles dilate; peripheral and skin arteries constrict. The liver secretes glycogen; peristalsis decreases; the pupils dilate; and we sweat. The parasympathetic branch of the ANS also consists of pre- and postganglionic fibers whose neurotransmitter is acetylcholine. Its action is, for the most part, opposite that of the sympathetic branch, dominating during quiescence and relaxation. Incidentally, most of the fibers of cranial nerve X, the *vagus*, are parasympathetic nerves that send impulses to the heart, lungs, and some visceral organs.

The ANS mediates numerous vasomotor reflexes which cause blood vessels to constrict or dilate. Their existence was first demonstrated by Claude Bernard in 1852, when he cut the cervical sympathetic nerve in the neck of a rabbit and observed dilation of blood vessels and warming of the ear on the same side (Bell, Davidson, & Scarborough, 1968). Although there are other brain stem centers, we generally consider the vasomotor center of the medulla to be the major source of control of this function.

When the spinal cord is cut in the cervical neck region, vasomotor impulses cease and blood pressure drops. But after several days, if life can be maintained, blood pressure rises, presumably as a compensatory function of spinal vasomotor reflexes in the lateral columns of gray matter. Electrical stimulation of the lateral and posterior parts of the hypothalamus, or the premotor cortex, produces vasoconstriction and increased blood pressure.

Other reflex mechanisms involve epinephrine (adrenalin) and norepinephrine (noradrenalin) which, likewise, affect arterial smooth muscle and cardiac function. The biosynthesis of norepinephrine begins with the amino acid *tyrosine* (also a precursor of *thyroxin*, a thyroid hormone). Tyrosine also yields *tyramine*, a "sympathomimetic" substance (stimulating adrenergic nerves) which resembles epinephrine but is somewhat weaker in its effects. Unlike other neurotransmitters, the final step in the synthesis of norepinephrine occurs in the synapse. The terminal boutons contain dopamine which is then converted to norepinephrine by the action of an enzyme, dopamine-beta-hydroxylase.

Persons treated for depression with monoamine-oxydase inhibitors (MAO) are cautioned to eliminate tyramine-rich foods (such as aged cheese) from their diet because of the risk of a hypertensive crisis. MAO inhibitors increase the availability of catecholamines which drive up heart rate and constrict peripheral arteries. Norepinephrine, among these, acts on two types of receptors: *alpha* and *beta*. Alpha receptors effect arterial smooth muscle contraction, resulting in increased blood pressure. Stimulation of beta receptors results in increased pulse rate and stroke volume, and relaxes bronchial smooth muscle. Beta-adrenergic agonists are, therefore, used to treat asthma in which bronchial constriction is a primary concern.

There are vasomotor reflexes regulating blood pressure other than those of the aortic arch and carotid artery. Hale, who first described blood pressure in 1732, reported that it fluctuates in synchrony with breathing. These fluctuations, subsequently designated as Traube-Hering waves, are thought to arise from the effect of the respiratory centers on the vasomotor centers. (Mayer waves, fluctuations in blood pressure of lower frequency, may appear in the presence of hypoxia.)

When blood pressure is low, baro- and chemoreceptors in the aortic arch and carotid arteries stimulate vasomotor centers. Consequently, blood pressure and respiration rise. The baroceptors respond to fluid pressure, while the chemoreceptors respond to gas concentration. The cycle represents the operation of a negative feedback mechanism. Vasoconstrictor nerves carry impulses from the medulla into the cord. They exit the thoracic and lumbar nerve region from the lateral horn of the gray matter through the ventral root, and by the white ramus communicans, to the sympathetic ganglion. Postganglionic fibers go directly to blood vessels

(Bell, Davidson, & Scarborough, 1968; Carlson, 1981; Ruch & Fulton, 1960; Tortora & Anagnostakos, 1984).

Abdominal organs are innervated by the splanchnic nerve, which is crucial to the maintenance of peripheral vasotonus, since electrical stimulation causes vasoconstriction and increase in arterial blood pressure. If this nerve is blocked or severed, there will be a rapid and profound but temporary fall in systemic blood pressure. There is also a vasodilator carotid sinus reflex. Light pressure on the neck may cause a decrease in cerebral arterial blood pressure sufficient, in some cases, to cause loss of consciousness. Forearm blood pressure will rise in a person lying down if the legs are elevated. This indicates a redistribution of blood flow because it occurs in the absence of change in systemic blood pressure. And there are vasoconstrictive reflexes. For instance, a strong noxious stimulus, loud noise, or rapid deep breath will cause vasoconstriction in the skin.

The aortic arch and carotid sinuses contain receptors for vasoconstrictive reflexes. These receptors are sensitive to pressure and blood gases. But there are also localized reflexes. For instance, stimulation of a right or left femoral nerve (femur, in the leg), results in vasodilation in the ipsilateral (same side) limb, and vasoconstriction in the contralateral (opposite side) limb (Loven reflex). The *valsalva maneuver* consists of a deep expiration with the glotis closed. Arterial blood pressure rises first, then falls. Cardiac output may fall to the point where it jeopardizes consciousness. Low pressure in the baroceptors in the aortic arch and carotid bodies causes vasoconstriction and increased pulse rate (tachycardia).

The Lymphatic System

Lymph flow is important to fluid balance and blood circulation in the human body. Because of the lymphatic system, fluid leakage into interstitial space is compensated. Among the factors that affect lymph flow are the pumping action of the lymph vessels and the interstitial fluid pressure. Lymph vessels (lymphatics) also contract rhythmically from their capillaries to the thoracic duct.

Breathing is essential in maintaining lymph flow. Respiratory movement creates a pressure difference between the intracellular (interstitial) space where the fluid pressure is higher, and the thoracic region where it is lower. A system of valves prevents lymph from flowing backwards in the lymphatics, and keeps it moving toward the junction of the thoracic duct and the jugular and subclavian veins, from where it reenters blood circulation.

There are lymph nodes along the lymphatics. They give rise to lymphocytes, elements of the immune system. The lymph nodes are also the origin of plasma cells which produce antibodies. The thymus gland, tonsils, and to a great extent, the spleen, contain and have many of the anatomical and physiological properties of lymphatic tissue.

The Heart

The heart is a fist-sized muscle that sits between the lungs in the chest cavity, most of its mass to the left of the body midline. It beats about 100,000 times per day and pumps blood through about 60,000 miles of blood vessels (Tortora and Anagnostakos, 1984). It has four chambers: The atria are the upper chambers, and the ventricles are the lower chambers. A segment of the atrium, the auricle, increases the surface of the atrium.

Figure 6 is a cross-section of the heart showing the relative location of the right and left chambers and valves, as well as some of the conduction fibers.

The right and left atria are separated by a wall, the interatrial septum. (In the fetus, there is an opening between the atria called the foramen ovale, which should close at birth.)

The heart is a pump. (I like to remind my students that the invention of the pump had to precede Harvey's description of the blood circulating by the pumping action of the heart.) The ventricles form the two lower chambers of the pump separated by the interventricular septum. The atria and ventricles are separated by muscle-tissue flaps which function as valves permitting blood flow in only one direction. The atrioventricular (AV) valves separate the atria and ventricles. The right AV is called the tricuspid. The AV between the left atrium and left ventricle is called the bicuspid, or mitral valve. In addition, two valves prevent blood from flowing back into the heart. These are the pulmonary and aortic semilunar valves, located where the blood exits the heart and enters systemic circulation.

The right atrium receives blood from all parts of the body, except the lungs, through three major veins: (a) the superior vena cava, with blood from regions above the heart; (b) the inferior vena cava, with blood from below the heart; and (c) the coronary sinus, with blood from the heart proper.

The heart muscle wall is composed of three layers: The external layer, or epicardium, is separated from the myocardium (which constitutes the bulk of the heart) by a fluid-filled cavity. The pericardial cavity and fluid prevent friction damage to the heart as it contracts. The endocardium lines the inside of the heart. The heart muscle bundles are comprised of striated

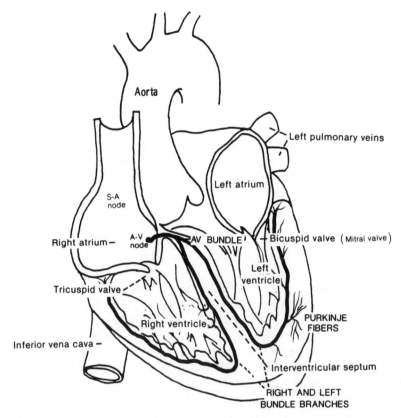

Figure 6. The heart.

muscle fibers, their cells oriented in the same direction. They contain multiple parallel rows of myofibrils, in which contractile units, sarcomeres, are joined end to end. Sarcomeres are the basic contractile units, containing contractile filaments and the proteins myosin and actin.

There are several theories about the exact nature of the contraction of the heart, centering principally on the structural and metabolic differences between the actin and myosin filaments: the thin filaments, actin, move inward along the fixed, thick myosin filament framework. Thus, the filaments do not shorten, but the sarcomere does (Sodeman & Sodeman, 1979).

Perhaps more than any other body tissue, heart muscle depends on aerobic metabolism. Myocardium requires a continuous supply of O_2, exceeding that of any other organ of the body. Extraction of O_2 from the heart is nearly maximal at rest (at rest, the heart consumes all the O_2 available in its blood supply). Increase in O_2 need is typically satisfied by increased coronary blood flow.

The heart is supplied with blood by the coronary arteries. In about one third of persons, coronary blood flow is balanced, that is, the right coronary artery supplies the right ventricle, while the left coronary artery supplies the left ventricle. In half the population, the right coronary artery predominates. In the rest, it is the left. Anastomoses between the right and left coronary arteries are common and the capillary density is greater than that of any other tissue. There is virtually a one-to-one relationship between capillaries and individual muscle fibers. In addition to veins, there is an auxiliary system of *thebesian* vessels which help to drain venous blood.

Blood flow in the heart does not vary in direct inverse proportion to heart rate, as one might expect. The amount of work performed and the availability of O_2 seem to be more significant factors. While the guiding principle is aortic blood pressure, it has been repeatedly noted that decreased O_2 availability (hypoxia) may increase coronary blood flow by as much as a five times. In the early stages of hypoxia, there is an increase in heart rate, blood pressure, and cardiac output. The duration of systole is shortened and respiratory minute volume (Vmin) increases, leading to HV. If persistent, this increased efficiency of the heart may lead to a "cardiovascular-respiratory crisis" with falling blood pressure, diminishing respiration, and failure of the heart cells terminating in death (Ruch & Fulton, 1961).

Electrical conduction in the heart (see Chapter 6) is largely regulated by sodium, potassium, and calcium ions. Sodium maintains resting potential of the cardiac cells. The "sodium pump" is the mechanism by which ionic pressure maintains the resting potential across cell membranes. Potassium likewise maintains resting potential. Increased intracellular concentration increases the resting potential of the cell so that it is less excitable—less likely to depolarize. Excess plasma potassium may block cardiac action.

Calcium increases excitability of heart tissue. The maintenance of the proper concentration of Ca inside and outside the cardiac cell, as well as that of arterial cells, red blood cells, nerve cells, and other muscles, is greatly influenced by the pH of the intracellular fluid. Increased pH (alkalosis) favors excessive calcium *in*flux, and reduced intercellular *e*flux. Increased pH may result from HV (respiratory alkalosis) due to hypoxia. As pH increases, compensatory kidney mechanisms also lead to increased sodium excretion. Thus, low O_2 availability may lead to an increase in the excitability of heart tissue by disturbing the ionic membrane balance.

Other factors being equal, when separated from the nervous system, the heart will beat more or less regularly. In the body, it receives (parasympathetic/inhibitory) impulses via the vagus from the medulla, and sympathetic innervation from the upper thoracic region of the spinal cord. There are also afferent "pain" nerves that follow the sympathetic nerves to the spinal cord. Impulses from the sympathetic nerves affect principally the S.A. node, resulting in increased heart rate, force of contraction, and shortened diastole interval.

A number of reflexes also govern the activity of the heart. Among these is that mediated by the cardio-aortic nerve in the left ventricle and aortic arch. The nerve endings appear to be baroceptors regulating pressure within the heart (Bell, Davidson, & Scarborough, 1968). The carotid sinus contains baroceptors which, when stimulated, result in reflex slowing of the heart and decreased blood pressure. The region of the bifurcation of the common carotid artery just above the carotid sinus, as well as the aortic arch, also contains chemoreceptors which respond to low PaO_2 and low $PaCO_2$.

Inflation of the lungs results in some degree of inhibition of brain respiratory centers (Hering-Breuer reflex), and, indirectly, slowing of the heart. But lung inflation causes predominating reflex acceleration of the heart directly through cardio-inhibitory centers. This increase and decrease in pulse rate as a function of lung inflation in breathing is termed "respiratory sinus arrhythmia" (RSA) (see Chapter 6).

The Regulation of Blood Pressure and the Kidneys

Blood courses through the circulatory system under pressure, flowing from the heart, where pressure is higher, to regions of the body where it is lower. The principal determinant of blood pressure is the amount of blood pumped by the left ventricle of the heart into the aorta each minute. This quantity is called the *cardiac output* (CO), and is determined by the product of stroke volume and heart rate. Typically, CO − 70 ml × 75BPM = 5.25 liters/min (Tortora & Anagnostakos, 1984). In the average healthy person, blood volume may be about 5 liters. Any change in blood volume will affect blood pressure. Thus, loss of blood through hemorrhage, or increase in blood volume through fluid retention, will affect blood pressure.

The friction caused by the irregularities in the surface of vessels through which blood courses causes it to slow down. This is called *peripheral resistance*. Vascular resistance may also be regulated by local effectors which respond to tonically active stretch (Folkow, 1955). It is affected by the viscosity of blood, and arterial vascular caliber. Viscosity, ability to flow, depends on the ratio of solids in the blood (red and other cells and proteins) to fluid. Red cell and platelet aggregation in diabetes and migraine, respectively, dangerously increase viscosity.

Arterial vascular caliber is determined by vasomotor reflexes which control the diameter of blood vessels, particularly arterioles. The medullary vasomotor center sends impulses to arteriolar smooth muscle resulting in an intermediate state of contraction called *vasomotor tone*. Vasoconstriction results from increased, and vasodilation from decreased, sympathetic impulses. Stimulation of aortic arch and carotid sinus receptors regulates cardiac output and arteriolar tone, through their influence on the medulla vasomotor center. Decreased blood pressure inhibits cardiac inhibition and stimulates acceleration, simultaneous with vasoconstriction. The net effect is increased blood pressure.

Chemoreceptors in the aortic arch and carotid bodies respond to decreases in circulating arterial blood levels of CO_2 and O_2. A number of chemical substances produced by the body affect blood pressure. Epinephrine and norepinephrine constrict cutaneous and abdominal arterioles, increase heart rate and cardiac output, and dilate cardiac and skeletal arterioles.

Blood pressure is also largely regulated by the action of the kidneys, whose primary function is to control the composition and volume of blood. They accomplish it by eliminating waste byproducts of metabolism, and control blood pH by reducing excess concentrations of ions to normal levels, excreting these in urine.

The kidneys. The functional unit of the kidney is the *nephron*, a renal tubule with its associated vasculature. There are two basic types made up of several membranes and tissue layers surrounding a capillary network, the *glomerulus*. One of these membranes, the endothelial capsular membrane, has open pores and permits filtering water and certain solutes in the blood.

The nephrons, pivotal in eliminating waste products and regulating the electrolyte composition of blood, are supplied with abundant blood vessels. The right and left renal arteries transport about one-quarter of the total output of the heart to the kidneys—about 1200 ml/min (Tortora & Anagnostakos, 1984). The entire volume of blood in the body is filtered by the kidneys about 60 times each day. Blood leaves the kidneys through the renal vein.

Nephrons perform three major functions. The first is filtration. Blood passes, under pressure, from capillaries through the layers and membranes of the nephrons, producing a filtrate consisting of all the materials in the blood other than blood cells and proteins excluded by the diameter of the filtration pores. Second, nephrons reabsorb much of the filtrate. Only about 1 to 2 liters a day, of about 180 liters a day of filtrate, is eliminated from the body as urine. The substances reabsorbed include water, glucose, amino acids, sodium (Na^+), potassium (K^+), calcium (Ca^{2+}), chloride (Cl^-), carbonate (HCO^-), and phosphate (HPO^{2-}). Most nutrients are reabsorbed. The elimination and reabsorption of sodium ion is of particular interest to clinical psychophysiologists concerned with treatment of hypertension, since it has been shown that it is affected by stress (Krantz & Glass, 1984). The rate of reabsorption of sodium ion varies with its concentration in extracellular fluid. When sodium concentration of the blood is low, blood pressure drops, triggering the *renin-angiotensin-aldosterone* mechanisms. The kidneys secrete renin, an enzyme which converts a liver product, angiotensin, to angiotensin I. Angiotensin I is, in turn, converted to angiotensin II in the lungs. Angiotensin II stimulates the brain to produce aldosterone causing increased sodium and water reabsorption in the kidneys.

The reabsorption of sodium ion increases the osmotic pressure of blood relative to the filtrate and consequently a quantity of water is reabsorbed to establish equilibrium. The balance of the water is excreted as a function of the permeability of nephron structures regulated by an antidiuretic hormone (ADH) produced by the thalamus. The third function of the kidneys, secretion, is relevant to the maintenance of the acid-base balance of the blood because it adds substances including hydrogen and potassium ion from blood to the filtrate (see Chapter 4).

Blood pressure is lowest in the capillaries. But blood flows discontinuously through them. Intermittent contraction and relaxation of the arterioles and precapillary sphincters occurs at a rate ranging between 5 and 10 per minute. This vasomotion is primarily affected by tissue O_2 concentration.

Blood and the Red Blood Cells

Introduction

Clinical psychophysiology requires competence in many therapeutic skills, including assessment of physical, mental, affective, and emotional states; biofeedback; and psychotherapy, which we may perform as strict behaviorists, cognitivists, or both. If we are physiologists, we tend to see the mind embedded in brain neurons; if mentalists, we believe a somatic disorder is due to faulty thinking, or the emotional outcropping of symbolic conflict jutting out of a quagmire of illicit urges; if behaviorists, it doesn't matter—everything yields to "modification" if you do it right. Given a hammer, we tend to treat everything as though it were a nail.

But there is a strong hint that blood constituents must somehow figure in the scheme of clinical concerns. For one thing, we know that we should encourage their circulation and we have developed biofeedback methods to that end. We study platelet aggregation in migraine, and erythrocyte aggregation in diabetes. But how and why do they aggregate? And why is this harmful? Doesn't it stand to reason that anything intended to be liquid that turns to mud will have difficulty coursing through vessels which have the additional unpleasant inclination to narrow as the mud thickens? This process leads to brain and body hypoxia.

But cognitivists can't see how hypoxia could cause aberrant thinking, and behaviorists don't deal with anything that can't be conditioned . . . excuse me, modified. Yet, psychologists familiar with *human factors* know that altitude affects cognition. By about 4000 ft, O_2 is sufficiently thin to seriously impair judgment.

Though clinicians recognize the benefits of deep-diaphragmatic breathing, they have not concluded that its major benefit is increased O_2, or decreased hypoxia—whichever way you look at it. They typically ascribe its benefits to the magic of relaxation. So how can you expect anyone to consider the possibility that depression, anxiety, and panic may be related to brain hypoxia, and that hypoxia may be a function of a disorder of the blood? What if you breathe funny because that's what your blood makes you do, and that makes you anxious or depressed?

It seems logical to me that if you are prepared to believe that depression may be due to malfunctioning chemoreceptor mechanisms in neural circuits, and that these have been shown to be adversely affected by hypoxia, you might be equally prepared to believe that it is something about blood which is responsible for the graded hypoxia.

Scientists willing to accept one thing are not necessarily going to accept another. Case in point: The medical anatomist William Hunter (1718–1783) said about William Harvey, the first to describe blood circulation:

> He lived almost thirty years after Asellius published the Lacteals, yet, to the last, seemed most inclined to think, that no such vessels existed. Thirty hours at any time, should have been sufficient to remove all his doubts.

It is enough to bring tears to the eyes.

> I have heard him say, that after his Booke of the *Circulation of the Blood* came out, that he fell mightily in his Practize, and that 'twas beleeved by the vulgar that he was crack-brained; and all the Physitians were against his Opinion, and envyed him; many wrote against him. (p. 164)

So said the biographer John Aubrey (1626–1697) about Harvey in *Brief Lives*. Who said, "If you build a better mouse trap, they'll beat a path to your door?"

The contention that brain cell oxygenation is not etiologic in clinical cases of depression where medication is indicated is illogical, since the effect of such medication is based on a model of the failure of neurotransmitter mechanisms that have been shown to be related to hypoxia (Blass & Gibson, 1979).

It would also bolster the theory that depression, for instance, is due to faulty, self-defeating cognitions, if it were shown that persons who do not have such depression are free of such cognitions. Depression, anxiety, and panic have yielded to medication, behavioral strategies, and "deep breathing," in numerous instances, independent of cognition (Aronson, 1966; Woods, Charney, Loke, Goodman, Redmond, & Heninger, 1986; Clark, Salkovskis, & Chalkley, 1985; Fried, 1987a, 1990; Fried & Golden, 1989; Grunhaus, Rabin, & Greden, 1986; Salkovskis, Jones, & Clark, 1985; van Dixhoorn & Duivenvoorden, 1986). If that doesn't convince you, how about the article by Mellman and Uhde (1989), "Sleep panic attacks: New clinical findings and theoretical implications," or the one by Sietsema,

Simon, and Wasserman (1987), "Pulmonary hypertension presenting as panic disorder."

In 1982, Katz asked, "Is there a hypoxic affective syndrome?" His interest arose from the observation that some forms of physical illness in which there is moderate (graded) cerebral hypoxia (low brain O_2) (such as heart failure, chronic obstructive pulmonary disease, and anemia), are also accompanied by depression. Katz reports that:

> A number of laboratories have studied the neurochemistry of mild to moderate hypoxia, focusing on those effects that occur before change in energy metabolism. Several of the enzymes of biogenic amine metabolism—tyrosine hydroxylase, tryptophan hydroxylase, dopamine-β-hydroxylase, and monoamine oxidase—are oxygenases: that is, they require molecular oxygen as a substrate and their activities can, in principle, be regulated by oxygen. (p. 849)

He continues:

> The effects of hypoxia on catecholamines and serotonin, together with the biogenic amine theories of depression, suggest that hypoxia can precipitate a depression, in the same sense as can reserpine; this together with psychogenic mechanisms may, in part, explain the increased incidence of depression in physical illness. (p. 850)

But it should be noted that:

> . . . apparent intractability of the serotonin receptor to changes after long-term treatment indicates a different post-synaptic regulatory mechanism than that found in catecholaminergic neurons. Furthermore, modification of serotonin receptor sensitivity is probably not relevant to the mode of action of antidepressant drugs. (Wirz-Justice, Krauchi, Lichtsteiner, & Feer, 1978, p. 1249)

Finally:

> . . . [it] is interesting to note that the initial observations on the activating and mood-elevating properties of the monoamine oxidase inhibitor iproniazid were in patients with pulmonary tuberculosis. (Katz, 1982, p. 854)

Not everyone is inclined to jump on the bandwagon; and while hypoxia is implicated in depression here, it has been even more strongly implicated in panic disorder where hyperventilation predominates.

Salkovskis, Warwick, Clark, and Wessel (1986) report that:

> . . . resting pCO_2 was consistently lower in patients experiencing panic attacks than in a group of age- and sex-matched controls, and that treatment resulted in the rapid restoration of patients' pCO_2 to normal levels. This suggests that these patients were hyperventilating chronically with resultant renal compensation (Brown, 1953), which maintains pH at normal levels. (p. 91)

Then again you might say, "Well, so what? At worst, hypocapnia causes minor vasoconstriction and since pH is normal in any case, there would be no shift in the OHb dissociation curve sufficient to warrant a suspicion of hypoxia." But if you read on, a different picture emerges:

As the sensations accompanying hyperventilation are mediated by an increased pH, such chronic hyperventilation does not produce symptoms. However, the adaptation of the blood-buffering system results in increased sensitivity to changes in pCO_2 such as those produced by stressors and exercise. This means that decreases in $paCO_2$ will result in relatively larger changes in pH and hence more rapid onset and greater intensity of the bodily sensations of hyperventilation. (p. 91)

Their point was well proven with the availability of blood samples—their subject was on dialysis. And many others have shown increased sensitivity to CO_2 (Pain, Biddle, & Tiller, 1988; Singh, 1984a; Woods, Charney, Loke, Goodman, Redmond, & Henenger, 1986). But such studies only indicate mechanisms that may cause cerebral hypoxia, not that they are activated by HV. Such evidence would have to come from direct observation of brain metabolism. And indeed it does. For, according to Granholm, Lukjanova, and Siesjo (1968), there is "evidence of cerebral hypoxia in pronounced hyperventilation":

At arterial CO_2 tensions below 25–20 mm Hg there was a progressive increase of the lactate concentrations and the lactate/pyruvate ratios in both CSF [cerebrospinal fluid] and brain tissue [in rats] . . . both the increased tissue and CSF lactate/pyruvate ratios, and the increased tissue NADH levels, indicated tissue hypoxia during pronounced hyperventilation with air. (p. IV:C)

But here is a study reporting that breathing retraining to relieve the effects of hyperventilation is not particularly useful in the treatment of panic disorder and agoraphobia, conditions even more strongly linked to breathing and hypoxia than depression. In a report by de Rutter, Rijken, Garssen, and Kraaimaat (1989) we are told that, "the limited effectiveness of breathing retraining in reducing panic . . . leads us to conclude that the role of hyperventilation in panic is less important than previously thought." All right, let's see how they arrive at this conclusion.

They compared (a) breathing retraining with cognitive restructuring (BRCR); (b) graded self-exposure *in vivo* (EXP); or (c) a combination of BRCR and EXP, in a group of persons suffering from agoraphobia as defined by DSM-III-R. Assessment of self-report measures centered on panic, phobic anxiety and avoidance, depression, general anxiety, somatic complaints, and fear of bodily sensations.

They report decreased breathing rate, and reduction in self-report of all symptoms except panic, and conclude that "Contrary to expectation, and at odds with findings from earlier studies, BRCR had no significant effect on panic frequency." What they are saying is that by slowing breathing slightly you can reduce just about any symptom except panic. In that, they are absolutely right.

According to the authors, "Four junior clinical psychologists served as therapists in the study. They all had some prior experience with psycho-therapy and were specially trained in the treatment used." What was the BRCR treatment in which they were "specially trained"?

> . . . [a] pacing tape was used. Breathing rate was adjusted for each patient and had to be slightly slower than his or her usual breathing rate.
> . . . diaphragmatic breathing was further encouraged by suggesting patients put one hand on their abdomen, and breathing "against the hand." (p. 649)

This is the kind of "breathing training" that one would institute in a study designed to fail. This is not how to do diaphragmatic breathing training. You certainly would not find it in an elementary pulmonary rehabilitation or physiotherapy textbook such as Haas, Pineda, Haas, and Axen (1979).

Second, that respiratory rate and end-tidal CO_2 were observed while the subject "was seated in a reclining chair while breathing normally through a mouthpiece for 10 min" indicates their total disregard for countless published reports that one cannot breathe normally through a mouthpiece (Tobin, Chadha, Jenouri, Birch, Gazeroglu, & Sackner, 1983). Gilbert, Auchincloss, Brodsky, and Boden (1972) reported, in an unam-biguously titled article, "Changes in tidal volume, frequency, and ventila-tion induced by their measurement," that respiratory frequency decreases, Vt rises, and Vmin changes variably with the use of a mouthpiece. Weissman, Askanazi, Milic-Emili, and Kinney (1984) published an article equally clearly titled, "Effect of respiratory apparatus on respiration," reporting changes in breathing, and so did Maxwell, Cover, and Hughes (1985), who found changes in Vt but no change in breathing rate. There are many other such reports (Bradley & Younes, 1980; Hirsh & Bishop, 1982; Milic-Emili, 1982; Sackner, Nixon, Davis, Atkins, & Sackner, 1980).

The data in the above-mentioned study (de Rutter et al., 1989) are equally noteworthy: Comparing pre- to posttest, mean respiratory rate decreased in the BRCR (15.1 to 12.7) and BRCR + EXP (16.6 to 13.9), and rose negligibly in the EXP group (15.6 to 15.9), indicating that if you tell people to slow down their breathing they usually will. Nonsignificance of differences between group means notwithstanding, anyone who has ever seriously done breathing retraining should be embarrassed to report an average decrease in breathing rate of only about 2 b/min, especially when it might be due to the apparatus. The largest drop was from 16.6 to 13.9 b/min, about 3 b/min—in subjects in a recliner!

Comparing pre- to posttest mean PCO_2, we find 39.8 to 37.1, 36.7 to 35, and 36.5 to 36.2 for BRCR, EXP, and BRCR + EXP, respectively. Paradoxically, PCO_2 *decreased* in each group! Yet no one has ever questioned that doing deep-diaphragmatic breathing should result in *decreased* breathing rate and *increased* PCO_2. Since panic is ascribed to low PCO_2 (in those studies in which it is ascribed to PCO_2 at all), it stands to reason that if PCO_2 does not increase, neither should you expect to see a reduction in panic. And that is exactly what they showed—quite correctly so.

It is astonishing that they did not fault their training procedure because they recognized the dilemma: "Treatments that included breathing retraining techniques . . . seemed to result in a decrease in respiratory rate, but not in an increase in alveolar pCO_2." They were probably "unable to replicate the significant increase in resting alveolar pCO_2 reported by Salkovskis and colleagues (1986)" because they didn't replicate the procedure.

It is on the basis of such studies that I recommend cautious reliance on the conclusion that HV is not etiological in anxiety, panic, and so on. It will become even more clear, as you read on, how pervasive and pernicious are the physiological effects of low CO_2 on O_2 delivery to the brain and the body.

Blood

The previous chapter described how blood is pumped by the heart through a circulatory system consisting of interconnected arterial, arteriolar, capillary, and venous components. The blood is under pressure controlled by vasomotor reflexes of the ANS, which is regulated by various sensors, and by action hormones and the kidneys.

Blood consists of fluid plasma and "formed elements," those that have form. It is about 91% to 92% water in which various components are dissolved, including proteins such as albumins; globulins, which include antibodies; and fibrinogen associated with clotting. Plasma also contains metabolic byproducts of protein, including urea and ammonia salts, and nutrients including amino acids, glucose, fatty acids, and glycerol. In addition, it also transports enzymes and hormones, O_2, CO_2, and electrolytes.

Electrolytes include cations (positive-charge ions) such as sodium, calcium, potassium, and magnesium; and anions (negative-charge ions), including chloride and bicarbonate. They help maintain (osmotic) tissue fluid pressure, blood pressure, and pH homeostasis.

Formed elements include red blood cells (RBC), or erythrocytes, involved in O_2 and CO_2 transport; white blood cells such as eosinophil and basophil cells that combat allergens; neutrophil phagocytes that "clean up"; lymphocytes involved in antigen-antibody immunity reactions; and finally, platelets (thrombocytes) involved in blood clotting. *Hematopoiesis* (from Greek: poiesis, production) is the process by which red and white blood cells and platelets are formed and mature. *Erythropoiesis* is red cell formation. Several basic characteristics of blood readily lend themselves to simple quantification and are commonly observed in connection with assessment of health status or disease progress.

Hematocrit. If a sample of uncoagulated blood is centrifuged at about 2000 RPM for 20 minutes, its constituents separate into two layers: The upper layer of clear plasma (roughly half the volume) contains mostly blood platelets, or thrombocytes; the lower layer contains red blood cells. A narrow band made up mostly of white blood cells, or leukocytes, separates the two layers. The hematocrit is the "packed-cell volume" and may be used as an indication of anemia, and the relative amount of fluid as an indication of hydration (Bell, Davidson, & Scarborough, 1968).

Erythrocyte sedimentation rate. Red blood cells form clumps, or aggregates, in blood to which an anticoagulant has been added. The cells in these aggregates stack, face to face, and gradually drift down in the fluid leaving clear plasma at the top. The sedimentation rate is the amount of clear plasma observed in one hour, above the sediment, or clumps of RBCs. It depends on the concentration of fibrinogen and the presence of various globulins in the blood. These substances increase in the presence of infection and disease.

Leukocytes

Unlike RBCs, white blood cells, or leukocytes, have a cell nucleus, but no hemoglobin. There are three basic types of leukocytes, two arising in bone marrow. The monocytic type is the largest cell circulating in blood. The myelocytic type has three varieties: neutrophil, eosinophil, and basophil. The *lymphocytes* are produced predominantly in lymphatic tissue. The principal role of leukocytes is protection from infection. They are capable of passing through vascular endothelial tissue to reach a site of infection. Depending on the type, their action may be *phagocytic*, that is, they engulf and devour a foreign microorganism, apparently chemically attracted to it (*chemotaxis*); or they may be the source of antibodies. Basophils, which are principally responsible for the production of antibodies, also release heparin, an anticoagulant, *histamine*, a vasoconstrictor, and serotonin, which contributes to platelet aggregation. Of special interest to clinical psychophysiologists concerned with immune function is that most types of leukocytes contain numerous mitochondria and their respiration rate (O_2 consumption) is high (Ruch & Fulton, 1960; Tortora & Anagnostakos, 1984).

Platelets

In 1982, Hanington published an article entitled, "Migraine as a blood disorder: Preliminary studies." In this article, she hypothesizes that "migraine is due primarily to abnormality of platelet function." Remarkably, Miller, Waters, Warnica, Szlachic, Kreeft, and Theroux reported a similar conclusion in the *New England Journal of Medicine* just the year before. Miller et al. (1981) went one step further:

> The prodromal phase of migraine is caused by inappropriate vasoconstriction of cranial arteries, and enzymatic markers of cerebral ischemia can be detected in the cerebrospinal fluid after the attack. As in variant angina, abnormal platelet function has been described in migraine. (p. 764)

What they are saying here is that migraine and variant angina, also known as *Prinzmetal's angina*, or "resting angina," are etiologically related to abnormal platelet function, and to each other. Furthermore, they support the notion that Raynaud's phenomenon is also another manifestation of this etiological root which is considered to be a generalized vasospastic syndrome:

> The high prevalence of migraine and Raynaud's phenomenon in variant angina raises the possibility that a common underlying defect or mechanism may partially account for all three conditions. If this should prove to be so, the single clinical syndrome of generalized arterial vasospasm could be diagnosed. . . . (p. 766)

They cite previous reports of significantly increased incidence of these three conditions in the same patients, leading Leon-Sotomayor (1974) to coin the term "cardiac migraine," and Bulkley, Klacsmann, and Hutchins (1978) to postulate "myocardial Raynaud's phenomenon." As you can see, a diversity of conditions which cut across medical specialties is connected to the same etiological component, namely platelet malfunction. Platelet aggregation is commonly observed in vasospasms associated with ischemia (reduced blood flow) and hypoxia (Amery, 1987), wherever it may be found to occur in the body.

Hanington (1987) reported a number of abnormalities in platelets of migraine sufferers, with a significant decrease in platelet monoamine oxydase (MAO), and a significantly increased tendency to aggregate, above that of nonmigraineurs. Why?

Blood platelets, or thrombocytes, are the smallest of the formed elements in blood. They have a life span of about 10 days and they are similar in structure to white blood cells. They may be round or oval, have no nucleus, but have mitochondria, and amoeba-like projections (pseudopods) which may be extended and withdrawn in response to the O_2 concentration in surrounding blood. Platelets are unevenly distributed in circulation, showing a greater concentration in pulmonary blood. Their formation is stimulated by lower blood O_2 concentration (hypoxia). In asphyxiation, there is an "outpouring" of platelets into the bloodstream (Ruch & Fulton, 1960).

They disintegrate at the site of a tissue injury, thus playing a significant role in coagulation and clot formation (*thrombus*) at the site of ruptured blood vessels and tissue injury. Their exterior surface is negatively charged, they tend to repel each other, and they are less inclined to adhere to vascular tissue whose exterior surface is similarly negatively charged.

Gastrointestinal mucosa ordinarily releases a considerable quantity of serotonin (5-hydroxytryptamine, 5-HTH), a strong local vasoconstrictor and hypotensive, into the bloodstream. 5-HTH is rapidly taken up by platelets and maintained in inactive form as they circulate through the bloodstream. When local blood vessel injury reduces their negative potential, they may clump together at that injury site. As they disintegrate, platelets liberate serotonin, and thrombokinase, which, in the coagulation process and the presence of calcium, initiates conversion of prothrombin to thrombin.

Serotonin, liberated by the disintegrating platelets in the presence of ruptured blood vessels, enhances local vasoconstriction and promotes a fall in systemic blood pressure, thus reducing blood loss (Bell, Davidson, & Scarborough, 1968; Ruch & Fulton, 1960; Tortora & Anagnostakos, 1984).

It has been shown that catecholamines likewise promote platelet aggregation (Bell, Davidson, & Scarborough, 1968). And of particular concern to clinical psychophysiologists is one of the so-called factors found in platelets, Factor 4, which antagonizes heparin, an anticoagulant. Thus, the viscosity of blood, and therefore, cardiovascular function and blood pressure, are related to platelet function.

Clearly, the platelet aggregating function is an essential life-protecting mechanism, and its bad press, derived from its role in migraine, is undeserved. It is, however, a further indication that many disorders show an inappropriate enlistment of otherwise essential functions.

The Red Blood Cells

Red blood cells (RBCs) develop continuously from bone-marrow cells (hemocytoblasts) and have a life span of about 90 to 100 days. They lack a nucleus and cannot reproduce. Their maturation and number depends directly on the availability of numerous substances, especially iron and vitamin B_{12} (cobalamin). Anemia, a reduction in the number of RBCs, lowers tissue oxygenation in proportion to its magnitude, while polycythemia, its opposite, is an increase in RBCs and may also compromise health.

The mature red blood cell, or *erythrocyte*, has a skeleton of sorts, the stroma, mostly protein, and lipid, with an internal filament network comprised of a protein, spectrin (Stryer, 1981). Spectrin strengthens and regulates the shape of the RBC, which is subjected to considerable mechanical stress and deformation in the blood stream due to the pumping action of the heart. Both surfaces of the RBC are concave (biconcave), thus increasing their surface area and facilitating diffusion of gases and other substances through the membrane.

The main constituent of the RBC is hemoglobin (Hb), which makes up about a third of its volume. Its function is to transport O_2 from the lungs to body tissues. The RBC has a limited metabolism which, among other things, maintains its electrochemical balance of sodium and potassium (Bell, Davidson, & Scarborough, 1968; Ruch & Fulton, 1960). If hemoglobin were not confined inside the RBC, it would dissolve in blood where its viscosity would interfere with circulation. It would then leak out of the blood because it is a relatively small molecule. The RBC also protects it from substances which would, in other ways, remove it from the blood.

There are two principal genetically determined types of RBC antigens (aglutinogens): (a) the ABO grouping; and (b) the Rh system. These blood groupings are part of the antigen-antibody defense response of the so-called immune mechanism and must be considered in connection with the transfusion of blood from one individual to another. A mismatch causes RBCs to clump (agglutinate).

Hemoglobin.   Hemoglobin is a complex molecule consisting of a protein molecule, globin, and an iron-based pigment, heme. In the lungs, each of the four iron atoms in the Hb molecule combine with a molecule of O_2 to form oxyhemoglobin (OHb). Adult Hb differs from fetal Hb in that it takes up O_2 and gives up CO_2 less readily (Bell, Davidson, & Scarborough, 1968; Oski, Gottlieb, Miller, & Delivoria-Papadopoulos, 1970).

Globin combines with CO_2 in body tissues to form carbahemoglobin (COHb). Whereas O_2 is for the most part transported by Hb. Only about one quarter of the CO_2 is transported this way; the rest of the CO_2 is in plasma in the form of bicarbonate, where it plays a crucial role in the acid-base balance of the blood.

Iron in hemoglobin is in the ferrous state, that is, the bivalent state (Fe^{++}). A small quantity of it is in the ferric, or trivalent state (Fe^{+++}), and combines with hemoglobin forming methemoglobin, to which O_2 does not bind. Ordinarily, methemoglobin constitutes about 2% to 10% of hemoglobin, but it can increase with the administration of drugs including phenacetin, a nonsalycilate analgesic. Ascorbic acid (vitamin C) reduces methemoglobin to Hb (Bell, Davidson, & Scarborough, 1968). Hb also combines reversibly with carbon monoxide (CO). Its affinity for CO is about 200 times greater than that for O_2, but small amounts of it are not directly harmful (Roughton, 1964).

There are several important RBC metabolites that affect Hb function, Principally, adenosine triphosphate (ATP) and 2,3-diphosphoglycerate (DPG).

Adenosine Triphosphate (ATP). ATP is indispensable to life. Found in all living organisms, this "energy reserve" of the cell is crucial in reducing sugar to simpler components (glycolysis), and in transporting potassium into the cell and sodium out of it. ATP is a "high energy" molecule because the total amount of usable energy is released when it is broken down by the addition of a water molecule (hydrolysis). Energy released from ATP is used by the cell to perform its basic functions. As it is expended, ATP must be replenished by the cell (Tortora & Anagnostakos, 1984).

ATP helps to maintain the biconcave shape of the RBC (Brewer, 1974), since as ATP decreases so does the cell deformability—the flexibility required for the RBC to squeeze through ever-narrowing capillaries, which in some instances may have a diameter less than the red blood cell. It regulates the O_2 affinity of Hb (Benesch & Benesch, 1976; Chanutin & Curnish, 1967) by binding to the same sites as does 2,3 diphosphoglycerate (see below), reducing the number of available binding sites for O_2. It also regulates glycolysis, regulation being highly dependent on pH and magnesium concentration.

2,3-Diphosphoglycerate (DPG). DPG is an intermediate by-product of glycolysis found in greatest concentration in RBCs. Because it is not a useful way of obtaining energy, its lack of any apparent function initially puzzled physiologists. Purified Hb has a higher O_2 affinity than Hb in intact cells. The mystery was more or less resolved when it was shown that DPG, when added to purified Hb, decreased O_2-Hb affinity to that of intact cells (Brewer & Eaton, 1971). This lends support to the belief that the function of the RBC is related to its metabolism. In fact, Oski, Gottlieb, Miller, and Delivoria-Papadopoulos (1970) showed that the RBC concentration of DPG is proportional to the degree of hypoxemia (chronic hypoxia). They conclude that:

> It is now apparent that the position of the oxygen-hemoglobin dissociation curve is not only influenced by changes in pH, PCO_2, and temperature but also by the organic phosphate compounds within the red cell. (p. 406)

Since the metabolism of the RBC is itself related to the amount of O_2 available to the system, it now seems that this also affects its function in O_2 transport to other tissues.

Clinical psychophysiologists have more or less ignored regional metabolic function, reserving the term "metabolism" to reflect the overall activity level of individuals. A microview of metabolism makes the picture enormously more complex. On the other hand, it integrates what we actually know about behavior and physiology in a more comprehensible manner.

RBC metabolism and the production and constitution of metabolites is altered during hypoxia in a direction which maximizes delivery of available O_2. This is a homeostatic functional adaptation. As DPG increases, the ratio OHb/Hb increases, liberating more O_2 to tissues (the process is pH related): DPG production increases with increased pH (alkalosis), which prevails where the concentration of CO_2 is greatest, in the tissues where O_2 need is also greatest. DPG binds to deoxyhemoglobin, the desaturated form of Hb, thereby competing with O_2. Conversely, O_2 tends to force Hb into the oxyhemoglobin (saturated) form, driving off DPG (Brewer, 1974). Consequently, variations in the concentration of DPG will shift the oxygen dissociation curve (ODC) (see below), affecting O_2 availability.

Blood DPG levels rise with stress, hypoxia of almost any type, anemia, altitude, and some forms of heart and pulmonary disease (Brewer, 1972). The effect of DPG on oxyhemoglobin dissociation is considered in detail by Brewer (1974):

> Four major factors influencing tissue oxygenation can be identified: *cardiac output,* *pulmonary oxygen exchange,* the circumstances affecting each individual's red cell's pickup and release of oxygen during *red cell oxygen transport,* and lastly, *hematologic parameters* such as red cell mass and the amount of hemoglobin per red cell. (p. 481)

Any one of these factors, and their subfactors, may compensate for a deficit in any one of the others. It might be helpful to keep in mind the complexity and diversity of this multivariate model of O_2 transport as well as its elasticity and functional limitations.

Acid-Base Homeostasis and Other Factors in Oxyhemoglobin Dissociation

In 1904, Bohr, Hasselbach, and Krogh reported the effect of change in CO_2 concentration on the Hb molecule (Bohr effect): Oxygenated hemoglobin (OHb) is a stronger acid than deoxygenated hemoglobin (Hb). Therefore, release of O_2 to body tissues, in arterial blood, makes Hb molecules a weaker acid and more likely to bind with hydrogen ions. This also contributes to the ability of arterial blood to bind and transport locally produced CO_2. Oxygenation of blood in the lungs makes it a stronger acid, reversing CO_2 binding and facilitating release. Thus, adding CO_2 to blood enhances O_2 release from hemoglobin (Comroe, 1974; Shapiro, Harrison, & Walton, 1982).

The Bohr effect is typically represented as the "displacement of the oxyhemoglobin (OHb) dissociation curve (ODC)" by a concomitant change in pH, and is twofold, consisting of an immediate and a sustained homeostatic process (Astrup, 1970). In the immediate process, the ODC is shifted to the right (see Figure 1). Within hours, the extent of the shift is reduced as DPG increases.

Astrup (1970) summarizes the reasons for postulating a mechanism whereby the O_2 affinity of hemoglobin is controlled by the pH dependence of DPG production in the RBC during hypoxia. The effect of such a mechanism is evident in the resulting ratio of oxygenated and reduced Hb, the Hb/OHb ratio. When the concentration of Hb increases, more DPG can be bound to Hb. Decreased concentration of DPG leads to its increased production to reestablish a "steady state." The duration of the Hb/Ohb ratio is a function of pulmonary O_2 uptake, cardiac output, total amount of Hb, and O_2 release in the tissues, but is not effective in all circumstances (Astrup, 1970):

> In individuals with respiratory insufficiency, the 2,3-DPG concentrations seem to be determined not only by the Hb-HbO$_2$ ratio but also by plasma pH. (p. 203)

High altitude increases plasma pH and DPG concentration (high altitude adaptation; see Winslow & Monge, 1987), but increasing CO_2 concentration will reduce DPG.

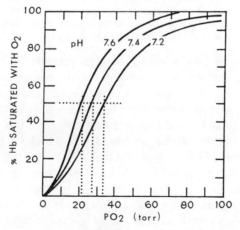

Figure 1. Oxyhemoglobin Dissociation Curve (ODC).

Astrup further states that:

> . . . the effect of pH on 2,3-DPG formation under various circumstances abolished the $Hb-HbO_2$ ratio effect, and one may therefore ask whether the regulatory mechanism in an oxygen affinity control system depends more on changes in red-cell pH than on $Hb-HbO_2$ ratios. . . . This connection between the effects of pH on the oxygen affinity of hemoglobin and their relation to a self-regulating adjustment of the oxygen release to the tissues might be one explanation for the maintenance of plasma and red-cell pH in the living organism within *extremely narrow limits*, a fact that so far has been puzzling to many. (p. 203) (italics added)

This report, as well as many others, confirms my contention that it is virtually senseless to engage in clinical respiratory psychophysiology without monitoring alveolar CO_2 concentration by capnometry. Astrup also pointed out in his article that:

> In addition to an effect of red-cell pH due to an increased $Hb-HbO_2$ ratio, a certain degree of hyperventilation, leading to slightly increased plasma pH values, usually exists with increased ratio. (p. 203)

The hazards of the left-shifted *oxygen dissociation curve* (ODC) have been demonstrated repeatedly in connection with numerous clinical disorders where ischemia jeopardizes O_2 delivery to a tissue system, and in particular in connection with cardiac function (Woodson, 1970, 1979):

> . . . several recent studies indicate that leftward ODC shifts, when occurring in combination with other abnormalities of oxygen delivery, produce or aggravate hypoxia. These data suggest that the brain and heart are the organs particularly at risk. (p. 368)

One factor cited here is hyperventilation:

> Patients with cerebral or coronary vascular disease may be at particular risk, because they lack the ability to increase local perfusion. Hyperventilation may likewise be hazardous, because, in addition to increasing oxygen affinity, it *appreciably reduces cerebral and coronary blood flow.* (p. 372) (italics added)

Although Woodson was referring here to patients being mechanically hyperventilated, any ordinarily prudent practitioner would conclude that, barring the absolutely guaranteed absence of cardiovascular or cerebrovascular ischemic disease, the HV-challenge is a form of Russian Roulette. I won't use it, and I recommend that you don't either.

The concentration of CO_2 in blood will affect its pH. When CO_2 concentration rises, pH decreases and the ODC is "right-shifted," favoring O_2 release. In contrast, when $PaCO_2$ decreases, pH rises and the ODC is "left-shifted," favoring O_2 retention. At a normal pH (7.4), the 50% saturation point P_{50}, is at about 27 millimeters Hg, as previously noted. If pH rises to 7.6, P_{50} drops to about 21 mm Hg. If pH drops to 7.2 P_{50} rises to about 33 mm Hg. What is the implication of this shift in practical terms?

What is alkalosis? The answer lies in an understanding of acid-base homeostasis. Although the formulas and computations in acid-base physiology may seem complex if you are uncertain about the basics of chemistry, the principles of acid-base homeostasis are quite simple, and understanding its basics does not require such computations. Thus, I mostly omit them here. Also, I must confess to the amazing discovery that after reading a sufficient number of initially nearly incomprehensible textbooks, by some mysterious means I began to get the drift. It is very much like learning a new language: it takes a little while and a little effort before you feel at ease with the vocabulary.

To summarize what I have learned, I recommend three books for their outstanding ability to convey acid-base lore in a manner most can understand:

Comroe, J. (1974): *Physiology of Respiration*, 2nd ed. Chicago: Year Book Medical Publishers.

Gamble, J.L. (1982): *Acid-Base Physiology*. Baltimore: Johns Hopkins University Press.

Shapiro, B.A., Harrison, R.A., & Walton, J.R. (1982): *Clinical Application of Blood Gases*, 3d ed. Chicago: Year Book Medical Publishers.

In the human body, the concentration of hydrogen ions is closely regulated, so that the pH will vary little from 7.4 (slightly alkaline); where neutral is 7.0, acid is below 7.0, and alkaline (base) is above 7.0. Less than 1% of the hydrogen generated each day is excreted by the kidneys; therefore, acid-base imbalance due to renal failure is not immediately life threatening. However, such an imbalance due to respiratory failure is critical within minutes.

Increase in blood CO_2 concentration increases hydrogen (H) concentration. This is called respiratory acidosis. Conversely, a decrease in blood CO_2 concentration results in a reduced concentration of H, or respiratory alkalosis (Shapiro, Harrison, & Walton, 1982). The body maintains this pH by a system of protein buffers with a high affinity for H (Comroe, 1974; Gamble, 1982). Proteins bind H to amino acids. In the RBC, the protein responsible for buffering is Hb.

The basis for evaluating the acid-base status of the body requires consideration of change in pH, concentration of plasma bicarbonate, carbonic acid, chloride, and sodium in extracellular fluid. Bicarbonate is present in considerable amounts in extracellular fluid, and it is estimated that it accounts for 97% to 98% of buffering there (Gamble, 1982).

The Role of Respiration in the Acid-Base Balance.   When CO_2 dissolves in water, it comes into equilibrium with carbonic acid, catalyzed by carbonic anhydrase. Equilibrium is rapid and the concentration of the acid is a fairly constant function of the concentration of $PaCO_2$ (Comroe, 1974; Gamble, 1982; Roughton, 1964).

CO_2 is a product of body metabolism and is expelled in the lungs. But its expulsion in the lungs is "rate-limited" by its concentration, or pressure (PCO_2), and respiratory rate. Any change in respiration rate, an increase or decrease, cannot be compensated by increase or decrease in CO_2 production because that is more or less independent of pulmonary expulsion. Thus, an additional buffer system must be considered: the Henderson-Hasselbach equation is a logarithmic expression of pH as a function of the ratio of two variables under separate physiological control. Gilman (1953) expressed it this way:

$$pH = constant\frac{(kidneys)}{lungs}$$

Figure 2 illustrates one way of quantifying the relationship between these variables.

Gamble (1982) points out that "pH is clearly targeted as the entity to be defended by the compensatory mechanisms [though] . . . change in pH does not supply the information most needed for quantitative assessment. . . ." But:

> . . . a difficulty is presented by the high sensitivity of pH to change in PCO_2. Ventilatory variation can make large changes in pH that can easily mask a primary metabolic disturbance. Thus a patient having enough metabolic acid to reduce bicarbonate . . . could have a normal pH if the PCO_2 were reduced . . . by hyperventilation. (p. 30)

I cautioned about this in *The Breath Connection* (1990a), and *The Hyperventilation Syndrome* (1987a). And I would remind the practitioner again that HV may be part of a protective homeostatic adjustment to metabolic acidosis as may be found in diabetes, heart disease, kidney failure, and so on, where bicarbonate is the primary buffer. Failure to anticipate this possibility may result in destabilizing an individual in compensated acidosis. In such a case, simply reducing breathing rate, and retaining PCO_2, could prove fatal because HV may be the compensatory homeostatic mechanism.

Ventilatory failure. Shapiro, Harrison, and Walton (1982) define ventilatory failure as the condition in which the lungs are unable to meet the metabolic demands of the body for meeting CO_2 homeostasis, as compared to respiratory failure which entails both oxygenation and CO_2 expulsion. Ventilatory failure leads to respiratory acidosis. Chronic ventilatory failure is not accompanied by acidemia (i.e., excess blood acid). In fact, chronic ventilatory failure is defined by the existence of metabolic compensation. Chronic respiratory acidosis is marked by elevated $PaCO_2$, with near-normal pH. A corollary of this principle is of particular interest:

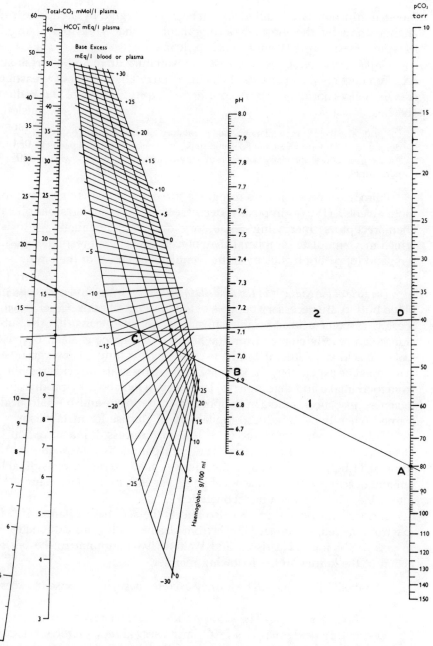

Figure 2. Sigaard-Andersen Alignment Nomograph. Reprinted with permission from P.L. Altman and D.S. Dittmer (1971): *Respiration and Circulation*. Bethesda: Federation of American Societies for Experimental Biology.

"cellular function is disrupted to a far greater degree by a sudden pH change than by the gradual development of that same pH change" (Shapiro, Harrison, & Walton, 1982, p. 106).

Respiratory alkalosis. An increase in respiratory drive above metabolic requirements results in alveolar HV, characterized by arterial CO_2 tension ($PaCO_2$) below normal levels. According to Shapiro, Harrison, and Walton (1982):

> . . . *acute* alveolar hyperventilation (*acute* respiratory alkalosis) is the occurrence of a decreased PCO_2 with alkalemia [elevated pH], and *chronic* alveolar hyperventilation (*chronic* respiratory alkalosis) is the occurrence of a decreased PCO_2 with a near-normal pH. (p. 107)

Pulmonary physiologists recognize three mechanisms that may promote alveolar HV: (a) hypoxia—decreased $PaCO_2$ stimulates peripheral chemoreceptors, increasing respiratory drive; (b) metabolic acidosis, which may stimulate peripheral chemoreceptors or brain respiratory centers; and (c) pathophysiology of the ventilatory centers of the brain.

The Role of the Kidneys in the Acid-Base Balance.   Intra- and extracellular blood buffers are necessary because of the presence of acids. Chief among these is carbonic acid, a volatile substance. Volatile means that the substance can readily change from the liquid to the gaseous state. Because carbonic acid is volatile, it can be expelled by the lungs. However, other acids must be expelled by the kidneys. Among these are (a) acids resulting from food intake and digestion; (b) lactic acid, a metabolic by-product that increases in concentration in proportion to hypoxia; and (c) keto acid, formed when there is reduced availability of glucose for metabolism.

Kidney excretion of H into urine is a slow process. It may take hours. Urine has its own set of buffers. The principal one is phosphate, in the form of H_2PO_4. Thus, though the kidneys may excrete a considerable amount of acid, urine pH may not change. For each hydrogen ion excreted into urine, blood gains a bicarbonate ion.

Intracellular potassium (K) also affects the acid-base balance. If K is lost from the cell, it is replaced by H from plasma, adding a bicarbonate ion to plasma. Shapiro, Harrison, and Walton (1982) summarize the buffer action of the kidney in the following manner:

> Metabolic alkalemia—The kidney excretes base in response to excess blood base.
> Metabolic acidemia—The kidney adds bicarbonate.
> Respiratory acidemia—As PCO_2 increases, kidney excretes H^+, adding base to the blood.
> Respiratory alkalemia—Decreased PCO_2 causes less H^+ excretion, adding base to the blood.

Protein metabolism results in the presence of small amounts of ammonia in the blood. In acidosis, however, considerable amounts of ammonia may be found in urine, though not in blood. The excess is formed in the kidney to neutralize acid (Bell, Davidson, & Scarborough, 1968; Ruch & Fulton, 1960).

The Oxygen Dissociation Curve (ODC) and O_2 Concentration

The total O_2 content of blood includes that in plasma and that bound to hemoglobin (OHb). Saturation depends, first and foremost, on the amount of O_2 available. This relationship is typically represented graphically in Figure 3.

Note that, normally, blood is 50% saturated (P_{50}) at a partial pressure of O_2 (PO_2) equal to about 27 torr (27 mm Hg). When PO_2 is high, the percentage of OHb increases. When PO_2 is low, hemoglobin will be only partially saturated. This means that there will be O_2 in plasma but a lesser proportion of saturated hemoglobin (OHb). Under these conditions, O_2 will be released principally from OHb. In the capillaries surrounding the alveoli of the lungs, PO_2 is high and most of the available hemoglobin will be saturated. But in the body tissues, there is lower PO_2, and so hemoglobin will release O_2 and it will diffuse into the tissues. PO_2 is not the only factor that affects O_2 dissociation. When blood temperature increases, saturation decreases.

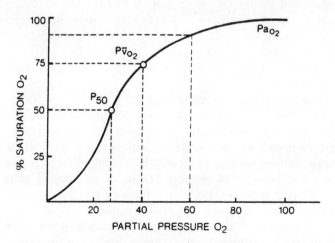

Figure 3. Arterial oxygenation. Reprinted with permission from B.A. Shapiro, R.A. Harrison, and J.R. Walton (1982): *Clinical Application of Blood Gases*, 3d ed. Table 9-3, p. 81. Chicago: Year Book Medical Publishers.

Some Pathophysiological Conditions of Blood Associated with Hypoxia and Hypoxemia

Fortunately, we seldom encounter clients with anoxia, a life-threatening medical emergency. Typically, we treat conditions commonly thought of as psychosomatic, or stress-related, in the broadest sense of that word. It is a major theme of this book that *all* of these conditions have one physiological thing in common, primary or secondary "respiration" impairment, and therefore chronic graded hypoxia with its physical and emotional sequelae. (Respiration is in quotes here to emphasize both of its meanings, respiration [O_2], and ventilation [CO_2].) In some instances, the impairment and its etiology may be relatively obvious such as in chronic diaphragm tension, when part of dysponetic bracing; or in the gasping and breath-holding common in asthma.

It is exceptionally imprudent for the clinician to dismiss any physical symptom as psychological, or psychosomatic, because in the end, all physical symptoms have an organic basis irrespective of their etiology, with consequences that cannot be ignored. Thus, while a client may obviously hyperventilate, an underlying diabetic, thyroid, cardiac, or seizure disorder may be etiological. Or it may be anemia. In some cases, it may be a food sensitivity, while in another case, the medication prescribed for an existing condition may be involved. Bumex (Roche), a commonly prescribed diuretic; Cardizem (Marion), a calcium channel blocker; Empirin with Codeine (Burroughs Wellcome); are among the many commonly prescribed medications which are known to directly affect breathing, their symptoms ranging from dyspnea to HV (Fried, 1990).

It is absolutely essential to look at the side effects of all medications, prescription or nonprescription, used by clients, and at family history for clues to food allergy or sensitivity. These are known to raise blood histamine levels and affect cardiac function, blood circulation, and breathing (Coca, 1956).

There are countless conditions with unclear etiology. For example, a client with hypertension seems to resist efforts to relax. Could it be pheochromocytoma, an adrenal medullary-tumor that secretes epinephrine and norepinephrine (Sodeman & Sodeman, 1979)? Or do we blame the client for failing to learn, or use the techniques for "secondary gain?" Do we ask a hyperventilating client about one or another of the many possible underlying causes such as cardiovascular, kidney, or pulmonary disease; anemia, or variant hemoglobin, including the genetic variety such as sickle-cell anemia, or thalassemia? Many clues to these disorders are apparent in family history.

Blood disorders, allergies, and many other conditions that explain the client's bizarre breathing can be accounted for in this way, and psycho-physiological treatment strategies can be more appropriately devised. You have already seen how metabolic acidosis and respiratory alkalosis may affect hemoglobin. There are numerous other conditions that affect O_2 transport as well (Berkow, 1982; Sodeman & Sodeman, 1979; Stein, 1983). Polycythemia, or erythrocytosis, is a condition of increased red cell mass where blood viscosity increases, causing sluggish circulation, despite vasodilation. Among its symptoms are headache, tinnitus, and dizziness. It has been associated with persons who are tense, and with chain-smokers ("stress-polycythemia"). Polycythemia has many forms, primary and secondary, and its etiology has been linked to hypoxia, pulmonary disease, and methemoglobinemia, among other factors. Of particular interest is that it has been reported to be secondary to sustained HV (Sodeman & Sodeman, 1979).

Anemia, lowered blood cell mass, results in blood adjustments which are intended to stabilize tissue O_2 levels near normal. Initially, anemic hypoxia increases the percentage of anaerobic metabolism. Consequently, blood level of lactic acid rises. The acidosis shifts the ODC to the right, favoring OHb dissociation and great O_2 release. DPG production increases and the system stabilizes as cardiac output increases to meet O_2 demand of body tissues. Symptoms include dermal vasoconstriction—there may be pallor—shortness of breath, tachycardia, leg cramps, and light-headed-ness (a symptom specific to hypoxia). There are many other forms of anemia and I can only alert you to the more common ones:

Iron deficiency anemia is predominantly the result of dietary defi-ciency, or blood loss in U.S. populations. Common symptoms include fatigue and pica. Megaloblastic anemia includes pernicious anemia due to vitamin B_{12} deficiency, and folic acid deficiency. Common symptoms of B_{12} (cobalamine: cobalt-derived) deficiency include glossitis (burning of the tongue), gastrointestinal signs, anorexia, weight loss, gait (ataxia) and neurological disturbances (paresthesia), mild depression, and acute para-noia (megaloblastic madness).

Folic acid anemia may result from its destruction by extended cooking of foods. It is also common when its absorption is inhibited by the use of alcohol, oral contraceptives, or anticonvulsants. Except for the neurologi-cal signs, its symptoms are similar to those of B_{12} deficiency. B_{12} and folic acid are co-enzymes in DNA synthesis. Likewise, copper and vitamin C deficiency may cause anemia. But unlike vitamin C (ascorbic acid), excess copper is injurious to RBCs.

There are also disorders of hemoglobin, and variant or mutant forms with unique ODCs: Some have high O_2 affinity (left-shifted ODC), imped-ing O_2 release in body tissues; some have low O_2 affinity (right-shifted

ODC), resulting in lowered OHb saturation and cyanosis (a bluish appearance, especially of the lips) (Berkow, 1982; Sodeman & Sodeman, 1979; Stein, 1983).

We do not typically have the means to detect blood based pathophysiology for disordered breathing, but it is a good idea to suspect them. And it often helps to ask the same question repeatedly over the course of treatment.

A case in point: I treated a client for dyspnea, fatigue, and anxiety attacks. The answer to the question, "Has anything unusual ever been reported to you in connection with a blood test?" was invariably "no." But though this client was referred because of serious HV, both PCO_2 and breathing rate were normal. With deep diaphragmatic breathing training, PCO_2 dropped precipitously and by 25 torr, training was immediately discontinued.

On the umpteenth repetition of the question, the answer turned out to be, "Why, yes. I didn't think it meant anything, but a large number of enlarged red blood cells were noted. No one thought much of it." "It" being, most likely, macrocytic anemia, perhaps of megaloblastic origin. Referral was made to a physician who suggested elimination of all salycilates from the diet. The client soon improved. The moral of this story is that you should not be set on what to expect: Li'l Abner found out improvidently that "It ain't necessarily Moe."

Chapter **5**

Capnometry and the Computerized Psychophysiological Profile

WITH JOSEPH GRIMALDI*

Introduction

The methods used to detect functional breathing disorders are different from those used in the diagnosis of lung disease. In lung disease, diagnosis hinges upon a first detection of changes in breathing force and volumes. These methods constitute the core of pulmonary function testing and are part of medical treatment. The presence of both functional and organic breathing disorders begins with a report of symptoms, typically dyspnea (i.e., difficulty breathing); inability to catch one's breath; wheezing; shortness of breath, and so on. We tend to view these as manifestations of tension, stress, or anxiety, unless the client reports a medical diagnosis.

Dyspnea

In an article titled "Behavioural breathlessness," Howell (1990) asserts that "part of the reason for uncertainty about the diagnosis of the hyper-

*University of Massachusetts Medical Center, Worcester, Massachusetts; Decision Institute, Worcester, Massachusetts; and Carmel Psychological Associates, Carmel, New York.

ventilation syndrome is that the condition has never been clearly defined" (p. 287). And by the very title of that article, he further confounds the issue by explicitly suggesting that the terms "breathlessness" and "hyperventilation" are synonymous. Not much later in that report, he seems to have overlooked this interchangeability and stated that ". . . I identified 31 patients with disproportionate breathlessness from my outpatient clinics on the basis of dyspnea grade III or more . . . and the absence of adequate respiratory, cardiovascular and other relevant disease" (p. 287). Here, he defined breathlessness on the basis of breathlessness. Are you confused? Table 1 of that article (p. 287) shows that his subjects who had "disproportionate breathlessness" had a $PaCO_2$ of 39.6 mm Hg—textbook normal; while those with "appropriate breathlessness" had a $PaCO_2$ of 50.6 mm Hg! These data can only be described as unusual. It almost seems as though there were a capnometer calibration error of about 15 mm Hg ($\pm$), because one might expect those with disproportionate breathlessness to have a mean $PaCO_2$ of about 25 mm Hg, and the other about 35 mmHg. Finally, the table should have been labeled PCO_2, and not $PaCO_2$, since he did not directly measure arterial gas tension.

But earlier, Campbell and Howell (1963b) suggested that breathing involves the action of "motor control mechanisms which adjust the tension developed by the inspiratory muscles so that they change in length by the amount appropriate to tidal volume demanded, despite changes in mechanical conditions" (p. 40). Thus, they postulated, breathlessness is associated with breathing difficulty in those conditions where there is a disturbance of the relationship between "information about length and information about tension."

Another approach to dyspnea is that of Tobin (1990) according to whom, ". . . there is no universally accepted definition of dyspnea . . . everybody has experienced the sensation and thus has an intuitive understanding of the phenomenon" (p. 1604). He describes several different grades:

(1) Awareness that there is a little increase in ventilation;
(2) A little shortness of breath;
(3) A pleasant or satisfying sensation with deep breathing;
(4) Sensation of hindered breathing;
(5) Sensation of suffocation with acute need for a deeper inspiration;
(6) The sensation at the breaking point of breath-holding. (p. 1604)

An important aspect of the Tobin article is that it emphasizes the subjective element in dyspnea and then systematically describes the probable mechanisms of its etiology: chemosensitivity, pulmonary receptor, respiratory muscle receptor, and respiratory motor command. Many of these mechanisms have been detailed in Chapter 2, but, briefly, respiratory efferent activity predominates over CO_2 chemoreceptor sensitivity, and vagal efferent information from the lungs projects to the cortex and can be directly perceived. Second, the respiratory muscles are a major source of dyspnea. Citing Campbell and Howell (1963a): "During normal breathing, there is an appropriate relationship between the tension developed by the respiratory muscles and the resulting displacement in muscle length." This is the so-called length-tension inappropriateness theory which is providing an excellent justification for breathing retraining. Third, again citing Campbell and Howell (1963b): "A respiratory physiologist offering a unitary explanation for breathlessness should arouse the same suspicion as a tattooed archbishop offering a free ticket to heaven." Finally, Tobin asserts that "dyspnea is a cardinal manifestation of respiratory and cardiac disease" (p. 1609). But White and Hahn (1929) would have strongly disagreed with this position, having previously stated that:

> For the diagnosis of effort syndrome, neurocirculatory asthenia, cardiac neurosis, nervousness and fatigue the symptom of sighing is a useful but neglected aid, especially differentiating these conditions from disability due to cardiovascular disease. (p. 179)

In other words, ". . . sighing is never due primarily to heart disease but always to fatigue and nervousness. . ." (p. 180). Is that reassuring? Their illustrations of this phenomenon, derived from *kymograph*-drum recordings, are reproduced below in an order somewhat different from that in their original illustration.

Figures 1a and 1b show respiratory tracings from two women with neither heart disease nor "nervousness." No sighing dyspnea is evident. Figures 1c, 1d, and 1e show tracings in three persons with organic heart disease. No sighing is evident here either. Figures 1f, 1g, and 1h show deep sighing: The tracings in Figure 1f and in Figure 1g were from persons free of heart disease but who displayed "nervousness." And the individual in Figure 1h had both heart disease and "nervousness." We may reasonably conclude that if sighing is absent, there is probably no "nervousness," but if it is present that does not preclude heart disease, contrary to the initial assertion. Thus, the presence of dyspnea does not preclude heart disease even if its absence precludes "nervousness."

Parenthetically, White and Hahn's venture into psychiatry in that article would have earned them no small reprobation today, with the allegation that "[sighing] was especially common as a frequent event in young women . . . and it is generally recognized that it is this sex at this age that shows the greatest degree of nervous instability" (p. 187).

Although clinical psychophysiologists are seldom trained to recog-

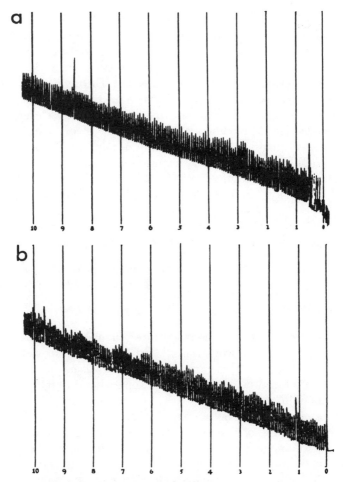

Figure 1 (a–h). Respiratory tracing of patients with heart disease and without heart disease. Respiratory tracing from two women with normal heart and with no effort syndrome or nervousness (a,b). No sighs are evident in either tracing though occasional deeper breaths occur. Respiratory rate ranges between 15 and 17/min, in 1a, and 14 to 17/min in 1b. (Figure continued on next page.)

nize it, nor are they typically predisposed to look for it, I agree with Gardner et al. (1992) who asserted that they certainly should suspect lung disease when dyspnea is reported, even when medical examination does not indicate it, because routine medical examination does not screen for it (Chernick & Raber, 1972; Discher & Steinborn, 1970; Morris, 1976). In fact, Morris (1976) proposes tests for vital capacity (VC); forced vital capacity

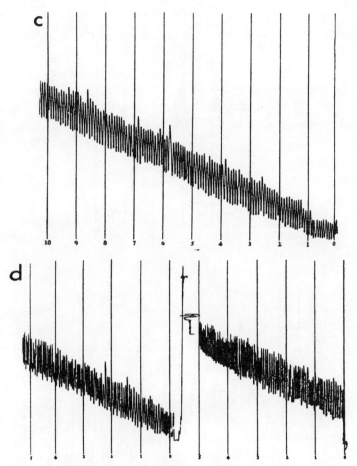

Figure 1 (continued). (c) Respiratory tracing from a young woman with organic heart disease (mitral stenosis) without congestive failure or nervousness—breathing rate is 12/min; (d) from a middle-aged woman with organic heart disease (hypertension, arteriosclerosis) with congestive failure—breathing ranged between 13 and 26/min, with severe dyspnea but no sighing. (Figure continued on next page.)

(FVC); one-second forced expiratory volume (FEV1); the ratio of one-second forced expiratory flow (FEF 200–1200), and forced midexpiratory flow (FEF 25%–75%); maximum voluntary expiration (MVV); total lung capacity (TLC); and forced end-expiratory flow (FEF 75%–85%), as part of routine general medical screening since the connection between breathing-related symptoms and general health impairment has been widely recognized.

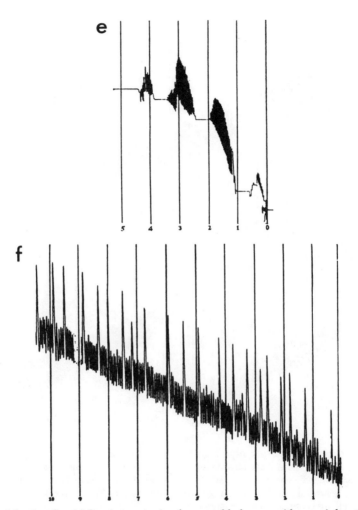

Figure 1 (continued). (e) Respiratory tracing from an elderly man with organic heart disease (hypertensive-arteriosclerotic type, with auricular fibrillation) showing congestive failure and Cheyne-Stokes respiration—hyperpnea alternates with apnea, but there is no sighing. Respiratory tracings from two women with effort syndrome and nervousness but no organic heart disease (f and h). Breathing rate ranged between 13 and 16/min in (f), and 8 to 13/min in (g). Marked sighing is evident. Respiratory tracing in a woman with both heart disease (rheumatic aortic regurgitation) and marked nervousness. Breathing ranged between 9 and 13/min (h). (From White and Hahn (1929): The symptom of sighing in cardiovascular diagnosis with spirometric observations. *American Journal of Medicine and Science.*)

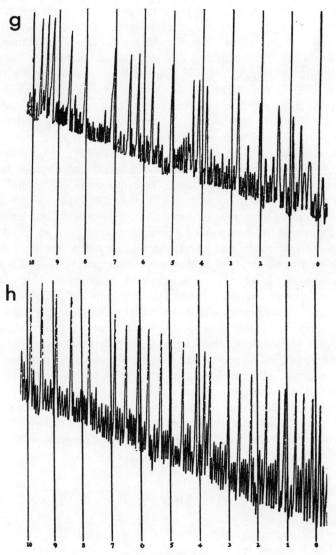

Figure 1 (continued).

Not only is pulmonary disease considered by some investigators to be more prevalent than generally thought, but it also shows a high correlation to loss of work days from other diseases (Rosser & Guz, 1981), including heart disease. In fact, because pulmonary function tests are so rarely performed routinely, a number of respiratory symptom questionnaires were developed and widely tested to affirm the role of breathing-related symptoms in general health and disease (Comstock, Stone, Tomascia, & Johnson, 1981; Helsing, Comstock, Speizer, Ferris, Lebowitz, Tockman, & Burrows, 1979; Samet, 1978). While these screening questionnaires concerned bronchitis, asthma, emphysema, sputum formation, and so on, none of them were concerned with functional disorders, and none addressed psychological or psychiatric variables.

Behavioral physiologists who recognize the inherently organic nature of HV, commonly regarded in medicine as a functional disorder, have also developed screening questionnaires. The Nijmegen Questionnaire is one example (Folgering & Colla, 1978; van Dixhoorn & Duivenvoorden, 1985). In either instance, the report of subjective breathing-related symptoms is intended to show the existence of a condition other than simply the mere presence of those symptoms. And it should be noted that virtually all of the pulmonary investigators cited above, who report the use of subjective questionnaires, strongly recommend routine conventional lung function diagnostic screening when respiratory symptoms are reported.

Whichever way you look at it, we'd better define terms and concepts in clinical respiratory psychophysiology, so that we can communicate with some degree of confidence the relationship of their parameters to those of stress and emotional disorders and specific pulmonary conditions that we treat. I have cautioned previously, in connection with HV, that we cannot afford to fail to tell the difference between stress-related tachypnea with hypocapnia and compensatory hyperventilatory alkalosis due perhaps to heart or kidney disease, diabetes, or another source of metabolic acidosis. Nor can we ignore the possibility of respiratory acidosis due to a ventilation problem, despite tachypnea.

The First Profile

A psychophysiological hyperventilation profile (PHVP) was first proposed (Fried, Fox, Carlton, & Rubin, 1984) on the basis of research on behavioral control of idiopathic seizures, conducted at the Rehabilitation Research Institute, ICD—International Center for the Disabled, N.Y. Although there were certainly enough symptom lists available in the literature, there seemed to be no efforts to standardize assessment protocols; thus the following physiological indices were chosen from among those that we found useful in noting pre- and posttreatment status: respiration rate and mode; percentage of end-tidal CO_2 ($PETCO_2$); cardio-respiratory synchrony (RSA); EEG; and peripheral (finger) temperature. These are practical objective indices from which the physiological impact of HV can be inferred.

Tidal volume and arterial blood pH were omitted. Though very illuminating, observing them is invasive and not generally practical. Ventilatory monitoring devices requiring a mouthpiece, such as the spirometer, were also rejected because they increase tidal volume (Vt), decrease respiration rate (f), and disturb breathing rhythm (Tobin et al., 1983). The latter recommended plethysmography, but it entails spirometric calibration prior to use; and impedance plethysmography is not sufficiently standardized (electrode type and placement are crucial variables) (Hamilton, Beard, & Kory, 1965). In any case, these methods are excessively elaborate and are more appropriate in research than in office practice. Eliminating them reduces the reliability of assessment but does not render it useless by any means.

The protocols were tested on three groups of clinical subjects, men and women ranging in age between 22 and 53 years; and an asymptomatic control group, 10 women and 5 men, health service professionals at the ICD, N.Y. There was a second clinical group consisting of 36 women and 28 men, psychiatric outpatient clients at the Payne Whitney Clinic, Cornell University Medical Center, and the Behavior Therapy Institute, New York, N.Y. In addition, many psychologists, psychiatrists, and other physicians in private practice, sent us clients for PHVP evaluation.

The patients presented with anxiety, panic disorder, migraine, vertigo, phobias, respiratory complaints, depression, chest pain, primary and secondary Raynaud's disease, and so on. None were psychotic. A third group of subjects, 11 men and 16 women with various idiopathic epileptic seizure conditions, and with chronic or severe episodic HV were used to evaluate the usefulness of the PHVP. These seizure sufferers were for the most part intractable to therapeutic serum levels of a number of different anticonvulsant medications, and were enrolled in the behavioral control of seizures study. The results were detailed in Fried et al. (1984, 1985) and Fried (1987a, 1990).

Briefly, it became clear that normal respiration rate is not an absolute quantity, but a range of accepted values, since ventilation can be achieved by different combinations of breathing rate and tidal volume (Otis, 1964). For a given metabolic demand, there is an optimal breathing frequency, when the work required of the respiratory muscles is minimal (Mead, 1960). At these times the system is at its most efficient. Normal breathing rate reported by various sources was found to vary considerably: 10 to 18 (Bell, Davidson, & Scarborough, 1968); 16 (Basmajian, 1978); 14 (Haas et al., 1979); and 13 (Finesinger, 1943).

Breathing is often considerably dysrhythmic, with rapid and unpredictable shifts in PETCO$_2$, a wide range of such shifts, and sighs, gasps, and spasms. Apnea is not infrequent. Kilburn (1965) reported tachypnea and hyperpnea as signs of compensatory ventilation, suggesting, as did also Hughes (1975), that these observations may indicate uneven ventilation of the lower lobes of the lungs and, quite possibly, loss of function of distal pulmonary vessels due to lung disease.

The mode may be observed by noting chest movement (i.e., expansion and upward excursion). Often it is subtle. In some cases, it is apparently absent. As predicted in previous research, the controls had a mean breathing rate of about 12. Both the psychiatric referrals and the seizure control group had a mean breathing rate of about 17. The differences between the means are statistically significant, as shown by an analysis of variance.

The relationship between peak- and mean-PETCO$_2$ can be used as an indication of rhythmicity. When they are similar, breathing is usually more or less rhythmic; if the peak and mean deviate sharply, aperiodicity is observed. When PETCO$_2$ is monitored in the resting state, peak-percentage changes may reflect habituation, while mean changes reflect adaptation (Fried, Korn, & Welch, 1966; Fried et al., 1967; Wilder, 1959). Asymptomatic controls show a greater degree of habituation than do the other two subject groups, consistent with the commonly accepted model of psychophysiological arousal and its relationship to anxiety states (Franks, 1961; Welch & Kubis, 1947a, 1947b).

The distribution of the cardiac interbeat interval may show a number of different patterns that have clinical implications. In some persons, one may observe the increase in heart rate with inspiration and the decrease with expiration, that is, respiratory sinus arrhythmia (RSA). RSA is controlled by breathing frequency and pattern (Angelone & Coulter, 1964; de Boer, Karemaker, & Strackee, 1985; Hirsh & Bishop, 1981; Porges, McCabe, & Yongue, 1982; Sroufe, 1971). It is rarely observed in persons with chronic HV and is absent when hyperpnea and tachypnea prevail in otherwise normal persons.

EEG is included in the PHVP because HV has been repeatedly shown to be accompanied by low-frequency, high-voltage brain-wave activity (*theta*) (Gibbs, Lennox, & Gibbs, 1940; Holmberg, 1953; Swanson, Stavney, & Plum, 1958). HV is routinely used in clinical EEG to provoke abnormalities (Blinn & Noell, 1949; Brill & Seidmann, 1942). The spectrum analyzer, with fast-Fourier analysis, permits analysis of EEG frequency composition (Engel, Romano, & McLin, 1944; Gibbs, Lennox, & Gibbs, 1940).

Figure 2 shows average power spectral composition of the EEG of asymptomatic control subjects compared to those of psychiatric referral clients and idiopathic seizure sufferers. There is, in all cases, an elevation at the very low frequency which represents the dc component. Power is depressed in the psychiatric group and in the idiopathic seizures group below that of the controls. Some psychiatric referrals showed *theta* elevations, but they invariably appear in persons with Raynaud's disease, migraine, and angina (i.e., vascular disorders). Finally, a record of peripheral (left) finger temperature at the beginning and end of an assessment or training session provided an index of peripheral vascular caliber and blood flow (Birk, 1973; Budzynski, 1983; King & Montgomery, 1980, 1981; Surwit, Shapiro, & Feld, 1976; Taub & Emurian, 1976; Wickramasereka, 1973).

This PHVP was a protocol for standardizing physiological parameters

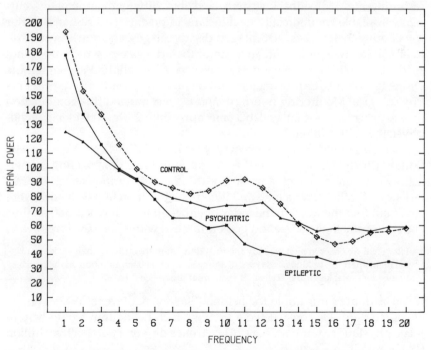

Figure 2. Average EEG Power Spectral Composition in asymptomatic control, seizure, and psychiatric subject groups.

of respiration, heart function, blood flow, and brain-wave activity. Based on combined reports of previous investigators, it was a beginning. Each of its measures was imprecise and limited in scope, but by analogy to psychometrics, the composite was thought to be useful for inferring various parameters, including autonomic arousal. Respiration rate, mode, and $PETCO_2$ permit, within limits, assumptions about arterial blood pH and Hb function; hand temperature, peripheral vasotone; ECG-RSA and vagal tone; and EEG *theta* elevation, cerebral ischemia, reduced blood flow, and oxygen deficit.

The Psychophysiological Profile

The PHVP of almost 10 years ago was a seedling, so to speak. In revising it, a broader range of physiological indices were considered, especially in light of advances in computerized physiological monitoring technology, and the availability of a reasonably priced capnometer. We considered and evaluated the features of virtually every physiological recording and biofeedback system, and four different capnometers currently available commercially to clinicians in practice and research. After considering their merits, advantages, disadvantages, and quirks, we chose to integrate two units into a state-of-the-art system which does not sacrifice simplicity of operation for power and versatility. We coupled the Ohmeda 4700 OxiCap oximeter/Capnometer with the J & J Instruments Physiological Monitoring Interface, and we recommend this combination to you for reasons that will become apparent as we consider psychophysiological profiling.

The American Heritage Dictionary of the English Language, New College Edition (1980), defines "profile" as "a graph or table representing numerically the extent to which a person or thing shows various tested characteristics." Profiles have a long and illustrious tradition in psychology, yet I could not find the word in the index of either an introductory, personality, or psychopathology college text book published within the past three years.

> How shall we observe men, classify them, and measure them? How shall we learn to tell them apart . . . as kinds and types of animals . . . and fasten attention on the basic, first-order variables of the science of individual differences? (p. 2)

If you attributed this quote to Sheldon (Sheldon & Stevens, 1942), you are of course right. He constructed a profile which he thought would help to relate physique to temperament. And, from a different perspective, Millon (1987) puts it this way:

> Several assumptions are made when the diagnostic focus is narrowed to a limited range of clinical behaviors. Most basically, it is assumed that specific clinical behaviors

will be shared by a distinctive group of patients. Further, it is assumed that prior
knowledge concerning the characteristics of these distinctive patient groups will
facilitate a variety of diagnostic and treatment goals. (p. 16)

Millon was considering populations with psychopathological characteristics. We are considering populations with somatic characteristics. However, his dictum provides a frame of reference for our own psychophysiological profiles and classification schemes:

If diagnostic placement simplifies clinical tasks such as alerting the diagnostician to
features of the patient's history and present functioning that have not yet been
observed, enabling clinicians to communicate effectively about their patients, guiding
selection of beneficial therapeutic plans, or assisting researchers in designing better
studies, the process of diagnostic identification will have served many useful purposes. (p. 17)

These are only two sources of concern about profiles, but they clearly indicate that we have a deep-seated belief that there are fundamental types to which one may add some degree of individual variation. Types may be thought to be uniparametric or multiparametric: The uniparametric view holds that there is one relevant continuum which has predictive validity for an inborn characteristic of concern. For instance, depending on how you score on a given symptom inventory, you may be a "hyperventilator." If that is true, does the inventory measure the behavior of a physiological type, or does it measure the physiology of a psychological type? Both, perhaps? The multiparametric profile is, in physiology, an analog of the well-known psychometric omnibus. It is based on multitrait or multifactor theories and attempts to provide a composite evaluation based on multimodal measurements. Is one preferable to another? It is hard to say. We typically teach our college students that many observations are superior to just one, but just one may be better than many, if it is the right one.

HV is technically defined as alveolar CO_2 concentration below normal (38 torr) (Comroe, 1974; Gardner et al., 1992). If you are simply interested in identifying hyperventilators, then $ETCO_2$ is clearly the only direct means to do it. A symptom inventory is not superior because (a) the definition of HV is based on $ETCO_2$; and (b) it is not invariably accompanied by the same set of symptoms. But there is really a submerged agenda in profiling: The use of HV symptom assessments, for instance, is not intended simply to identify HV, but type of hyperventilator. This "type" is (a) a chronic hyperventilator who (b) may be expected to have a specific set of somatic symptoms, and (c) psychological symptoms. Being able to identify such a type appears to lend diagnostic validity to arguments about which method of treatment may be expected to be most effective: medical/psychiatric (drugs), psychological/psychotherapy (cognitive), biofeedback, breathing training, and so on. You will find a more detailed discussion of types in Chapter 7. With this in mind, let's get on with physiological profiling.

Parameters of the Profile

The parameters of the profile are:

(a) Breathing:
- respiration rate in breaths per minute
- respiration mode (nasal vs. mouth, thoracic vs. abdominal)
- respiration pattern (I/E ratio, spasm, etc.)
- tidal volume
- alveolar CO_2 concentration (PCO_2, $ETCO_2$)

(b) The heart:
- pulse rate (HR)
- blood pressure
- ECG
- rotation
- RSA

(c) Circulation:
- percentage of OHb (SaO_2)
- hand temperature
- head-apex temperature

(d) Muscle:
- EMG
- muscle microvibration

(e) CNS:
- EEG

Apparatus*

We recommend an infrared capnometer (Ohmeda 4700) which collects end-tidal breath exhaled through the nose, then transmits an electrical analog of CO_2 concentration to a computer, which analyzes it and displays it as a trace on a video monitor and records it as "hard copy." In addition, biopotentials from various skin surface sources, as well as other transducer information, are simultaneously gathered, analyzed, displayed, and/or stored for later analysis and data summaries by a J & J I-330 Physiological Monitoring Interface System of modules and software (i.e.,

---

*For information about Ohmeda capnometers, or the J & J physiological monitoring system, please write to Robert Fried, 1040 Park Avenue, New York, NY 10028-1032.

the USE Physiological Programming Language, and many prepro-grammed software applications).

The profile employs one or more of these modules: Isolation amplifier (I-801); plethysmograph (p-401); temperature/EDG (T-601); respiratory pneumograph (R-301); electromyograph (M-501); EEG/EMG (E-201).

The J & J I-330 will operate with any computer having an RS-232 port. The software was written for IBM-compatible PS2, PC AT, and XT computers. We used an AGI 286-12 MHz computer with an Everex VGA monitor.

The J & J I-330 Physiological Interface comprises interchangeable modules, commonly preamplifiers, for physiological monitoring of muscle biopotentials (EMG), temperature, heart rate (pulse, RSA), electrodermal (EDG) or galvanic skin response, EEG, etc. (Fig. 3).

Method

In a typical session, the client is seated in a comfortable recliner chair facing a video monitor placed at eye level. The trainer sits to the client's right, about six feet away, and has a keyboard and a parallel monitor. The trainer is seated in such a way that she or he can see across the client as well as see the monitor screen.

PCO_2. A nasal catheter, $6'' \times \frac{1}{8}'' \times \frac{1}{32}''$, is inserted about ¼ inch into a nostril and held in place, taped to the upper lip. The distal end of this nasal catheter inserts over a fitting on the distal end of the capnometer intake-catheter. The proximal end of the capnometer intake-catheter is coupled by

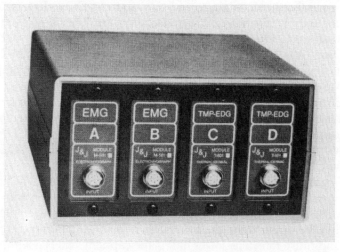

Figure 3. J & J I–330 Physiological Interface System Modality Modules.

a twist-type male-fitting to a corresponding female counterpart on the capnometer. Presterilized flexible latex surgical tubing, packaged in 50 foot rolls and precut to 6 inch lengths, is used as the nasal catheter. Caution: *This tubing must be immediately discarded after each use. It is never to be reused.*

SaO_2. The client's left index finger is inserted into the oximeter sensor.

Thoracic (chest) and abdominal pneumograph. The pneumograph sensor belts are attached with Velcro strips, one around the upper thorax, at approximately armpit-level; the other one is attached around the abdomen, at about navel-level.

Pulse rate and interbeat interval. The right index finger of the client is inserted into the plethysmograph sensor (J & J, PS-400).

Thermal monitoring. Two thermistors are used. One is taped under the surface of the pinky (little finger) of the subject's nondominant hand; the other is attached to the head apex, placed over the scalp (parting the hair if necessary) with a small cotton wad placed squarely over it. Two bobby-pins fasten the pad down. If the client is bald, tape may be used to hold the thermistor in place.

Blood pressure. A cuff is placed over the right bicep and left deflated except when measurements are taken.

Spirogram. Volume measurements are not usually made except where the client has asthma, or some other organic airway impediment. An incentive-inspirometer, incentive-expirometer, or peak flow meter may be used.

Monitoring Breathing: The Capnometer

The nasal catheter conducts end-tidal air to an Ohmeda 4700 OxiCap. Its analog output is conducted to an Isolation Amplifier (I-801) in the J & J I-330 interface modules (channel 1). Screen time is arbitrary but in this application, it is 30 seconds. The capnometer measures CO_2 by infrared analysis of a mixture of gases, of which CO_2 is a proportional component. We chose the Ohmeda 4700 OxiCap for the same reason that we chose the J & J I-330 System. They are versatile, user-friendly, and reliable units, and are available at reasonable cost. The Ohmeda 4700 Oxicap, shown in Figure 4, comprises both an oximeter to measure arterial blood OHb saturation (PaO_2), and a capnometer to measure alveolar, or end-tidal CO_2 (PCO_2).

The Ohmeda 4700 OxiCap is a programmable, free-standing, infrared CO_2 gas analyzer. It can be used with the I-330 System, or by itself. For most operations, its display screen is preprogrammed on four screen quadrants. The upper left quadrant displays systolic-diastolic pulse waveform, and the upper right quadrant shows OHb saturation (percentage of SaO_2) and pulse rate. The lower half is the capnometer. The left quadrant

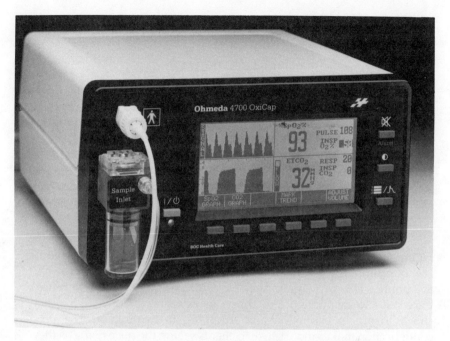

Figure 4. Ohmeda 4700 Oxicap Capnometer and Oximeter unit.

displays inspiration and expiration as an $ETCO_2$ waveform, by virtue of which one can view the breathing pattern, and the lower right quadrant displays either percentage of end-tidal CO_2 ($PETCO_2$) or partial pressure (PCO_2) in torr (mm Hg), depending on how it is instructed to report this value. Programs, easily reached by push-button on the front panel, permit presetting various functions such as screen-sweep time, threshold limits, and so on. Selection of appropriate settings and values may be made before the information is fed to the computer. Either a finger-type or earlobe transducer may be used with the 4700 OxiCap oximeter.

The ISA can be adjusted by pin-switches and a setscrew in the rear of the housing so that peak-$PETCO_2$ on the 4700 OxiCap matches the value produced by the computer.

Capnography. The capnograph is a hard copy tracing of the distribution of CO_2 over real-time obtained by computer printout of the analog trace on the video monitor. There are several important and often confused terms common in capnography. These are usually represented by symbols:

(a) Carbon dioxide (CO_2);

(b) End-tidal CO_2 (ETCO$_2$): the concentration of CO_2 in expired air; alternately, alveolar CO_2 concentration (PCO$_2$); usually expressed in mm Hg, or torr;

(c) Percentage of end-tidal CO_2 (PETCO$_2$);

(d) Arterial blood CO_2 concentration (PaCO$_2$): the concentration of CO_2 in arterial blood; usually expressed in mm Hg, or torr;

(e) For conversion of percentage to torr:
PETCO$_2$ × 760 = torr (for instance: if PETCO$_2$ is 5%, then .05 × 760 = 38 torr);

(f) For conversion of torr to percentage:
$\dfrac{torr}{760}$ = percentage (for instance: if ETCO$_2$ is 38 torr, then

$\dfrac{38}{760}$ = .05, or 5%).

Figure 5 shows a capnograph obtained from a young woman volunteer, free of pulmonary disorders. A hard copy was made with an Epson LQ 850 printer. This capnogram may be said to be upside down because the trace rises to inspiration and drops to expiration. Conventionally, it is shown rising to expiration and dropping to inspiration. The present configuration makes more sense to clients seeing the trace rising as they fill up with air, and drop as they expel it, since we tend to connect filling with

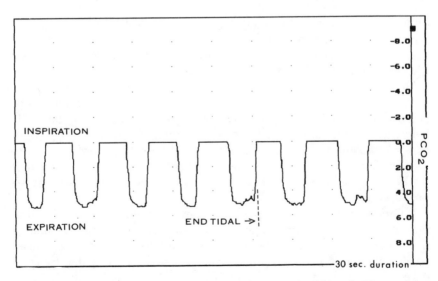

Figure 5. Capnograph: 30-second tracing of percentage of end-tidal breath CO_2 concentration (PETCO$_2$) shown on an inverted scale (right).

going up, and emptying with going down. It is also simpler for the trainer when the trace is inverted because it is easier to imagine what the client is doing when inspiration goes up, rather than down.

Therefore, in the scale on the right, negative values are above positive ones. As the person exhales, CO_2 rises (upside down) over time until it reaches peak around 4.5%. When inhaling, the trace is zero because she is breathing "against" the pump. Little air, if any, now reaches the capnometer and it therefore reads CO_2 at atmospheric pressure (i.e., near zero).

Counting complete inspiration and expiration cycles, depending on screen duration, yields breathing rate, though both the capnometer and the computer will yield the same values. In this capnograph, breathing rate is about 14 b/min, with $PETCO_2$ at about 4.5; $ETCO_2$ is 34.2 torr. *Caution: $PETCO_2$ means percentage of end-tidal CO_2. Therefore, $PETCO_2$ is 4.5, not 4.5%.*

According to Hess (1989), in a normal capnograph (right side up) PCO_2 is zero during inspiration and zero at the beginning of expiration. The capnograph rises sharply, as alveolar gas mixes with air in the anatomical dead space; then the curve rises to the alveolar plateau during expiration. At the end of the alveolar plateau PCO_2 is end-tidal CO_2 ($ETCO_2$). You may note in Figure 5 that the 3rd, 4th, and 6th expirations show a sort of plateau, but the others show halting and relatively rapid expiration with slightly longer inspirations. There are other deviations from the normal capnograph but they are not invariably pathophysiological. For instance, Figure 7 illustrates cardiac oscillations which are quite normal and occur in expiration in deep slow breathing, when the heart beats against the lungs forcing out small quantities of air. In this figure, the capnograph gain was increased to enlarge the pattern. Cardiac oscillations have mistakenly been taken as evidence of hysteria and other psychoneurotic states (see Chapter 7).

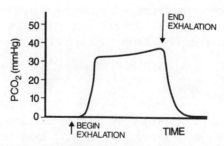

Figure 6. Normal capnograph. From D. Hess (1989): *A Guide to Understanding Capnography.* Louisville, CO: Ohmeda—The BOC Group, Inc. Reprinted by permission.

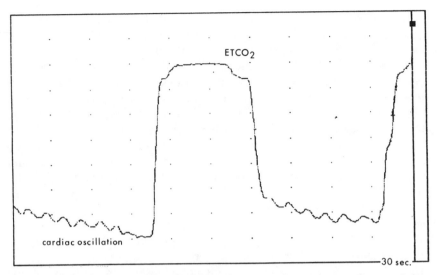

Figure 7. Thirty-second capnograph showing "cardiac oscillation" (saw-tooth pattern) during exhalation in deep diaphragmatic breathing.

You are also cautioned that the length of the catheter will effect a delay in transmitting air from the client to the capnometer, which will appear as a delay in the trace. This delay may, in some cases, be dismaying to the client watching the trace on the video monitor. It is advisable to explain the latency to the client. But do not alter the catheter length, since unit calibration depends on it.

Ordinarily, the digital readout below the trace window will register peak CO_2 per trial epoch, arbitrarily preselected. But this value may be inaccurate if breathing is relatively rapid, because computation depends on sampling duration. The concentration of CO_2 sampled during a trial will depend on whether the peak occurs during the trial sampling interval. When breathing becomes deeper with training, a trial may be shorter than a breathing cycle. Then, it is advisable to use the numeric display on the capnogram and to note $PETCO_2$ or $ETCO_2$ for later recording on the hard copy.

The Respiration Ratio: I/E

The respiration ratio (I/E) is the relative duration of inspiration and expiration. In Figure 5, breathing seems to favor inspiration. This is common when abdominal breathing does not prevail in a person without pulmonary disorder. Many clients present with unusual I/E ratios and report having acquired their peculiar type of breathing from books or in yoga classes. Idiosyncratic breathing maneuvers without any basis in scientific fact, or without merit, for that matter, have been touted as healthful: inspiration twice as long as expiration, or vice versa; explosive expiration; and so on. When breathing is natural, the I/E ratio is approximately 1.00 (Fried, 1987b, 1990a).

Monitoring Blood O_2: The Oximeter

The Ohmeda 4700 OxiCap tells us about the level of blood O_2. Whereas the capnometer applies infrared technology to measuring the concentration of CO_2 in gas form, the oximeter uses infrared technology to measure oxygen bound to hemoglobin. You are probably aware that oxygenated blood is reddish, whereas deoxygenated blood tends to be bluish. That is what we mean by cyanosis (from Greek: kuanosis, i.e., blue) when an individual has bluish lips.

Generally, oximetry estimates available arterial blood O_2 (SaO_2) by determining percentage of saturated hemoglobin (OHb). But in clinical psychophysiology, we do not ordinarily see individuals in anoxic crisis. What is the usefulness of the oximeter, then? First, we have found that persons who have severe allergies tend to show a 2% to 3% decrease in SaO_2, ranging from the normal limits of 95% to 98% down to a percentage in the upper 80s (i.e., 87% to 92% in some cases; see also Chapter 9, Asthma). Such a small decrease in SaO_2 does not constitute a significant medical datum. But it is graded hypoxia and contributes to lactic acidosis by increasing the percentage of anaerobic metabolism. This change, small though it may seem, will significantly increase breathing rate and will be accompanied by an exacerbation of what clients report when they say, "I just don't feel well."

Second, when PCO_2 is normal, there will be an increase in SaO_2 with deep-diaphragmatic breathing. As air pressure in the lungs increases, there will be a corresponding increase in profusion and SaO_2 will rise. This is normal. But when there is severe episodic HV and PCO_2 is well below 30 torr, you may observe high SaO_2, 99% to 100%, indicative of a left-shifted ODC. Then, when deep-diaphragmatic breathing normalizes PCO_2, you may observe what must appear to be a paradoxical decrease in SaO_2 to the normal limits range, as increased OHb dissociation liberates O_2 to the tissues. Figure 8 shows a capnograph with a superimposed SaO_2 trace.

SaO_2 is taken from the analog output of the Ohmeda 4700 OxiCap and connected to a second isolation amplifier (I-801) in the J & J I-330 interface. Note that PCO_2 is 4.9%, and that SaO_2 is 98.6%, with a

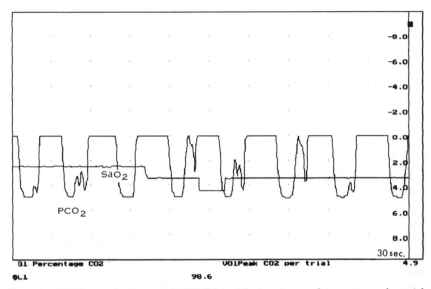

Figure 8. Thirty-second capnograph (PETCO$_2$) with superimposed percentage of arterial blood hemoglobin (Hb) saturation (SaO$_2$)—L1 = 98.6%

breathing rate of about 14.5 breaths per minute, with inspiratory and expiratory gasps.

The 4700 OxiCap displays only in whole integers, but the analog output is translated by the J & J I-330 system into 10ths of one percent. The readout on the oximeter may differentiate between 96.0% and 97.9% only as a 1% change (i.e., from 96% to 97%). But the I-330 translation would clearly show it as being almost 2% (1.9%). In breathing training, small changes in SaO$_2$ may reflect considerable changes in graded hypoxia, and these changes can be quite dramatic when they reflect increased pulmonary profusion as they follow the breathing cycle.

So far the profile shows that breathing rate is at the upper limit of normal (about 14.5 b/min), though the pattern is choppy. Inspiration tends to be somewhat longer than expiration, with some gasps and abdominal/thoracic shifts which are observed as interruptions in the inhale and exhale phase. PETCO$_2$ is 4.9 (PCO$_2$ is about 37 torr), or near-normal.

Breathing Mode: Abdomen versus Chest

To reduce the number of figures illustrating this book, we have combined abdominal and thoracic pneumography with the ECG/RSA trace along with the PCO_2 and SaO_2 traces on Figure 9. So let's look at just the pneumographic traces now.

To obtain these traces, we used the J & J I-300 interface (respiratory) pneumograph module (R-301) with the abdominal and thoracic pneumographic sensor "belts." Despite absolute pressure in the sensors, the baselines were so placed that, given the same value in each, they will not superimpose on the screen. Thus, the fact that they are not at the same level on the screen does not directly indicate pressure differences at rest. You have to look at the digital values below the tracings window.

The thoracic trace was set above that of the abdomen for logical consistency, since the chest is located above the abdomen. The chest and abdomen may be seen to move more or less together during the breathing cycle and with about the same degree of expansion, slightly favoring the chest, as indicated by the deflections in the traces. Several aspects of this profile deserve special attention.

First, note that although abdominal and chest excursions appear quite smooth, the $PETCO_2$ trace does not. It is composed of some incomplete, brief, sharp interruptions in inspiration. Then, about two thirds of the way through the profile, there is a stretch of virtually imperceptible abdominal

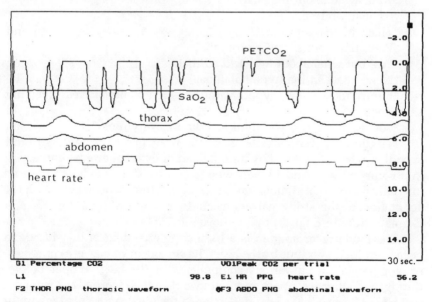

Figure 9. Thirty-second capnograph with superimposed SaO_2 (L1); ECG tachometer (E1) showing consecutive interbeat intervals (IBI); and thoracic (F2) and abdominal (F3) pneumographic excursion tracings.

and thoracic excursion, yet airflow appears to be, if anything, smoother. It may be concluded from this observation, which is by no means rare, that observable movements of the chest and abdomen may not necessarily reflect air flow into and out of the lungs.

Second, abdomen and chest excursions don't seem to exactly fit airflow in and out of the lungs. Remember that pneumography is virtually instantaneous while capnography is not. There is a delay in transmission of air through the catheter—all traces on the profile are a little ahead of $PETCO_2$. "How much," you ask; it depends on the length of the catheter. You will have to establish that empirically by timing the delay.

The Heart

In Western tradition, the groom places the wedding band on the fourth finger of the bride's left hand. During medieval times, that finger was thought to have a vein tying it to the heart. "How romantic," you say, "the heart is the seat of emotions." No, in those days, the heart was considered to be the organ for thinking; emotion sat elsewhere. The idea was to control thoughts, not emotions.

"Well, what about the heart?"

"It's just a pump."

"That's it? Just a pump?"

"Well, that's not exactly nothing!"

"Yes, but what about love and all that?"

"Naw! That's in the hypothalamus."

"Funny, never saw hypothalamus-shaped Bonbonierres given for Valentine's day."

"You science-guys, you think you know everything."

For clinical psychophysiologists, the heart is a behaving organ, responding when stimulated by internal and/or external events, interacting in a complex way. And its behavior "feeds back" to modulate both its internal and external stimulation. Much of this first came to light with the adaptation of the string galvanometer to electrocardiography (EKG in German; ECG in English) by Einthoven in 1903.

The modern cardiogram is a hard copy recording of the change in voltage emitted over time by the heart. Its change in voltage is a composite of biopotentials from various components of the heart proper before, during, and after its contraction. By convention, it is recorded at 25 mm per second, and set so that a 1 cm deflection of the trace represents 1 mv input to the amplifier. Thus, the ECG is a (milli-)voltmeter.

With electrodes on various body surfaces, electrical sources within the heart and the course or path of the bioelectrical innervation around and through the heart can be identified. The most common such observation is made with bipolar limb leads from the right and left arm, and the left leg. The path between the right and left arm is designated *I*; between the right arm and left leg, *II*; and between the left arm and left leg, *III*.

The lead-*I* trace configuration, at the bottom of Figure 10, identifies the trace components with letters standard in medical electrocardiography. Their duration in the normal heart is shown at the top of the figure. The sequence of events together with valve action and the blood pressure consequences of contraction are also shown in this figure.

The P-wave indicates atrial depolarization (i.e., the spreading of excitation from the SA-node), stimulating contraction of the right and left atria. The large upward deflection in the QRS-complex, the R-wave, is due to depolarization as the electrical impulse spreads through the ventricles; the T-wave indicates ventricular repolarization. Atrial repolarization is masked by the QRS-complex (Tortora & Anagnostakos, 1984; Ruch & Fulton, 1969).

The heart differs from other muscles in that it has a conduction system of specialized muscle fibers that initiate and propagate electrical impulses throughout the organ, causing sequential contraction. The conduction system begins at nodes which are aggregates of conducting cells. The SA-node (sinoatrial) in the right atrial wall initiates each cardiac cycle. It is said to be the cardiac pacemaker. Contraction of the atria coincides with the depolarization of the AV-node (atrioventricular). Fibers from the AV-node divide into the right and left bundle-branches which innervate the ventricles via ramifications called Purkinje fibers. The coordinated action of the conducting system results in a normal heartbeat in which the atria contract simultaneously (systole), while the ventricles relax (diastole).

The Effect of Diaphragmatic Breathing on the Heart

Two aspects of heart action are of primary interest to us in the study of the relationship between breathing and the heart: rotation and sinus rhythm. Goldman (1967) describes a standard 12-lead ECG (Figure 11), which reflects the effect of deep breathing. He states that:

Deep inspiration and expiration can appreciably alter the appearance of the individual electrocardiographic leads. With deep inspiration the heart position becomes more vertical and there is greater clockwise rotation. With deep expiration the heart becomes more horizontal and there is greater counterclockwise rotation. Variations in right and

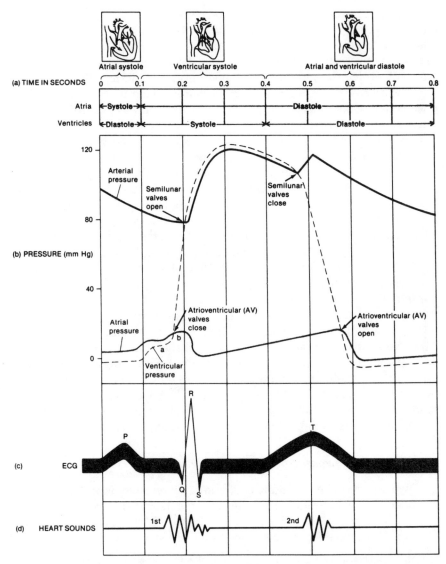

Figure 10. Cardiac cycle. (a) Systole and diastole of the atria and ventricles related to time. (b) Atrial, ventricular, and arterial pressure changes along with the opening and closing of valves during the cardiac cycle. (c) ECG related to the cardiac cycle. (d) Heart sounds related to the cardiac cycle. From G.G. Tortora and H.P. Anagnostakos (1984): *Principles of Anatomy and Physiology*, 4th ed. Cambridge: Harper & Row. Reprinted with permission.

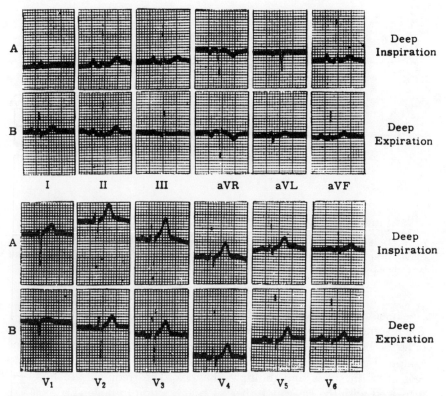

Figure 11. Effect of deep respiration on the electrocardiogram. (A) Deep inspiration. (B) Deep expiration. In deep inspiration the frontal heart position is vertical; this becomes semi-vertical in deep expiration. In the latter phase the voltage increases in I, V_4, V_5, and V_6 and decreases in aVF. From M. J. Goldman (1967): *Principles of Electrocardiography*. Los Altos: Lange Medical Publications. Reprinted with permission.

left heart stroke volume during inspiration and expiration also play a role in these electrocardiographic changes. (p. 80)

We used a capnometer, an ECG preamplifier, and an E & M Physiograph (polygraph) to produce the two traces in Figures 12 and 13, illustrating the rotation phenomenon during deep-diaphragmatic breathing: Figure 12 shows the ECG and capnometer trace in a 52-year-old man in treatment for mild anxiety, tension headaches, and moderate hypertension (inspiration is upward-excursion, expiration is downward-excursion). Figure 13 shows rotation in a 22-year-old woman treated for severe primary Raynaud's disease and colitis.

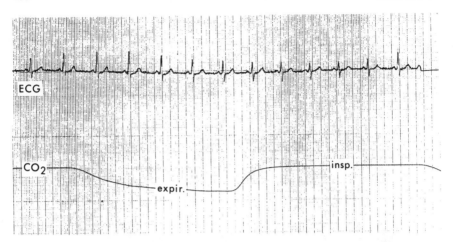

Figure 12. ECG "rotation" (upper trace) over the breathing cycle and ETCO$_2$ (lower trace), during deep-diaphragmatic breathing training in a 52-year-old man with mild anxiety, borderline hypertension, and headaches.

In some instances, a simple ECG such as lead-*I* is helpful, especially when someone with anxiety reports "skipped" heart beats. Typically she or he has been told, "It's anxiety . . . all in your mind." Figure 14 shows the "skipped beat" (ventricular premature contraction, VPC) in a 43-year-old woman with stress and multiple allergies. The frequency of her VPC increased with the severity of her allergic reaction to pollen.

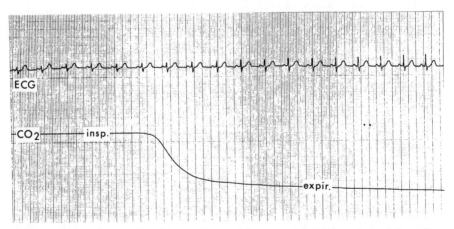

Figure 13. ECG rotation and ETCO$_2$ in a 22-year-old woman with anxiety, primary Raynaud's disease, and colitis, during deep-diaphragmatic breathing training.

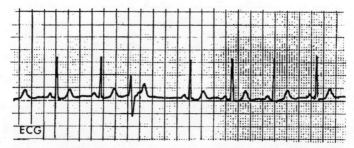

Figure 14. Cardiac ventricular premature contraction (vpc) in a 40-year-old woman with stress, panic, and "skipped beats."

Cardiac Interbeat Interval and the RSA

The heart is also innervated by the ANS which can accelerate or inhibit its action. This action together with cardiopulmonary reflexes may be observed in the time-distribution of pulses. Figure 9 shows an additional trace labelled heart rate (HR), obtained by placing the plethysmograph sensor (J & J PS-400) over the left index finger of the individual. The sensor is coupled to the J & J I-330 plethysmograph module (P-401). The P-401 module may be used to monitor heart rate on a beat-by-beat basis, blood volume pulse, and pulse waveform for instantaneous cardiovascular function monitoring.

The height of the HR trace in Figure 9 represents pulse rate based on interbeat interval (IBI). For a given rate, the IBI will have a given duration. If pulse rate is 60 beats per minute, the IBI will be about 1 second. Thus, a 1-second time interval between two consecutive pulses would indicate that the heart, if it were to continue at that IBI, would have a rate of 60 beats per minute. Rarely are IBIs exactly evenly paced. For instance, it is possible for pulse rate to average 60 per minute, with considerable IBI variation. That is exactly what is observed in all ECGs, but the IBI distribution will show predictable rhythmic variation in respiratory sinus arrhythmia (RSA).

Unfortunately, the term "arrhythmia" suggests that IBIs should be equal, and their inequality suggests pathology. Actually, the reverse is true (Hinkle, Carver, & Plakun, 1972; Hrushesky et al., 1984): We noted that in all cases where RSA reappeared with deep-diaphragmatic breathing training, mean pulse rate remained the same. Figure 9 shows what appears to be an increase in pulse rate coinciding with inspiration. But in Figure 15, RSA is considerably more profound and pronounced with deep-diaphragmatic breathing. You may note, again, that HR peaks appear to be a little ahead of inspiration. Earlier we cautioned you to control for delay in

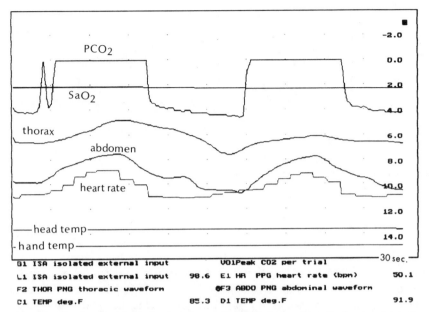

Figure 15. Psychophysiological respiration profile (PRP) during deep-diaphragmatic breathing, showing PETCO$_2$; SaO$_2$ (L1); thoracic (F2) and abdominal (F3) pneumograph; ECG tachometer (E1); and hand (C1) and scalp (D1) temperature.

transmission of end-tidal breath in the catheter to the capnometer. The timing virtually coincides with the pneumographic traces which now show breathing rate at 4 breaths per minute, and greater abdominal excursion, as compared to the thorax (chest). RSA is determined primarily by breathing frequency and pattern (Angelone & Coulter, 1964; de Boer, Karemaker, & Strackee, 1985; Grossman, 1991; Grossman, Karemaker, & Wieling, 1991; Hirsh & Bishop, 1981; Porges, McCabe, & Yongue, 1982; Sroufe, 1971).

Breathing and Thermal Monitoring

Since Taub & Emurian detailed it in 1976, it has been some time since anyone questioned the wisdom of controlling peripheral blood flow by self-regulation of skin (finger) temperature (King & Montgomery, 1980). But biofeedback techniques which rely on the conditioning of autonomic responses within what looks, at first blush, to be an operant paradigm often yield statistically significant, but unimpressive, changes unless they are accompanied by voluntary activities (King & Montgomery, 1981).

The idea of controlling circulation is hardly new. Olsten proposed the following in 1902:

> All will, no doubt, agree to the ability of the reflex action to influence the circulation in a part. But when the claim is made, as I unqualifiedly make it, that the conscious mind has the power to direct and control the cells of the spinal cord and cause them to carry out its dictates—thus controlling the caliber of any certain artery—objection is raised and doubts arise. (p. 146)

Clearly these persist since conditioning was chosen over voluntary control of peripheral circulation. Olsten continues:

> I treated a lady who was having trouble with the circulation of her lower limbs. She told me that she feared some calamity because her limbs were never warm and this caused her not only grave apprehension but considerable suffering.
>
> I gave her one treatment a day for about a week. The treatment consisted simply of telepathic suggestions to her subjective mind instructing it to open the arteries and give free and continuous circulation to the limbs. Before the week was past the circulation was continuous and it remained so. Another person was a great sufferer from pains in the back. He said it was always cold. In treating him I would simply put my hands upon his back and, coming into close rapport with his subjective mind, I trained the arteries to respond to the instructions so that his back would become warm from the increased circulation. I then trained him to do the same for himself; with the results that he could, by placing his hands upon his back and directing his attention for a few minutes to the desired results, cause the part to become warm and the pain to disappear. (pp. 148–149)

"Hypnosis!" you say? Well let's read on:

> I have a friend who can, by attention, rush the blood to his feet and warm them when they are cold. This is simply a matter of training. The subjective mind has the power to dilate the arteries to any part, or to contract them. The success of such efforts depends simply upon the obedience of the subjective mind. *That obedience is acquired by training.* (p. 149) (italics added).

You may call it autosuggestion, or self-hypnosis, but that does not explain the nature of the connection between "subjective mind" and vasomotor reflexes. I have used this method to treat chronic pain due to muscle and vascular damage in one case of ankle injury, in another where a back injury was sustained in an industrial accident, and in yet another where there was inflammation due to mandibular-joint arthritis (Fried, unpublished). Teaching the client to raise local temperature by focusing on breathing and imagining warming at the location increased local temperature and reduced pain.

Repeated multiple site thermal monitoring was accomplished with an optical infrared thermometer (Minolta/Land Infrared Thermometer; Model, Cyclops Compac 3). This is a small, hand-held device that permits temperature measurements at a distance from the surface or object being observed. In the case of the arthritic right jaw location, one looks through the instrument, locates the target on the face, presses a button, and a digital temperature readout is obtained within a fraction of a sec. Thus, hundreds of such measurements can rapidly be used to pinpoint hot or cold spots as locations of regional impaired blood flow, or sites of inflammation. Paradoxically, irrespective of whether the site is initially hot or cold, warming it reduces pain; and one of the fastest ways to warm hands, if not the fastest, is by deep-diaphragmatic breathing (Fried, 1987a; 1990a).

Typically, peripheral temperature is obtained with a thermistor attached to the surface of the skin—commonly the fleshy undersurface of the fifth finger (pinky) of the nondominant hand. Figure 15 shows two thermal traces. They have been set apart so that, were they to represent the same temperature, they would not be superimposed. Thus, location of head temperature above hand temperature does not, ipso facto, mean that that temperature is higher. The actual temperature (Fahrenheit) can be read as C1, hand-temperature, and D1, head-temperature. Hand temperature is standard in biofeedback, but head temperature is added to the profile for the two reasons indicated below.

Temperature at the Apex of the Head

Much is now known about the vasomotor mechanisms which control blood circulation in the head and in the limbs (Bazett, Love, Newton, Eisenberg, Day, & Forster, 1948; Blair, Glover, & Rodie, 1961; Donhoffer, Szegvari, Jarai, & Farkas, 1959; Folkow, 1955; Fox, Goldsmith, & Kidd, 1959, 1960, 1962; Froese & Burton, 1957; Gaskell, 1956; Hertzman, 1959; Hertzman & Roth, 1942), and these findings are also consistent with our observation that reducing hypocapnia in our clients increases hand temperature. But it would not be desirable to draw blood away from the head, inadvertently, when warming the hands. Therefore we included scalp-apex temperature in the profile.

How can we justify the belief that scalp temperature rises as brain-mass metabolism increases? How else can we explain it? There are no known constrictive vasomotor reflexes in the human forehead and scalp (Fox, Goldsmith, & Kidd, 1962; Hertzman & Roth, 1942; Royer, 1965), only dilatory. The reduced ANS activity of counter-arousal strategies could not induce scalp warming—and certainly not unilaterally. Thus, Zajonc's (Murphy, Zajonc, & Ingelhart, 1989) "facial efference theory" is without basis in physiology.

We have repeatedly observed differences between right and left scalp temperature that coincide with EEG. Just recently, in a 48-year-old woman with idiopathic left-side muscle weakness, scalp temperature was noted to be significantly lower on the contralateral side with diffuse elevated *theta*, while the left side was normal (Fried, unpublished).

Second, observing pulsatile variation in cerebral impedance (rheo-encephalography, REG) led Tachibana, Kuramoto, Inanaga, and Ikemi (1967) to report that:

> It was concluded from an analysis of simultaneous recordings of blood flow, tempera-ture, and EEG from the same hypothalamic site that the blood flow response to arousal coincides with the local temperature rise due to increased metabolic heat production and with the prior EEG activation . . . it seems highly likely that any sort of mental activity will elicit the characteristic (hypothalamic) blood flow increase, pre-sumably indicative of increased neuronal activity at the site. (p. 296)

These findings were replicated by Jacquy, Dekoninck, Piraux, Calay, Bacq, Levy, and Noel (1974), among others. The methodology is logical insofar as there is an illustrious previous history of the use of embedded thermocou-ples to measure regional blood flow which correlated it to EEG (Gerard, 1938; Schmidt & Hendrix, 1938). In fact, more recently, Sandman, O'Hal-loran, and Isenhart (1984) report that "Temporal similarities between response of the cerebral vasculature and the electrical response of the brain suggest common generating mechanisms," (p. 1357) in connection with a hypothetical cerebral vascular response.

It is not unreasonable to hypothesize that scalp temperature is a measure of local blood flow to the same degree that EEG spectral composi-tion correlates with it. Thus, it was empirically determined (Fried, in preparation) that when deep-diaphragmatic breathing rapidly raised hand temperature, the temperature at the scalp apex (paradoxically, we thought at first) rose as well. This was documented in the 1st and 4th weekly breathing training sessions in 7 clients with anxiety-related and psycho-physiological disorders. Both rose during biofeedback-assisted deep-diaphragmatic breathing training (using beach imagery), and also from session 1 to session 4 (see Figure 16).

On day 1 (A), hand temperature rose 4.8°F, from 87.06° to 91.86°F. Head temperature started out at 3.21°F above hand temperature (90.27°F), and rose 2.07°F. At the end of the training session, the difference between hand and head temperature decreased from 3.21°F to 0.48°F (ANOVA supports rejection of linear, parallel trends). On day 4 (B), hand tempera-ture rose 2.94°F, from 89.26°F to 92.2°F. Head temperature rose 1.18°F, from 90.59°F to 91.77°F. By the end of the training session, hand and head temperature, which were 1.33°F apart, were now 0.43°F apart (ANOVA supports nonrejection of linear trends). Hand temperature rose more than head temperature from the 1st to the 4th session, limited, as it were, by the Law of Initial Value (Wilder, 1959). Room temperature did not differ

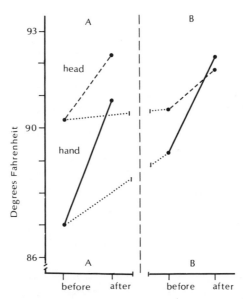

Figure 16. Average change in hand and scalp temperature in 4 subjects, before and after deep-diaphragmatic breathing training on the 1st and 4th days of training.

significantly between the 1st and 4th training sessions: it averaged 72.9°F (SD = 4.82°F), and 72.3°F.

In this type of clinical population, one often finds some degree of peripheral vasoconstriction, as evidenced by hand temperature in the 87°F region and, as relaxation with deep-diaphragmatic breathing progresses, vasodilation is suggested by an increase in hand temperature averaging about 4°F. This increase in hand temperature, accompanied by an increase in the temperature at the apex of the head, is evident from the very first breathing training session, and appears to be the beginning of an upward trend.

If the hypothesis that head-apex temperature reflects blood flow in the vascular bed of the brain is correct, then it follows that breathing training reduces cerebral vasoconstriction and increases brain blood flow, just as it seems to reduce peripheral vasoconstriction and increases peripheral blood flow in the hand. And, as previously shown (Blinn & Noell, 1949; Brill & Seidmann, 1942; Cobb, Sargant, & Schwab, 1938; Darrow & Graf, 1945; Davis & Wallace, 1942; Gibbs, Lennox, & Gibbs, 1940; Gibbs, Williams, & Gibbs, 1949; Gotoh, Meyer, & Takagi, 1965; Holmberg, 1953; Kooi, 1971; Lennox, Gibbs, & Gibbs, 1938; Liberson & Strauss, 1941; Meyer & Waltz, 1961; Morrice, 1956; Penfield & Jasper, 1954; Raichle, Posner, &

Plum, 1970; Robinson, 1944; Swanson, Stavney, & Plum, 1958; Tower, 1960; Whittier & Dhrymiotis, 1962), cerebral $PaCO_2$, SaO_2, and *theta* EEG intercorrelate.

One may reasonably conclude that a scalp thermistor can provide about the same information about local blood flow and metabolism as a set of EEG electrodes. Then again, we know this and that is why we use thermographs of the brain. Funny that no one thinks that *those* reflect the local scalp temperature.

For the present client population, there is a solid link between HV, common in anxiety, and cerebral vasoconstriction (Granholm, Lukjanova, & Siesjo, 1968). Meyer and Gotoh (1960) reported that HV produces rapid reduction in alveolar CO_2 in the first 5 to 10 breaths, and the resulting hypocapnia reduced cerebral arterial diameter by as much as 50%, with attendant EEG slowing. Darrow & Graf (1945), in mechanically hyperventilated cats, reported transient ischemia to have the appearance of "sausage links." Similarly, Penfield and Jasper (1954) referred to "blanching" of the ischemic arteries. If hypocapnia causes cerebral vasoconstriction and reduces blood flow to the brain, how could there not be lowering of brain temperature? By the same token, if breathing deepens, as these subjects shift to diaphragmatic breathing in the 3 to 5 b/min range, one would expect restoration of brain arterial caliber, increased blood flow as $PaCO_2$ normalizes, and increased brain temperature.

Based on these preliminary findings, we recommend adding head-apex temperature to the psychophysiological profile used in connection with assessment of status or change in status of peripheral and cerebral circulation as part of self-regulation and biofeedback procedures.

Monitoring Muscle Activity

Motion is an essential human function, accomplished by the action of muscles which are attached to the skeletal framework of the body. This action consists primarily of contraction and relaxation. Muscles have excitability, that is, they respond to stimulation by contracting. They can stretch (extensibility), and they can return to their original shape after contraction or extension (elasticity). This makes us move, maintain posture, and generate heat (Tortora & Anagnostakos, 1984).

Muscles are classified by location, structure, and source of control: Skeletal muscles are microscopically observed to be made of bands (striation), and respond to voluntary control. Visceral and arterial muscles are smooth, lacking the bandlike structure, and are typically not under voluntary control. Paradoxically, cardiac muscle is striated and involuntary.

In rehabilitation, we train striated muscle action by (a) self-regulation of impaired function or motility due to congenital or trauma-related muscle abnormality, damage, or atrophy leading to chronic or spasmodic contraction, and/or diminished capacity; and (b) tension and dysponesis.

Muscles may take the form of fiber aggregates as bundles, or as sheets (i.e., fascia). The superficial fascia are subcutaneous layers varying in thickness depending on their location, thick over the abdominal region and thin over the back of the hand. The deep fascia line the body wall and hold muscles together. Unlike the superficial fascia, the deep fascia do not contain fat. There is an additional type, the visceral fascia, which form part of the serous membranes of the viscera (Tortora & Anagnostakos, 1984).

Movement is produced when skeletal muscles exert force on tendons attached to bones. A muscle is typically attached to one bone, reaches beyond a joint, and is attached to the articulated bone. When contracting, it draws the articulated bone towards the one to which it is attached which, also typically, remains more or less stationary. Thus, the force of contraction, the degree of contraction or angular displacement of the articulation, and the amount of work the muscle can do (force exerted over time) can be monitored as mechanical events by an ergometer or other appropriate device. But under ordinary circumstances, muscles are also contracted to a degree even when they are not performing work. Muscles have piezo-electric property, that is, contraction results in biopotentials, so we record their tension as a function of their resting (micro-)voltage.

Muscles are constantly in motion. In respiratory alkalosis, and other clinical conditions, especially excess blood or tissue levels of calcium (hypercalcemia), or insufficient magnesium (hypomagnesemia), there will be a tendency toward tremors (i.e., latent tetany, or spasmophilia) (Altura & Altura, 1978; Durlach, 1969; Seelig, 1980). The findings of Kotowicz (1974), in connection with the observation of these bursts of electro-myographic activity (i.e., "latent tetany") are noteworthy: In 200 "neuro-tic" subjects, 187 of whom showed Chvostek's sign (of HV), 61% showed latent tetany, 38 out of 50 seizure sufferers showed Chvostek's sign, and 54% showed latent tetany.

The normal tonic activity of muscle, as well as latent tetany, may also be observed mechanically as minor tremor, or microvibration.

Microvibration (MVB)

Minor tremors, or microvibrations, are little known in the United States, though they have been investigated extensively in Germany and Japan. They may be, to a degree, normal tremors, or mechanical vibrations of muscles which range in amplitude predominantly between about 0.5 and 5.0 microns, and in frequency between about 5 and 20 Hz. They are typically observed with a variety of transducers, and are thought to originate in skeletal and smooth muscle vascular networks (Rohracher & Inanaga, 1969).

Their clinical correlates appear to be relevant to self-regulation and we strongly urge you to consider this modality on the basis of the interesting studies of MVB which have appeared in the past few years (Hosaka, Shirakura, Iga, Ohsuga, Noji, & Nezu, 1987; Jitsuiki & Bauer, 1973; Ozaki & Konda, 1968).

Rorhacher and Inanaga (1969) illustrate a number of means by which MVBs may be observed. Their "Abb.1" is reproduced below (see Figure 17). Figure 18 shows a piezoelectric transducer consisting of a modified crystal phono-cartridge, the needle of the cartridge replaced by a common pin which had a small spherical plastic head, a standard item in the "5 and 10¢ store." A plate electrode provides both a relatively stable base and reduces ambient electrical fields by grounding the skin surface in the vicinity of the transducer. The transducer may then be taped down or held by an elastic strap with the pinhead adjusted so it rests on the skin.

In Figure 19, the recording shown (made on a 54-year-old man at the upper surface of the left forearm, midway between the wrist and the elbow) shows the MVB baseline at rest. The frequency ranges between about 6 Hz and 7 Hz, and the waveforms do not appear to be sinusoidal. The second strip shows the effect on the left forearm of squeezing the right hand. Amplitude and frequency increase, and then return to a stable trace in 5 to 6 seconds. The third strip shows the effect on the left forearm of pulling the right ankle up and contracting the right calf muscle. The disruption of the trace is similar to that above, returning to baseline at about the same time.

The reported frequency composition of microvibrations is typically derived from the same electromagnetic pen recorded techniques usually restricted to frequencies below 50 Hz. There is, however, absolutely no evidence that this is their true upper limit. Ozaki and Konda (1968) report reaching equipment limit at about 1 KH. MVB have been studied in connection with examination stress (Bircher, Kohl, Nigg, & Koller, 1978), and microvibration biofeedback has been successfully applied to the reduction of functional tremors (Hosaka, Shirakura, Iga, Ohsuga, Noji, & Nezu, 1987). It is most likely related to arterial pulsation (Fried, 1989; Jitsuiki & Bauer, 1973).

Electromyography (EMG)

We believe that evolution shaped our genetic predisposition for certain individual and social behaviors by chance, but many of these evolutionary changes led to successful adaptations in our predecessors, who

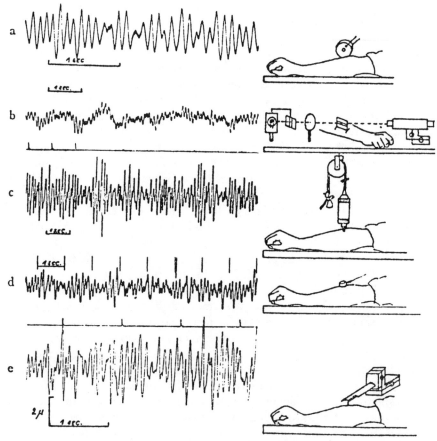

Figure 17. Methods for observing microvibration on the forearm by (a) induction; (b) split optical comparison; (c) Phillips motion detection; (d) Kohden piezoelectric transducer (Japan); and (e) H. Steinringer's strain gauge. Reprinted with permission from H. Rohracher and K. Inanaga (1969): *Die Mikrovibration*. Bern: Hans Huber. Reprinted with permission.

survived to become part of succeeding generations. Basic survival mechanisms, such as protection from threat or attack, or flight from danger are performed more or less automatically. In higher-order organisms, these "fight-or-flight" mechanisms are complex, stereotyped, and may comprise many interdependent internal activities.

But sometimes it may be more advantageous to neither flee nor fight. It may be better to hide, wait, and carefully assess the situation before deciding on a course of action. It is not clear whether this defensive-

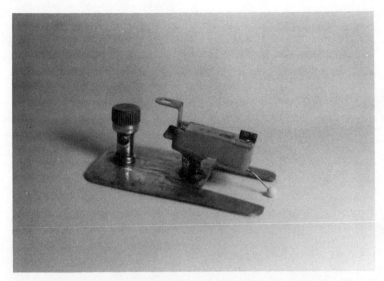

Figure 18. Phonograph crystal microvibration transducer: The phonograph "pickup" crystal is epoxied to a silver plated, slotted, "ground" electrode.

vigilant or freeze-vigilant condition is part of the "fight or flight," or a separate response (Miller, 1989; Thayer, 1989).

In fact, we now rarely fight or flee. Threats in modern society are more typically psychological than physical, and it is even frequently the case that action may be inappropriate or counterproductive. Therefore, we may be more likely to encounter inhibition of action than its overt expression. In the defensive-vigilant state, sensory, somatic, and motor functions are inhibited (Lacey, 1956; Lacey, Kagan, Lacey, & Moss, 1963). According to Thayer (1989), when we experience threat, we crouch and wait, making ourselves smaller, and moving so as to prevent detection. We may momentarily hold our breath, but then it becomes shallow and rapid at the same time that we prepare to act.

This positive adaptation to a threatening situation illustrates the link between patterns of muscle tension and HV. The breathing changes are, for the moment, biologically beneficial. Breath-holding is part of the somatic and motor inhibition which promotes heightened sensory awareness, and also conserves CO_2, favoring increased O_2 release to the tissues. HV in which excessive CO_2 is lost from the body leads to alkalosis, which favors reflex hyperexcitability, for quick reaction. The muscle tension which produces it prepares you for action. This muscle tensing, or "bracing," that is part of this defensive-alarm state is also advantageous in the

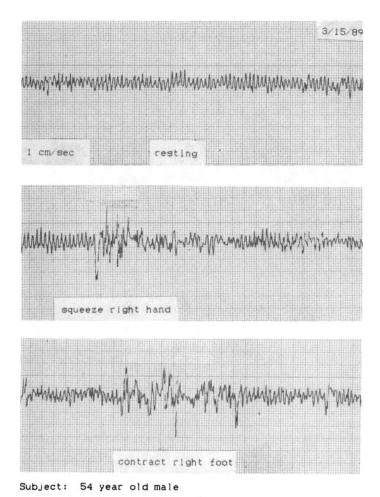

Figure 19. Microvibrations recorded from the left upper forearm using the crystal phonograph-pickup transducer mounted as shown in Figure 18.

short run in that it promotes a physiological shift towards sympathetic arousal (Gellhorn & Loofbourow, 1963). But that which is adaptive in the short run may be maladaptive in the long run: Frequent elicitation of this muscle bracing may lead to a chronic condition termed dysponesis by Whatmore and Kohli (1979).

Chronically elevated muscle tension has been causally implicated in a variety of disorders including muscle-contraction headaches, temporo-mandibular-joint disorder (TMJ), a wide variety of musculoskeletal pain syndromes, chronic anxiety, and panic disorder, to mention just a few. These and other conditions which we typically treat with counter arousal and biofeedback methods have been detailed elsewhere (Basmajian, 1989; Schwartz, 1987). We recommend these sources for more specific electro-myography techniques. Because of the physiological normalizing effects of deep-diaphragmatic breathing on blood circulation and on both smooth and striated muscle tone, breathing evaluation and training may be an important component of an integrated approach to EMG biofeedback procedures.

Electromyography is the observation and recording of the electrical activity that arises from muscle tissue. In some instances, that activity is the composite of resting potentials associated with muscle cell metabo-lism. In other cases, it is the piezoelectric output of contracting muscles at work. In EMG biofeedback, surface electrodes are placed over the skin, covering a targeted muscle mass to measure underlying electrobiopoten-tials thought to arise there. An analog of the amplitude changes of those biopotentials is displayed to the client as a visual or auditory cue.

Amplifiers with appropriate filters ensure that the cue is reasonably devoid of contaminating signals such as those that arise from the heart. The latter are commonly, though inexplicably, called "artifacts," inexplica-bly because, according to The New College Edition of *The American Heritage Dictionary*, artifacts are defined as, among other things "object(s) pro-duced or shaped by human workmanship; especially a simple tool, weapon, or ornament of archeological or historical interest." Maybe they mean "factitious."

Interpreting EMG signals is complex. It is difficult to isolate their exact source when obtained with surface-electrodes, as muscles are multi-layered and overlap, especially though not exclusively in the trunk. In some instances, it is justified to specify very exact electrode placement, but for generalized muscle-tension reduction, the most effective placements are those that include the largest muscle mass.

The two placements that we have found to be most clinically useful are those that involve (a) the head and face, especially the common frontalis placements; and (b) upper body musculature, by wrist-to-wrist electrodes. The frontalis placement consists of two active electrodes on the forehead, roughly one over each eyebrow, with a "ground" electrode between them (in line with the nose). This is adequate for collecting information about tension of the head muscles, especially the face. In the wrist-to-wrist configuration, one active electrode is placed on each wrist, and the ground electrode, wherever it is convenient, commonly on the wrist next to one of the active electrodes.

In a client resting quietly, this placement is useful for monitoring trunk musculature, especially the upper trunk; and it is extremely useful when working with clients who suffer back pain. Another option is the ankle-to-ankle placement; it targets the muscles of the lower body. But the head-and-face and the wrist-to-wrist placement are the two most useful placements in clinical practice involving counter-arousal and tension reduction.

When working with these two sites, you will quickly observe that they provide different but related information. Head EMG is very labile, easily disrupted, and difficult to control in clients with high stress levels. Those who are most able to quiet their thoughts may gain the greatest reduction in head and face muscle tension. This is most likely the case because facial muscles are intimately involved in expressing emotions (Zajonc, Murphy, & Inglehart, 1989).

In fact, they are very sensitive to thoughts that involve effort, even absent emotions and thoughts such as "What will I prepare for dinner?" or "I must remember to drop the clothes off at the cleaners." Some clients may show a differentiated response such as lowering of upper body tension without a concomitant change in head and face tension. But experience has taught us that those persons who are most successful at simultaneously lowering both achieve the deepest state of relaxation. The more the two systems appear coupled, the more readily generalized tension reduction is achieved.

Parameters of the EMG. Muscle electrobiopotentials appear to have most of their energy concentrated at frequencies ranging between 10 and 500 Hz (Basmajian & De Luca, 1985), with most of the activity, as observed in power-density curves, below 100 Hz. The majority of our skeletal muscle fibers are of the "slow-twitch," or slow-firing variety. Consequently, there is little justification for using a 100 to 200 Hz bandwidth filter.

Except in special circumstances, larger electrodes are preferable to smaller ones: This is particularly true if you follow our recommendation to use placements that sample activity from as large a mass of muscle as possible. The wrist-to-wrist placement which, for the most part, measures the electrical activity of the skeletal muscles of the trunk, will also include the electrical activity of the heart (ECG). The latter is extraneous to our effort to lower the activity level of the trunk muscles.

In a person at rest, heart electrical activity is stronger than that of other muscles and therefore the ECG waveform overrides the EMG signal, partially masking it, and making for a busy, difficult-to-interpret compo-

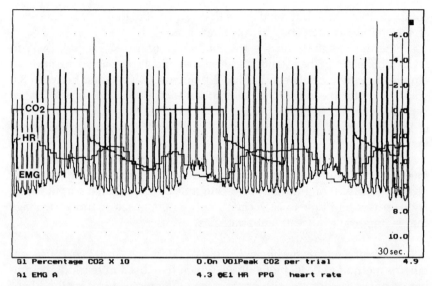

Figure 20. PETCO$_2$; ECG tachometer (HR) showing successive IBI; and unfiltered EMG showing the strong low-frequency cardiac signal. The EMG baseline voltage rises and falls with thoracic impedance: Decrease in thoracic impedance, as shown by rise in EMG baseline, corresponds to decreased pulse rate as shown by ECG tachometer (Hering-Breuer reflex).

site. Figure 20 shows a capnograph and ECG-tachometer (pulse rate) tracing with a superimposed unfiltered wrist-to-wrist EMG. Note that breathing rate is about 3 per minute, at 4.9% ETCO$_2$; RSA is prominent. The unfiltered EMG shows prominent elevations which correspond to the R-wave of the cardiac QRS-complex, in the lead-I configuration.

Unfiltered biopotentials obtained with wrist-to-wrist placement include arm, shoulder, neck, trunk, and cardiac muscle components. While the first four have relatively high frequency signals, the heart itself is basically an amplitude modulated signal with a frequency little above 1.0 per second, but with a voltage considerably greater than that of any of the others, in a person at rest.

The baseline voltage of this ECG/EMG is in step with both breathing and RSA. It rises with exhalation as the heart slows, and drops with inhalation as the heart accelerates. In fact, Pinciroli, Rossi, Vergani, Carnevali, Mantero, and Parigi (1986) have used the ECG to reconstruct the respiratory waveform (see also Grossman [1991]). These changes in baseline voltage have been calibrated to measure tidal volume, which varies linearly with thoracic impedance changes (plethysmography). So it makes little sense to refer to ECG in the EMG as "artefact." It is a proper component of EMG, but not the one that you wish to look at when looking at skeletal muscle tension, so you filter it out.

Filtering is simple on the J & J I-330 System (see Figure 21). With wide-filter setting, head-and-face EMG should be expected to have an amplitude ranging between 1.0 and 2.0 microvolts (uv), and between 8.0 and 10.0 uv for the wrist-to-wrist configuration in persons at rest. But in very tense clients, or in those with pain syndrome, head-and-face readings of 10.0 μv or more, and 40 μv or more for the wrist-to-wrist configuration, may be observed.

The meaning of intermediate EMG readings is unclear and cannot be interpreted as a precise quantity. But with successful training, one may observe a pattern of gradually lowering muscle biopotential amplitude. It is this pattern, unique to each client, rather than absolute (micro-)voltage that is important in treatment strategies.

Myofeedback with Breathing Exercises. Johnston and Lee (1976) detailed a method of EMG biofeedback which they used in teaching breathing exercises to patients with emphysema. Elements of this method have been applied with other client populations (see Chapter 9) because it tends to reduce the use of accessory muscles in breathing, a phenomenon typical in chest breathers. Persons with emphysema are said to have a low and flat diaphragm with limited excursion. The chest is relatively fixed in the inspiratory position, resulting in increased functional residual capacity

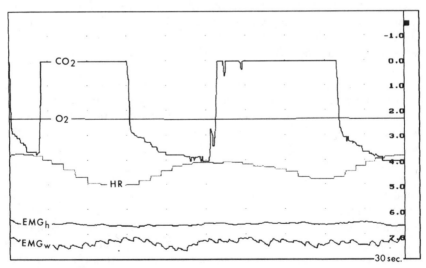

Figure 21. PETCO$_2$, SaO$_2$, heart rate, and filtered head and wrist-to-wrist EMGs.

(FRC), decreased expiratory capacity, and decreased pulmonary ventilation. According to Johnston and Lee:

> In an attempt to ventilate their lungs, the patients will frequently use accessory respiratory muscles, namely the scaleni, the pectoralis major, the shoulder girdle muscles, and the sternocleidomastoid muscles. Collectively, these muscles elevate the first two ribs and the sternum to produce an increased inspiratory volume. (p. 826)

In a sense, this action is similar, though to a somewhat lesser degree, in hyperventilators.

> Instead of attempting to improve pulmonary ventilation by increasing the patient's inspiratory capacity, Hofbauer, in 1925, introduced a breathing pattern designed to improve pulmonary ventilation by increasing the expiratory capacity. This breathing pattern involves an active contraction of the abdominal muscles during each expiration. . . . (p. 827)

This is, of course, deep-abdominal breathing. But the method is thought to be too difficult for these clients to execute.

Using audiofeedback, Johnston and Lee taught their patients to recognize and increase abdominal muscle activity. Three placements were used: (a) over the external oblique; (b) over the upper rectus abdominis; and (c) over the lower rectus abdominis. A ground electrode was placed over the sternum. In teaching the patients not to use accessory muscles, electrode placement was over the sternocleidomastoid, with instructions to reduce the feedback signal. Similar methods have been used in teaching breathing exercises to asthmatics (Peper, 1988) (see Chapter 9).

Electroencephalography (EEG)

A number of science fiction films dating from the late 1930s featured brains alleged to be alive, sitting, as it were, intubated in a saucepan or similar dish: A sort of sci-fi *cerveau isolé*. Just loved those films like *Donovan's Brain*. Sometimes, the brains were even alien, transported to earth and instructing their local agents in good or evil deeds. What struck me most about these representations was that the brains invariably pulsated, proof that they were alive.

Few of us realize that the brain does, in fact, pulsate, quite apart from arterial pulsations. Cooper, Moskalenko, and Walter (1964) contend that the phenomenon is due to "complicated hydrodynamic equilibrium." In other words, they don't know why it pulsates either. It is not the only thing about the brain that we don't understand.

We mentioned rheoencephalography (REG) in a previous section (Cowen, 1967, 1974, 1976; Cowen, Ross, & McDonald, 1967; Goldensohn,

Schoenfeld, & Hoefer, 1951; Jacquy, Piraux, Noel, & Henriet, 1973; Lechner, Geyer, Lugaresi, Martin, Lifshitz, & Markowich, 1969; Lugaresi & Coccagna, 1970; Waltz & Ray, 1967). Unlike EEG, which assumes that bioelectric brain phenomena are frequency modulated, REG looks at current changes in the brain, which are amplitude-modulated. What do we learn from this technique? First, the constant-current rheogram can be shown to reflect cross-sectional changes in the vascular bed of the brain, as well as the number of red blood cells per unit volume and their velocity, and therefore global brain blood flow. According to Lechner, Geyer, and Rodler (1967):

> . . . by including constant current rheography [one is in the position] to understand not only the arterial but also the capillary and venous participation in the blood flow. . . . The effect of CO_2 breathing on the cerebral circulation was demonstrated; in the rheogram an increase of blood flow, which has already been established by other methods, was also seen. The increase of blood flow showed itself in the classical rheogram in the well known way and in the constant current rheogram by a rise of baseline. (p. 85)

Parenthetically, studies of the transcephalic dc circuit by Cowen (1967) provide the only physiological correlate of yawning that we have ever encountered:

> . . . stimulation of those afferents which are mainly interoceptive (by deep inspiration, yawning, breath holding, and the Valsalva maneuver) promotes the predicted positive inhibitory frontal DC shift. . . . It does appear that voluntary respiration involves less cortical inhibition than does yawning. (p. 266)

So, the answer to the frequently asked "What is yawning?" may well be that it contributes to cortical excitation in attention homeostasis.

Jacquy, Dekoninck, Piraux, Calay, Bacq, Levy, and Noel (1974) reported that brain pulsations are independent of arterial circulatory pulsations since the latter did not cease with carotid ligation. But, as these authors noted, "respiratory artefacts make mandatory the use of an averager" (p. 510). In other words, breathing somehow ties in to brain pulsations, while heart-pulse does not seem to do so. Isn't that curious? What do you suppose the intervening variable(s) might be?

You are wondering, I suppose where this all leads. Here is the point: the fundamental frequency of the EEG is linearly related to $PACO_2$: (a) *theta* prevails during hypocapnia (low $PaCO_2$), and the fundamental frequency of the EEG rises toward *alpha* as $PaCO_2$ rises toward normocapnia (Lennox, Gibbs, & Gibbs, 1938) (see Chapter 3); (b) constant-current REG shows a linear baseline shift with brain blood flow and, therefore, metabolism; and (c) brain pulsations, which show idiosyncratic relationships to other body variables, seem to vary with breathing and oxygen availability (Cooper et al., 1964). Putting it all together, one might be tempted to conclude that in whatever tongue the brain speaks, it seems to make utterances about O_2 availability, blood flow, and metabolism.

The alternating cerebral dominance called the "ultradian rhythm," as evidenced by correlated EEG changes (Werntz, Bickford, Bloom, & Shannahoff-Khalsa, 1983), and in cerebral blood flow (Prohovnik & Risberg, 1979), is very closely tied to breathing, specifically to right/left dominance in nasal air flow. It has a periodicity estimated at 2 to 3 hrs in waking persons (Keuning, 1968), and is thought by Werntz et al. (1983) to be under the control of the autonomic nervous system. In fact, Werntz, Bickford, and Shannahoff-Khalsa (1987) demonstrated that "forced nostril breathing in one nostril produces a relative increase in EEG amplitude in the contralateral hemisphere" (p. 165). And they propose the method as a noninvasive means of treatment of "lateralized cerebral dysfunction."

It therefore follows that the EEG should be helpful in monitoring these variables which are breathing-related, in cases where cerebral brain blood flow and O_2 delivery may be suspected to be impaired. If so, the use of the EEG in clinical psychophysiology begins to make sense.

The EEG in Migraine

Many factors have been implicated in migraine, ranging from platelet aggregation to histamine and serotonin release, and so on. But, as Hanington (1982, 1987) pointed out, the final common pathway is hypoxia: Brain hypoxia typically results from cerebral vasoconstriction mediated by hypocapnia (low $PaCO_2$). That being the case, one would expect migraine to be accompanied by elevation in *theta*, typical in the EEG of a person with hypocapnia and hypoxia.

Figure 22, a typical average power spectrum, comes from Kooi (1971): Power decreases from dc (0 to 1 Hz) through *delta* and *theta*, then rises from about 7 Hz to about 11 Hz (*alpha*). It drops again to about 13 Hz and continues to decrease through *beta*—except for the elevation at about 20 Hz.

Figure 23 compares four individual EEG power spectra obtained by the methods described in Fried (1987a). There are 20 ordinates, beginning at 1Hz. The topmost is that of a normal 26-year-old woman, and is very similar to that in the EEG textbook of Kooi. The second is also from a normal, asymptomatic 34-year-old woman; but *alpha* is absent. The third is that of a 43-year-old woman suffering frequent grand mal seizures, and the fourth, that of a 38-year-old woman with frequent severe migraine. In both cases, there are significant elevations in *theta*.

Certainly this EEG pattern makes sense if one accepts the contention that both seizure disorder and migraine are vascular events related to

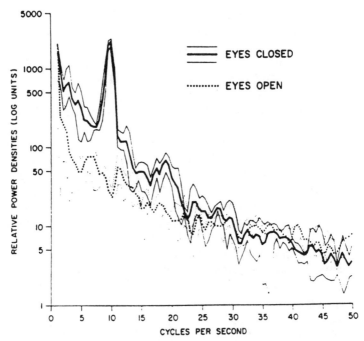

Figure 22. Reproduced with permission from K.A. Kooi (1971): *Fundamentals of Electroencephalography*. New York: Harper & Row, Fig. 5.1, p. 52. Reprinted with permission.

regional cerebral blood flow impaired by hypocapnia (Lauritzen, Olsen, Lassen, & Paulson, 1983), which has been consistently associated with an increase in EEG *theta*. Towle (1965), in fact, demonstrated increased *theta* production in migraine sufferers after 3 minutes of HV.

Barolin (1966), however, concluded that despite their interconnection, migraine and epilepsy were different entities, as did Gowers (1905) before him. However, Barolin reported that 50% of migraine sufferers showed an abnormal EEG, with focal signs in many instances. Weil (1962) noted that about 25% of his sample had "dysrhythmic EEG" sensitive to hypocapnia. Selby and Lance (1960) reported about 30% abnormal EEGs; Hoefer (1967), 52%; Goldensohn (1976), about 27%. Failure to make wider use of the EEG in migraine may perhaps be attributed to assertions such as those in the Summary by Townsend (1966):

> More abnormalities are observed to occur in the EEGs of sufferers from migraine than in the EEGs of comparable control populations. The difference, however, is *only statistically significant and is not of diagnostic importance.* (p. 20) (italics added)

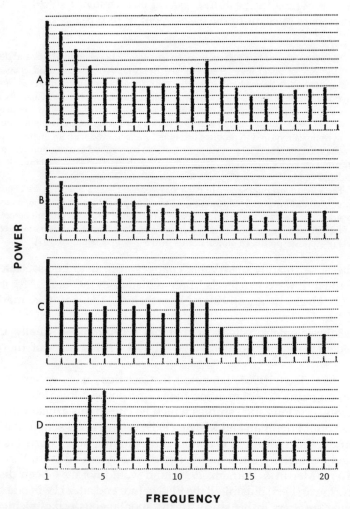

Figure 23. EEG power spectra (20 ordinates from 1.0 to 20.0 Hz) of four women: (a and b) asymptomatic normal EEG; (c) seizure sufferer with EEG power elevation at 6 Hz (*theta*); and (d), migraine sufferer with elevated *theta* (3, 4, 5, and 6 Hz, peaking at 5 Hz).

It boggles the mind. Parenthetically, Heyck (1969) reports 19% abnormal EEGs; Smyth and Winter (1964), 43%; and Hockaday (1978), from 62% to 71% in children, depending on the type of migraine.

Brewis writes in the *British Journal of Anaesthesia* (1969) in "Clinical measurements relevant to the assessment of hypoxia":

Cerebral Responses.

   The symptoms of hypoxia show much variation between individuals and depend upon the rate of onset and severity of the hypoxia. Age, disease and anaesthesia profoundly modify these changes, further reducing their reliability in the assessment of hypoxia. Restlessness, a sensation of faintness, pallor and sweating, usually occur below an arterial saturation of 75 percent and it is possible to demonstrate reduction in discriminative performance and learning ability (Ernsting, 1966). The minimum degree of hypoxia required to produce this effect was achieved with an inspired oxygen tension of 108 mm Hg (15.2 percent) calculated to correspond to a cerebral venous PO_2 of 32 mm Hg. Performance falls off rapidly below an inspired PO_2 of 70 mm Hg when calculated cerebral venous PO_2 falls between 21 and 23 mm Hg.

   The electroencephalogram (e.e.g.) has received some attention as a possible means of measuring and anticipating cerebral hypoxia. Ernsting (1966) noted the appearance of waves in the 18 to 16 c/s band where none had been present before to be the first sign of hypoxia. In his study hypoxia was always brief and the more profound levels of hypoxia produced slower waves in the 2–4n c/s band. (p. 747)

But, because "readily observable changes appear to be associated with dangerously low oxygen levels," Brewis dismisses the "e.e.g." for monitoring PO_2 levels in anesthesia. Nevertheless, the point is made here that brain O_2 levels are reflected in the EEG, a fact glaringly obvious to anesthesiologists, yet—with notable exceptions—virtually undocumented in neurophysiological and clinical EEG studies of the past 50 years.

In fact, Towle (1965) lamented the fact that "more recent studies of EEG in migraine do not mention the HV response." It is possible that the numerous previous such studies which he cites in his article were simply ignored after Friedman and Merritt (1959) categorically stated that HV did not produce significant EEG abnormalities in migraine. Merritt is usually credited with the clinical validation of phenytoin (dilantin) in seizure disorders (Merritt & Putnam, 1938), and would not have been dismissed lightly. Towle (1965) illustrated the EEG before and after HV in one of the 43 migraine sufferers in his study. In the spontaneous wake-tracings, there was little *theta* activity, while it predominated after 180 seconds of HV. This EEG activity was absent in the controls. In addition, the migraine sufferers showed much less dominant (defined as present in all leads) *alpha* in the wake state than did the controls. He concluded that:

   The lowered arterial CO_2 resulting from overbreathing may act on the cerebral vessels to produce vasoconstriction and decreased cerebral blood flow (Darrow & Graf, 1945;

Kety & Schmidt, 1946). This is apparently not a neurogenic autonomic effect, but a direct chemical vasomotor action (Schmidt, (1960). The resulting brain cell hypoxia would be responsible for the EEG changes. (Meyer & Gotoh, 1960)

It is noteworthy that he cites the same references for his conclusions as I usually do—EEG theta is caused by brain hypoxia resulting from cerebral ischemia induced by low arterial blood CO_2. Regrettably, I have never encountered a single instance when those opposed to these conclusions even knew of the existence of these studies. It is usually, "Can't be, it isn't proven."

A very strong link is forged in the report between EEG *theta* and reduced cerebral blood flow (CBF). Lauritzen, Olsen, Lassen, and Paulson (1983) further detail the relationship between CBF and CO_2. They report that regional CBF (rCBF) is reduced during HV-provoked migraine, first in the posterior part of the brain, then progressing anteriorly at a rate of 2 mm per minute. Their Table 1 and Table 2 are reproduced in Table 1.

After 1 minute of HV, mean $PaCO_2$ dropped 10.9 mm Hg (SD = 4.14 mm Hg). By comparison, administration of angiotensin 1 to induce hypertension resulted in a mean change of 0.5 mm Hg (SD = 1.38 mm Hg). They concluded that CBF was impaired by HV, that the impairment was localized to hypoperfused regions, and that the oligemia (blood volume deficiency) was due to a local phenomenon. They further stated that:

The relationship between CBF and $PaCO_2$ in the range of 20 to 55 mm Hg can be roughly described by two exponential functions, with a gradual decrease in slope taking place at $PaCO_2$ of 30 to 35 mm Hg . . . probably because of the imminent hypoxia produced by the dual action of low $PaCO_2$: vasoconstriction and decreased oxygen release to the tissue. The CO_2 reactivity of the oligemic region declined by close to half the value of the neighboring normally perfused brain, a reduction similar to the decreased reactivity obtained during hyperventilation below 30 mm Hg. (pp. 571–572)

I have often heard the naive argument that there is no way that breathing can effect such changes as would account for a shift in frequency from *alpha* to *theta*. It wasn't my idea after all, and the mechanism has been pretty well doped out.

How does this all fit together? The facts suggest that the abnormal EEG is coincident to migraine: Whatever causes migraine also causes this EEG phenomenon. And it should be pointed out that the observations are virtually identical to those in seizure disorders: HV causes cerebral arterial vasoconstriction and a left-shifted ODC promoting O_2 retention by Hb. Cerebral vascular ischemia causes regional oligemia and, potentiated by reduced O_2 availability, regional hypoxia. Since the vasoconstriction in migraine affects brain vessels as well as those external to the skull, why

Table 1. *The Effect of HV-Provoked Reduced CO_2 Level on rCBF in Migraine, Compared to the Effect of Angiotensin-1-Provoked Hypertension on rCBF.*

Regional Cerebral Blood Flow during Classic Migraine Attacks: Effect of Hyperventilation

Patient no.	$PaCO_2$ (mm Hg)			CPF in hypoperfused area (ml·100 gm^{-1}·min^{-1})					CBF in normally perfused area (ml·100 gm^{-1}·min^{-1})					Mean cerebral blood pressure (mm Hg)	
	Rest	Test	Change	Rest	Test	Change	k	Reactivity (%)	Rest	Test	Change	k	Reactivity (%)	Rest	Test
384	44	39	5	34	29	5	0.032	3.3	53	36	17	0.077	8.0	128	110
449	42	27	15	34	24	10	0.022	2.2	49	28	21	0.038	3.9	113	106
	41	27	14	35	23	12	0.030	3.0	49	25	24	0.048	4.9	113	119
450	42	34	8	37	28	9	0.035	3.6	56	34	22	0.062	6.4	113	120
452	38	26	12	34	26	8	0.022	2.2	55	27	26	0.056	5.8	88	100
457	40	25	15	33	20	13	0.033	3.4	56	24	32	0.056	5.8	20	100
470	46	39	7	30	28	2	0.001	1.0	50	37	13	0.043	4.4	110	110
Mean ± standard deviation			14 ± 1					2.7 ± 0.93					5.6 ± 1.37		

Regional Cerebral Blood Flow during Classic Migraine Attacks: Effect of Hypertension

Patient no.	Mean arterial blood pressure (mm Hg)			CBF in hypoperfused area (ml·100 gm⁻¹·min⁻¹)		CBF in normally perfused area (ml·100 gm⁻¹·min⁻¹)		PaCO$_2$ (mm Hg)	
	Rest	Test	Change	Rest	Test	Rest	Test	Rest	Test
384	128	140	12	34	34	53	51	45	44
449	113	142	29	39	34	55	49	44	41
450	113	150	37	35	36	51	54	43	43
452	88	111	23	37	40	58	64	37	37
457	100	125	25	33	35	55	56	40	40
470	105	135	30	30	38	50	54	46	47
Mean ± standard deviation			24 ± 7						

CBF = cerebral blood flow; PaCO$_2$ = arterial carbon dioxide tension; k = slope of the natural logarithm CBF: PaCO$_2$ relationship. From Lauritzen, Olsen, Lassen, and Paulson (1983): *Annals of Neurology*, 14:569–572. Reprinted with permission.

doesn't everybody so predisposed get both migraine and seizures? There is no ready answer to this question, but one may hypothesize the failure of a protective mechanism in seizure sufferers, GABAergic perhaps.

I recently submitted an article on EEG in migraine. The editors flatly refused it on the grounds that there is no firm evidence of the connection—numerous prior publications cited notwithstanding.

Michael and Williams (1962) noted 3 Hz to 6 Hz EEG activity in children with migraine and allergies, and medicated them with, among other things, antihistamine—histamine is a powerful vasoconstrictor. Chobot, Dundy, and Pacella (1950) even reported abnormal EEG in children with allergies who did not suffer migraine. They found a 33% higher incidence of abnormalities, typically bursts of slow waves (*theta*), in allergic versus nonallergic children. EEG abnormalities varied directly with duration of the allergic symptoms and were also apparent in family members of the children, as allergies are inherited. Abnormalities correlated with elevated blood histamine.

Many investigators, including Meyer, Hata, and Imai (1987) have reported the adverse effects of histamine on the vascular system; and histamine has been prominently implicated in migraine. Remarkably, Chobot et al. (1950) conclude that:

> We were unable, in any case except one, to alter the abnormal pattern by use of Trimeton. It is likely that the occurance [*sic*] of an abnormal pattern without any clinical allergic manifestation should be regarded in the same light as a positive skin reaction without clinical correlation. (p. 338)

This clearly contradicts Townsend (1966), cited earlier, where EEG abnormality is *prima facie* evidence despite the absence of clinical symptoms. Abnormal EEG patterns in adults and children with migraine were also reported by Brill and Seidmann (1942), and Jay (1982), providing good reasons for us to monitor the EEG (epilepsy is probably the least of them).

For instance, we can report having applied the same procedure as Fried et al. (1984a) and Fried (1987b) in monitoring EEG during self-regulation of PCO_2, by $PETCO_2$ biofeedback, to reduce putative hypoxia in 4 women ranging in age between 27 and 42. Symptoms included unilateral and bilateral moderate to severe head pain, varying degrees of gastritis, nausea, prodromal and other altered states of awareness; frequency ranged between "a few days just before my period," to daily. Figure 24 shows average EEG power spectral composition in these clients before 10 minutes of breathing training, and afterwards. Before training, *theta* was sharply elevated at 4 Hz and 6.8 Hz. Subsequently, mean *theta* dropped with an elevation at 7 Hz, and alpha is elevated from 8 Hz to 10 Hz.

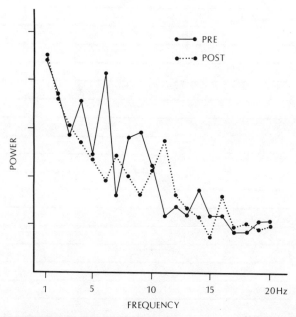

Figure 24. Average EEG power spectra in 4 migraine sufferers before 10 minutes of deep-diaphragmatic breathing training and after. Average pretraining spectrum shows marked *theta* elevation at 4 and 6 Hz. Posttraining shows a significant decrease in *theta* with a lesser elevation at 7 Hz.

Figure 25a shows the capnographs of a 34-year-old woman with tension, anxiety, nervousness, and mild depression, in addition to migraine. She reported unilateral head pain with mild gastritis and aura, four to five times per month. Her pretraining breathing rate was 18 b/min, with $PETCO_2 = 4.36$. Posttraining rate was 4.5 b/min, with $PETCO_2 = 5.32$. Figure 25b shows pretraining and posttraining EEG (left side). Pretraining shows *theta* elevation and no discernible *alpha*, while posttraining shows a considerable decrease in *theta* with a distinct, coherent *alpha*. Her migraine symptoms were reported to be less severe after breathing training.

Again, Figure 26a is the capnogram of a 42-year-old woman with migraine, depression, panic attacks, joint pain, and secondary Raynaud's disease. She reported pain, visual and smell auras, altered awareness, gastritis and nausea, virtually every day. Pretraining breathing rate was 16.5 b/min, $PETCO_2 = 4.25$. Postbreathing rate was 3 b/min, with $PETCO_2$ at 4.55, and diaphragmatic "flutter."

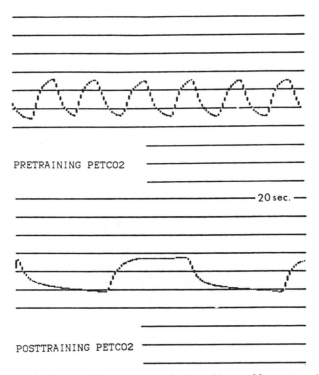

PRETRAINING PETCO2

POSTTRAINING PETCO2

Figure 25a. Pre- and posttraining capnographs in a 34-year-old woman with tension, anxiety, nervousness, depression, and migraine.

Figure 26b (bilateral EEG) has bilateral pretraining elevations in *theta*, peaking at 6 Hz, left side, and no discernible *alpha*. Posttraining EEG shows typical decreased *theta*, with a coherent bilateral *alpha* higher on the right than on the left side. Major reduction in head pain was reported to follow breathing training but lasted only briefly.

Before training, these two typical migraine sufferers had low $PETCO_2$, and abnormal elevated *theta*. Afterwards, $PETCO_2$ and EEG normalized, with a reduction in symptom severity. But, there is nothing published that reports a high incidence of dyspnea or spontaneous HV in this client population, though in our experience, it is a rare migraine sufferer who breathes normally. Furthermore, where deep-diaphragmatic breathing normalizes the EEG in migraine sufferers, the prognosis for symptom reduction in frequency and severity is excellent. Consequently, one may conclude that the only reliable diagnosis of migraine is the type of

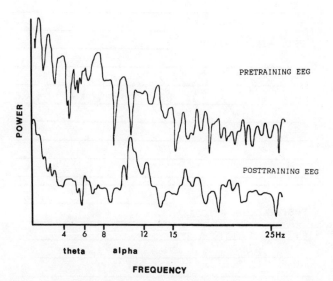

Figure 25b.   Pre- and posttraining left-sensorimotor EEG power spectra corresponding to the capnographs in Figure 25a. Average *theta* is markedly elevated pretraining, decreasing posttraining, with a distinctly elevated *alpha*. Posttraining EEG is normalized (see Figure 21, after Kooi).

EEG *theta* elevation described here. Where it is absent, the headaches are probably not due to migraine.

EEG in the Psychophysiological Profile

It would be extremely useful to include EEG power spectral composition in the psychophysiological respiration profile (PRP). However, certain aspects of these data make this unlikely in the near future. Brain biopotentials are continuous data distributions. By "freezing time," one can only record voltage as a discrete value at that point in time. To determine frequency requires an expanded point in time (a contradiction in terms). Thus, there is a critical resolution function for a given set of data (i.e., a minimum sampling time required to yield frequency). It so happens that EEG sampling time typically exceeds it, but it is nevertheless a small period.

In the case of the H-P spectrum analyzer (Fried, 1984, 1987), it is possible to update every 0.3 second. The computer can translate slope functions, do fast-Fourier analysis, and display its components about three times per second. Pretraining breathing rate may average 15 per minute in a typical client. With 200 possible updates, there would be about 13 per

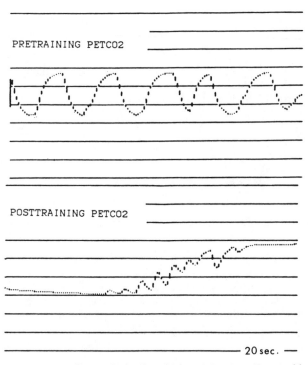

Figure 26a. Capnograph before and after breathing training in a 42-year-old woman with migraine, depression, panic attacks, and secondary Raynaud's disease. Note cardiac oscillations.

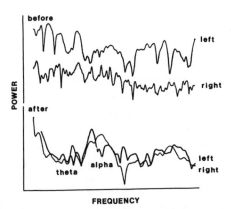

Figure 26b. Pre- and posttraining bilateral sensorimotor EEG power spectra corresponding to capnographs in Figure 26a. In pretraining, *theta* is elevated on both sides with baseline separation showing higher voltage (activity) on the left side. Posttraining shows "normalization" and reduced left hemisphere dominance with reduced *theta* and distinct elevated *alpha*.

breath, certainly enough to give you a picture of what's going on in the EEG during breathing. But to get more than a momentary picture, one may preset the H-P spectrum analyzer to average four consecutive 15 second samples. At 45+ seconds per average, there will be fewer than two samples per minute. That was the procedure used to obtain the previous, illustrative power-spectra.

Figure 4a (see Chapter 9) also illustrates the EEG and breathing pattern in migraine. Before training, this young woman showed an erratic capnograph, little RSA is evident, and the EEG had *theta* elevations at 5 Hz and 7Hz, with some *alpha* at 14 Hz. You may compare this to that of the control (Figure 4b, Chapter 9).

The J & J I-330 does not presently provide an EEG sufficiently rapid to be applicable in biofeedback. Consequently, we combined the PRP obtained with the J & J hardware and software, and the OxyCap 4700, with the H-P Spectrum Analyzer (3582A). Figure 27a shows breathing to be 6 per minute, $ETCO_2 = 3.7\%$, $SaO_2 = 97.4\%$, and PR = 89.3, with distinct RSA, in a 38-year-old woman with depression, headaches, thyroid insufficiency, and diffuse bilateral EEG abnormalities. Note in particular that hand temperature (C1) was 93.6°F, and head-apex temperature, 88.9°F.

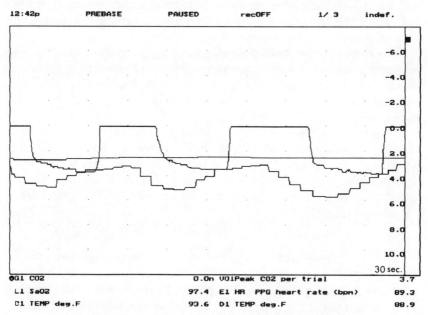

12:42p   PREBASE   PAUSED   recOFF   1/ 3   indef.

Figure 27a. Capnograph before breathing training.

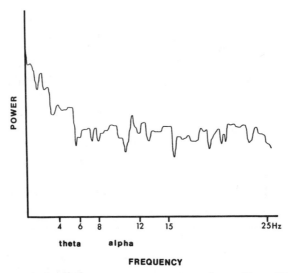

Figure 27b. EEG power spectrum corresponding to Figure 27a.

This is an unusual configuration. Typically, head temperature is higher than hand temperature no matter what the absolute values. The EEG obtained at the same time as the PRP shows much of the *theta* range elevated above *alpha* (see Figure 27b).

The third of three brief deep-diaphragmatic breathing training sessions over a period of about 20 minutes is shown in Figure 28a. Breathing is 5 per minute, $PCO_2 = 4.4\%$; SaO_2 decreased slightly to 96.4%, RSA is still prominent; and both hand and head temperature rose (94.7°F and 89.0°F, respectively). It might not be unreasonable to suspect that this client has some degree of ischemic impairment of cerebral blood flow, which would certainly account for her symptoms. Further tests may shed light on this hypothesis. But in keeping with a major theme in this book, deep-diaphragmatic breathing and consequent elevation of $ETCO_2$ were observed to result in decreased amplitude of the *theta* band to a level below that of *alpha* (Figure 28b).

Breathing and So-Called Alpha/Theta Training

There are recent studies which, it would seem paradoxically, emphasize increased rather than decreased *theta* amplitude, some during meditation (Ochs, 1992, personal communication), others featuring breathing similar to that described here and autogenic training. These are generally

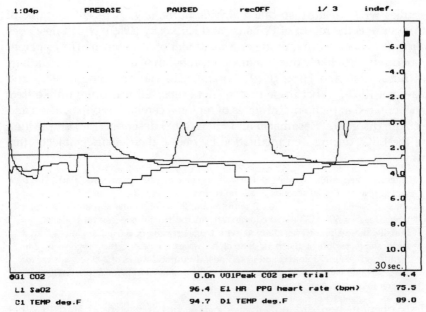

Figure 28a.   Capnograph after breathing training.

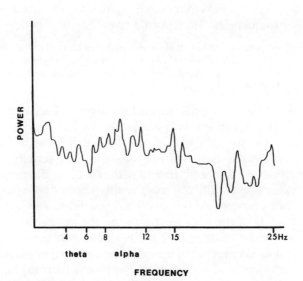

Figure 28b.   EEG power spectrum corresponding to Figure 28a. Note that as $PETCO_2$ rises, *theta* declines.

studies which feature so-called *alpha/theta training*. A recent example of this genre is the report of Peniston and Kulkosky (1989), which describes *alpha/theta* brain wave training as a treatment of alcoholism. The apparent paradox is most likely due to a misinterpretation of the pioneering findings of Kasamatsu and Hirai (1969), Anand, Chhina, and Singh (1961), and Banquet (1973). What these investigators reported was quite unlike *theta* encountered in pathological states of regional cerebral hypoperfusion and seizure disorders. Kasamatsu and Hirai (1969) described the composition of the EEG, during Zen meditation by one of their *disciple*-subjects, this way:

> After Zen meditation has started, the well-organized alpha waves of 40–50 uV., 11–12/ sec. appear within 50 seconds in all the regions and continue for several minutes in spite of opened eyes. . . . After 8 minutes and 20 seconds, the amplitude of alpha waves reaches 60 to 70 uV. predominantly in the frontal and central regions. . . . Initially, these alpha waves alternate with the short runs of activating pattern, but a fairly stable period of the persistent alpha waves ensues on the progress of Zen meditation. After 27 minutes and 10 seconds, rhythmical waves of 7–8/sec. appear for 1 or 2 seconds. . . . And 20 seconds later, rhythmical theta train (6–7/sec., 70–100 uV.) begins to appear. (pp. 209–210)

This phenomenon did not always occur, but it was replicated in other disciples during meditation. This *theta* is clearly unlike that evident in most pathological states which they studied, including anoxia, epileptic seizures, and other neurophysiological disorders, and they show in detail that it is also unlike that in sleep, and in hypnosis. Banquet (1973), in a spectral analysis of the EEG in meditation, likewise observed a shift from *alpha* to lower frequencies. He reported that:

> A dominant theta pattern (unlike that of drowsiness) was observed in the second stage of meditation. Within 5–20 min after the beginning of meditation short bursts of high voltage (up to 100 uV) theta frequency at 5–7c/sec occurred during 1 or 2 sec, simultaneous in all channels. . . . (p. 146)

Here again, so far as can be determined, *theta* did not accompany a brain pathological state. In concert with our thesis, the EEG frequency spectral composition in the subjects who showed elevated *theta* (in the Banquet study) had very rapid transient high voltage *theta* activity, sometimes singly, sometimes in rhythmic trains, within an overall attenuated *theta* band. This cannot be readily observed without online *fast-Fourier analysis* (FFA) capability. There would be no way to know what is happening in the different segments of the EEG frequency spectrum.

There is a world of difference between elevated *theta*, which corresponds to decreased brain blood flow and metabolism, as previously cited studies have shown, and a decreased *theta*-band with rapid, transient, high-voltage *theta* activity, which occurs in deep meditation. We raise this issue here to alert you to the difference between these two distinct types of *theta* phenomena in diagnosis, and in so-called *alpha-theta* training, gaining popularity in the treatment of such disorders as attention-deficit hyperactivity disorder (ADHD) (Lubar, 1991), and substance abuse (Peniston & Kulkosky, 1989).

We have no quarrel with the outcome of the study by Peniston and Kulkosky (1989). Although we would find it difficult to replicate it from their *method* section, their conclusions are not startling. Several factors come to mind. First, alcohol addicts were shown to have cerebrospinal fluid *beta*-endorphin levels threefold lower than nonalcoholic controls (Genazzani, Nappi, Fachinetti, Mazzella, Parrini, Sinforiani, Petraglia, & Savoldi, 1982). Second, consumption of alcohol raises *beta*-endorphin levels (Triana, Frances, & Stokes, 1980). Third, in men at risk for alcoholism, consuming alcohol decreases mean *alpha* frequency (Pollock, Volavka, Goodwin, Mednick, Gabrielli, Knop, & Schulsinger, 1983). And fourth, the endorphin antagonist, naltrexone, was recently shown to significantly reduce alcohol craving (Volpicelli, Alterman, Hayashida, & O'Brien, 1992). Taken together, these facts tell us that in alcoholics, both *beta*-endorphin levels and EEG *alpha* voltage are low. Drinking alcohol raises *beta*-endorphin level, but does not increase EEG *alpha* production. Training alcoholics to increase *alpha* production, especially since that procedure also increases *beta*-endorphin levels, may, therefore, logically be thought to contribute to reduced craving for alcohol. In other words, alcohol and opiates must, at the very least, share binding sites. No wonder administration of endorphin antagonist reduces the drive to drink alcohol.

But there is a twist to the story. According to Peniston and Kulkosky (1989), the subjects were given temperature biofeedback-assisted autogenic training, "and rhythmic breathing techniques in an effort to induce relaxation of the body and quiet the mind" (p. 273). The subjects were taught meditation! No wonder they produced the EEG patterns typical of that state. So far so good, but then the authors speculate that temperature training (of the dominant hand and foot) to 95°F "stimulates the production of the '*theta*' state" (p. 273). And here is where we find the source of the confusion: Which kind of *theta* does the training promote? Clearly Peniston and Kulkosky did not know that this question needs to be asked, and so their instrumentation—band-pass filters—was not designed to differentiate between kinds of *theta*. This mutation has, unfortunately, been inherited by their followers.

Why is it critical to differentiate? Lou, Henriksen, and Bruhn (1984), using the three-dimensional PET scanning technique, found regions of hypoperfusion in the white matter of the frontal cortex of the brain in 11 children with ADHD. Seven of these children also had hypoperfusion in the caudate nuclei. They also found regional cerebral hypoperfusion in children with dysphasia.

It must be considered risky to teach someone to increase *theta*, where *theta* might signal cerebral vasoconstriction and hypoperfusion. It would certainly seem imprudent to do so where, the literature tells us, hypoperfusion has been well documented. It is clearly naive to treat *theta* as though it were a singular event, and just another operant in the black box.

Chapter 6

Some Functional Relationships between Hyperventilation and the Endocrine, Cardiovascular, and Nervous Systems

Introduction

Regardless of specific cause, the effects of disordered breathing typically encountered in behavioral physiology are those of hyperventilation: hypocapnia, low alveolar CO_2 (PCO_2); hypocarbia, low arterial blood CO_2 ($PaCO_2$); and compensated alkalosis. These are integral to psychophysiological, emotional, and affective disorders because they adversely affect cell metabolism and function through a common final pathway: hypoxia (Fried, 1993a).

Homeostasis is energy costly and given the proper mix of circumstances, and individual predisposition, leads to stress and symptoms. HV, and systemic and cerebral physiology, impact on each other in numerous ways, many beyond the scope of this book, but all are known to affect the endocrine system, the heart, the peripheral and central nervous systems, the muscles, and the sensory organs.

Therefore those salient features are chosen which best help to explain the physiological basis for some of the more commonly encountered clinical problems.

HV affects all cell functions and metabolism, hemodynamics, the O_2 and CO_2 transport system, and muscles and nerves. It affects physiological "body economy" (Lum, 1978–79). Consequently, this chapter focuses on those aspects of HV in the endocrine system, the cardiovascular system, the heart, and the nervous system, which may have clinical significance to the practitioner; she or he is likely to encounter these aspects in persons whose symptoms are either caused by or aggravated by HV and/or dyspnea.

The Effect of Female Gonadal Hormones on Breathing

A decrease in alveolar PCO_2 during the luteal phase of the menstrual cycle has been reported. The average drop in PCO_2 is 8 torr (England & Farki, 1976), representing a decrease of about 25%. It could raise blood pH by about 0.1. Typically it does not, because of compensation by the kidneys. In fact, it was shown that the changes in base excess parallel those in PCO_2 with no detectable phase difference between the two over the course of their study. Figure 1 shows the chronological relationship between hypothalamus and pituitary hormone production, change in blood levels of estrogen and progesterone, and the menstrual cycle. Figure 2 illustrates the relative blood concentrations of principal reproductive hormones.

England and Farki (1976) conclude that compensation is so complete that they cannot determine with any degree of certainty whether the disturbance is primarily metabolic or respiratory. They propose, however, that it is more likely that the effects of progesterone are respiratory because (a) $PaCO_2$ is at its lowest level in the cycle when blood progesterone is at its peak; (b) a significantly decreased $PaCO_2$ is found in pregnant women; and (c) administration of progesterone to men or women lowers PCO_2 (alveolar). The decrease in PCO_2 and base excess is considerable.

On the other hand, Damas-Mora, Davies, Taylor, and Jenner (1980) contend that progesterone leads to primary metabolic acidosis, compensated by HV. Taking this one step further, Gault (1969) stated emphatically that "all pregnant women hyperventilate" (p. 1067); and, considering the current controversy over the extent of a "premenstrual syndrome," Damas-Mora et al. (1980) state that:

> Increased ventilation has consistently been found in the luteal phase of the menstrual cycle in normal women. Our results, similar to many others, show that carbon dioxide concentration starts to decrease early in the luteal phase and the lowest values are premenstrual.
>
> These findings suggest that women are more vulnerable to psychosomatic symptoms during the premenstrual phase, when stress would increase ventilation at a time when carbon dioxide levels are already low. (p. 495)

They further report that the CNS sensitivity increase noted before and during menstruation has implications for the interpretation of the EEG,

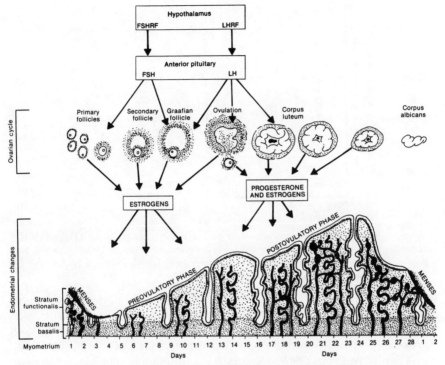

Figure 1. Correlation of menstrual and ovarian cycles with the hypothalamic and anterior pituitary gland hormones. In the cycle shown, fertilization and implantation have not occurred. Adapted with permission from G.G. Tortora and H.P. Anagnostakos (1984): *Principles of Anatomy and Physiology.* New York: Harper & Row, Fig. 28-16, p. 716.

particularly since HV is an integral procedure in electroencephalography. In those of my clients who show EEG low-frequency, high-voltage activity (*theta*), I have observed an increase in that activity when their blood progesterone levels would be expected to be highest.

   In another study of women with normal menstrual cycles, it was shown that reproductive hormones act directly on the respiratory system to cause HV (Goodland & Pommerenke, 1952; Goodland et al., 1953) and to promote low frequency EEG activity (Cogen & Zimmermann, 1979; Damas-Mora et al., 1980). They found that PCO_2 varies within the menstrual cycle: CO_2 rises from onset of menstruation to ovulation; it then decreases until the next menstruation. And they reported the effects of the injection of progesterone and estradiol as compared to a control substance, using adult men as subjects. The control substance produced no significant physiological effect, but progesterone significantly increased basal body temperature and decreased alveolar PCO_2. It also produced a

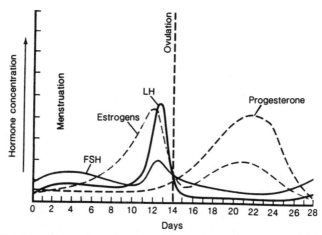

Figure 2. Relative concentrations of anterior pituitary hormones (FSH and LH) and ovarian hormones (estrogens and progesterone) during a normal menstrual cycle. Adapted with permission from G.G. Tortora and H.P. Anagnostakos (1984): *Principles of Anatomy and Physiology.* New York: Harper & Row, Fig. 26-17, p. 717.

somewhat variable increase in metabolism. Two successive daily injections of estradiol benzoate lowered the alveolar PCO_2. Administration of both progesterone and estradiol prolonged the suppression of alveolar PCO_2.

Similarly, Lyons (1969) showed that administration of progesterone to women lowers alveolar CO_2 tension and is probably responsible for the same effect during pregnancy and the luteal phase of the menstrual cycle. Progesterone appears to increase minute ventilation (Vmin) and raises the sensitivity of the CO_2 respiratory brain centers. Progesterone is a respiratory stimulant and acts differently on respiration than does estrogen; estrogen has a catabolic action and raises respiration by increasing metabolism. When women clients show an unusual increase in breathing rate over the course of training, it is probably a good idea to determine which phase of their menstrual cycle prevails before assuming that the change is mental.

Increase in basal body temperature, shown to accompany increased blood levels of progesterone, should not be discounted either. Increased temperature also contributes to an unfavorable left-shift of the O_2 dissociation curve (ODC) affecting tissue O_2 availability.

Hyperventilation and the Cardiovascular System

Breathing rate and rhythm are intimately involved in cardiovascular dynamics. They affect blood pressure, heart rate, and stroke volume (Bell,

Davidson, & Scarborough, 1968). Breathing also affects the cyclical pattern and distribution of heart rate—the so-called respiratory sinus arrhythmia (RSA) (Porges, McCabe, & Yongue, 1982). Each active inspiration increases venous return to the heart (Grossman, 1983), and cardiac output is altered by changes in heart rate and stroke volume related to breathing rhythm.

HV may result in vasodilation in the forearm (Roddie, Sheperd, & Whelan, 1957) and in a change in venous tone (Browse & Hardwick, 1969). It is thought that the afferent source of the venomotor reflex is the chest wall of the diaphragm, and there is also a reverse effect of change in vasotone on breathing. Painful unanesthetized arterial puncture has been noted to produce transient HV. However, Morgan et al. (1979) showed that this transient HV may have little effect on the accuracy of measurement of resting values of arterial pH and PCO_2.

Hyperventilation and Blood Pressure

Predictable variations in arterial blood pressure accompany breathing (Bell, Davidson, & Scarborough, 1968). They depend on respiration rate. When breathing is within normal range (see Chapter 1), blood pressure falls during most of inspiration. But when it is low, inspiration is accompanied by a small rise in blood pressure.

During HV, blood flow to the forearm and the large muscle groups is increased and blood flow to the intestines, brain, hands, and feet is decreased (Burnum, Hickam, & McIntosh, 1954; Harris & Heath, 1962; Pollack et al., 1964; Richardson, Wasserman, & Patterson, 1961). Conversely, systemic blood pressure affects breathing. Cerebral blood flow varies directly with systemic blood pressure and, within limits, respiration rate varies inversely with cerebral blood flow (Schmidt, 1928).

The relationship between blood pressure and breathing is well known. L.G. Tirala (professor of medicine, University of Munich) published *The Cure of High Blood Pressure by Respiratory Exercises*, circa 1935. Though this book is out of date, the concept merits consideration. I have frequently observed a dramatic decrease in systemic blood pressure in clients undergoing breathing training, and have made it a practice to make sure that they do not have hypotension before training begins. The decrease in blood pressure with slow, diaphragmatic breathing may be due to hypoarousal which this type of breathing tends to promote.

It is an apparent paradox that HV may also cause some persons to experience a sudden dramatic decrease in blood pressure. In these persons, this drop in blood pressure may cause syncope, or fainting. In some instances, this syncopal attack may be mistaken for an epileptic seizure (Lechtenberg, 1982; Riley, 1982).

Hyperventilation and Syncope

In vaso[de]pressor syncope, falling arterial blood pressure leads to unconsciousness accompanied by large high-voltage *theta* EEG activity (Engel, Romano, & McLin, 1944). This type of syncope may, also be caused by sudden, or strong, vaginal distention.

Vasopressor syncope is very similar to HV-syncope because hypocapnia has a vasoconstrictive effect. In fact, falling blood pressure and alveolar PCO_2 resulting from the breathing training alluded to above are not to be taken as evidence of HV. When the respiration rate is in the three-to-five b/min range (Fried, 1990b), $PETCO_2$ a little over 4.5 is not unexpected. This is more likely to be hypometabolism than hypocapnia. Thus, slow, rhythmic, diaphragmatic breathing may result in lowered blood pressure close to that observed in syncope, but the tell-tale sign of impending syncope is the predominance of high-voltage *theta* waves in the EEG, whereas in breathing training, *alpha* predominates.

I have observed this phenomenon in persons with a tendency toward metabolic insufficiency due to organic conditions such as thyroid deficiency. Thus, it is useful in monitoring blood pressure changes in persons undergoing breathing training, as well as monitoring the EEG.

According to Lechtenberg (1982), most persons with syncope do not suffer from cardiovascular problems. Their fainting spells are due principally to HV. But the precise mechanism by which HV causes syncope is not understood. It is variously attributed to hypocapnia or alkalosis (Lowry, 1967). But loss of consciousness is ultimately due to cerebral anoxia when cerebral blood flow drops. Raichle and Plum (1972) reported a *2% decline in CBF with every 1-torr decline in $PaCO_2$!*

There is a markedly similar change in EEG in HV and in orthostatic (postural change) hypotension-induced syncope, with the EEG showing elevated mean *theta* (attributed to anoxia and not to any epileptic or preepileptic condition [Brill & Seidmann, 1942; Withrow, 1972]).

The Effect of Hyperventilation on the Heart

There is a tendency by many (though usually not the client) to dismiss chest symptoms, and sometimes pain, as neurotic, anxious, or otherwise psychosomatic evidence of irrational oversensitivity and worry. But the effects of HV on the heart are real, and have been thoroughly documented. Missri and Alexander (1978) reported the following: reduction in myocardial oxygen supply; ECG changes unrelated to hemodynamics; depression of the S-T segment; flattening and inversion of the T wave; sinus tachycardia; increased cardiac output; and increased heart rate. Impairment of myocardial O_2 supply has also been described by Neill and Hattenhauer (1975) who concluded that HV increased $PaCO_2$ and OHb affinity (the Bohr effect) in proportion to the degree of alkalosis. With a higher pH in systemic capillaries, OHb dissociation will lower PO_2, resulting in a decrease in capillary blood PO_2, which may impair diffusion into the tissues. With respect to the heart, they caution that:

> In the coronary circulation, where vasomotor regulation is influenced prominently by the needs of the myocardium for O_2, decreased capillary blood PO_2 might be expected to result in compensatory vasodilation and increased coronary blood flow, as in anemia. Hypocapnic alkalosis, however, increases vascular resistance and decreases blood flow in some tissues. Voluntary hyperventilation has been reported to increase resistance, decrease blood flow and lower venous concentration in the normal coronary circulation of human subjects. If increased blood affinity and coronary vasoconstriction also occur in patients with ischemic coronary heart disease, voluntary hyperventilation might result in myocardial hypoxia. (p. 854)

Certainly, this may be taken as another good reason for not using the HV-challenge without a careful consideration of the physical condition of the client.

A number of investigators have also described the chest pain that accompanies HV and have attributed it either to the heart (pseudoangina) (Evans & Lum, 1981), or to the chest wall. Wheatley (1975) described chest pain as consisting of three distinct types:

> (1) Sharp, fleeting, periodic, originating in the anterior left chest, radiating into the neck, left scapula and along the inferior rib margins. Intensity is increased by deep breathing, twisting and bending.
> (2) Persistent, localized aching discomfort, usually under the left breast (lasting for hours or even for days, not varying in intensity with activity or motion of the chest wall). Chest wall is tender at the site of the pain (a local anesthetic provides relief).
> (3) Diffuse, dull, aching, heavy pressure sensation over the entire precordium or substernum which does not vary with respiration or activity (may last for minutes or days and is often confused with angina). (p. 197)

The role of HV in cardiovascular function has also been detailed by Freeman and Nixon (1985); and by Nixon (1989), who alerts us to the fact that:

> Hyperventilation should be considered in effort syndrome, DeCosta's syndrome, mitral prolapse, anxiety states, panic attacks, phobias, burnout, and posttraumatic stress disorders, and among patients "who have never been the same" since an event or accident "changed the course of their lives." (p. 80)

He asserts that HV associated with a high arousal state is probably the major cause of angina pectoris, myocardial ischemia (i.e., reduced blood flow to the heart due to constriction of coronary arteries and their branches), and infarction. He also implicates sudden coronary death, in the absence of an atheromatous element or its presence in a degree too slight to contribute to mortality. Nixon (1989) implicates a number of other conditions with HV:

- chest pain with loss of capacity for sustained effort;
- chest pain with ECG irregularities, including supraventricular tachycardia, with normal conducting system;
- Wolff-Parkinson-White Syndrome; Rosenbaum's right ventricular ectopy;
- arterial constriction: Raynaud's or arterial insufficiency of the foot. (p. 81)

He further cautions that one consider "wakening at 3 or 4 A.M. with angina pectoris as part of the chronic hyperventilation syndrome in person with organic coronary disease."

Numerous clinicians have also reported a connection between HV, pseudoangina (Prinzmetal's form of variant angina), and vasospastic phenomena, which they attribute to HV-induced ischemia and hypoxia in myocardial tissues (Miller et al., 1981; Yasue et al., 1978). Parade (1966) stated that the precipitation of angina pectoris-like symptoms is HV, while Levine (1978) referred to the cardiac manifestations of the HVS as "mimics of coronary heart disease." He reported that there is an accompanying "air hunger, light-headedness, paresthesia, syncope and atypical chest pain."

Evans and Lum (1981) also reported that HV may be a cause of chest pain mimicking angina. They showed that typical physical examination may reveal little about the cause of the presenting symptoms, that examination of the breathing usually shows exaggerated thoracic movement, and that abdominal breathing is rarely encountered in such patients. They attributed the symptoms to "lability of $PaCO_2$" (i.e., CO_2 sensitivity), rather than to hypocapnia. (More about CO_2 sensitivity later.) Arrhythmias, especially sinus tachycardia, have also been noted frequently in the HVS.

Hyperventilation and the Electrocardiograph. Christensen (1946) produced distinct electrocardiographic signs of myocardial hypoxemia in normal men during voluntary HV. These included sinus tachycardia, a slight reduction in conduction time, uncharacteristic changes in the height of the R wave, depression of the S-T segment, and inverted T waves. Such signs have also been reported by Gardin et al. (1980); Lum (1976); Thompson (1943); Wildenthal, Fuller, and Shapiro (1968); Yu and Yim (1958); and Yu, Yim, and Stansfield (1959). In the Christensen study, these signs disappeared rapidly after ending voluntary HV. Nevertheless, he cautions that "these electro-cardiographic changes are highly indicative of coronary insufficiency" (p. 884).

Lawson, Butler, and Ray (1973) concluded that:

- development of arrhythmias in the presence of alkalosis is independent of preexisting heart disease;
- heart disease patients on digitalis are more susceptible to alkalosis induced arrhythmias;

- blood pH at onset of arrhythmia (in their study) was elevated above 7.55 and sometimes reached 7.6 or more;
- restoration of normal rhythm invariably occurred at a pH below that at which arrhythmias occurred;
- arrythmias, principally consisting of *escape* mechanisms were "singularly refractory" to customary therapy;
- all patients (in their study) responded well to alteration of ventilation which restored normal $PaCO_2$ and pH;
- prevention and treatment is well served by "the control and proper management of ventilation." (p. 961)

They conclude with the warning: "Perhaps the major hazard of alkalosis is that it invites iatrogenic disease. . . . The persistent use of conventional methods of therapy on these refractory arrhythmias may be harmful."

Thompson (1943) also concluded that alkalosis is etiological in cardiac arrhythmias. He reports that:

> . . . patients with anxiety neuroses and the hyperventilation syndrome frequently exhibit marked electrocardiographic abnormalities. . . . The abnormalities disappear when recovery from the syndrome takes place, but may be reproduced by voluntary hyperventilation if recovery has not been too firmly established. (p. 389)

The $PaCO_2$ lability factor reported by Evans and Lum (1981) is corroborated by an earlier study (Lewis, 1964). Normal subjects and chronic hyperventilators seem to respond differently to rapid changes in $PaCO_2$. Lewis (1957) is a strong supporter of the "bag over the nose and mouth," the CO_2 rebreathing diagnostic technique. Yet, to Demany and Zimmermann (1966), who also reported T-wave changes, HV versus chest pain of coronary origin frequently seemed to be a diagnostic dilemma.

ECG and EEG. Holmberg (1953) reported the inverse relationship between the EEG and heart rate: the slower the EEG activity, the higher the pulse rate. That is, increased *theta* corresponds to increased heart rate. Darrow and Pathman (1944) demonstrated the same relationship of heart rate to slow waves in the electroencephalogram during overventilation. They suggest, as one possible mechanism responsible for this observation, that increased alkalinity of the brain milieu augments the breakdown of acetylcholine by cholinesterase. It is remarkable that there have been no studies of the role of pH and hypocapnia in cerebral physiopathologies where acetylcholine deficiency apparently prevails. Senile psychosis of the Alzheimer's type comes to mind immediately.

Darrow and Pathman (1944) erroneously contended that the connection between cardiac and cerebral events during hypocapnia suggests a vagal mechanism. Apparently, they were unaware that the autonomic nervous system does not affect cerebral arteriolar caliber and brain blood flow.

Eckberg, Drabinsky, and Braunwald (1971) reported that cardiac function, regulated by the sympathetic branch of the ANS, is frequently found to be profoundly deranged in congestive heart disease, a pulmonary disorder. Hymes and Nuernberger (1980) studied breathing patterns found in heart attack patients and described these patterns for 153 patients in the critical care unit of a hospital in the Minneapolis-St. Paul area. Chest breathing predominated in patients with myocardial infarction: 76% showed mouth breathing (compared to 71% in controls); none of the nose breathers showed open-mouth snoring or apnea, but 70% of the mouth-breathers showed open-mouth snoring.

Wilkenthal, Fuller, and Shapiro (1968) reported the case of a patient who hyperventilated during emotional stress and developed atrial arrhythmias. However, they contended that the arrhythmias were not due to alkalosis, contradicting Thompson (1943) who, unlike Christensen (1946), did not hold to the view that HV-related changes in the ECG are an indication of cardiac insufficiency, though they are frequently so interpreted.

Respiratory Sinus Arrhythmia. The relationship between cardiac function and breathing is still only marginally understood by many clinicians despite the considerable evidence linking the two physiological variables to each other, and to the so-called stress-related disorders. A study by Bass et al., published in the *Lancet* (1983), pointed out that HV may go unrecognized in patients with a presumptive diagnosis of angina. Lum has been reporting since 1976 that HV must be considered in chest pain. There are other cardiac functions relating to breathing that may have an important diagnostic value. One of these is the distribution of interbeat interval (IBI).

Hinkle, Carver, and Plakun (1972) reported that men who showed little evidence of phasic variation in heart rate with respiration, and no evidence of the random abrupt sinus slowing that occurs with sighing, frequently had cardiac abnormalities and experienced significantly more sudden cardiac deaths than would be expected by chance. Cardiac IBI duration is determined, in healthy persons, by an increase in heart rate with inspiration and a decrease with expiration. This normal periodic acceleration and deceleration is known as *respiratory sinus arrhythmia* (RSA). Figure 15 in Chapter 5 illustrates this cardiac pattern, together with a tracing of end-tidal CO_2 (capnograph) that shows the breathing pattern. It is because of the evidence of its connection to breathing and putative value in assessing the effects of (vagal) sympathetic arousal, and stress, that the RSA has been included in the diagnostic protocols described in Chapter 5. It is rare, in my experience, that a client with dyspnea will show any RSA. Likewise, in virtually every case where breathing retraining was accompanied by a reduction in symptoms, RSA reappeared.

A substantial number of different mechanisms are involved in RSA. They are generally thought to involve vagus-mediated modulation of heart action with pulmonary and diaphragmatic afferent input and central (brain) efferent control. The phenomenon is thought to be principally breathing rate related (Melcher, 1976).

The RSA was first attributed to pulmonary reflexes by Hering in 1871. Melcher (1976), Porges, McCabe, and Yongue (1982), and McCabe and colleagues (1985) provided systematic descriptions of current knowledge about the physiology of this phenomenon. It appears to involve the following components:

(a) *Timing sequence*: The heart rate accelerates during inspiration, reaching a maximum three seconds after beginning, and falls to a minimum seven seconds later (Melcher, 1976).

(b) *Amplitude of the RSA*: Strength of the RSA is primarily determined by pulse rate (Porges, McCabe, & Yongue, 1982).

(c) *Pulmonary reflexes*: There is no evidence that reflexes from the lungs or thoracic wall are the main cause of the RSA (Melcher, 1976), but the higher the intrapulmonary pressure, the higher the maximum value reached by the RSA (Manzotti, 1958).

(d) The shape and amplitude of the RSA may reflect the response of the heart to rhythmically changing intrathoracic pressure (Hrushesky et al., 1984).

(e) *Hemodynamics*: Variations in systemic arterial mean blood pressure are positively correlated with heart rate (Melcher, 1976); RSA is correlated with blood flow through the pulmonary circulation in such a way that, for a decrease of flow, there is an increase in the heart rate, and vice versa (Manzotti, 1958).

(f) The greater part of the phenomenon is probably due to afferent impulses from vasoreceptors, on the left side of the heart, as a result of changes in blood flow that accompany respiratory movement (Davies & Neilson, 1967).

(g) *Cardiac*: Variations in venous return and diastolic pressure, with respiration by distention of the heart, elicit the reflexes that control rate (Melcher, 1976).

(h) *Central*: Chemoreceptors in the respiratory center respond to $PaCO_2$ and to central integration of baroceptor afferents, which results in vagal modulation (Manzotti, 1958; Melcher, 1976).

There is little consensus on the importance of any single variable identified in connection with RSA. They are all important, but no clear picture emerges about which one, or which set, is the regulatory mechanism.

According to Porges, McCabe, and Yongue (1982), the amplitude of RSA is related to vagal efferents to the heart "gated" by respiration. Thus, measuring the RSA is a noninvasive assessment of cardiac vagal tone. But Grossman (1991) cautions us that this assessment is reliable only if breathing rate and tidal volume are controlled. He proposed that HV is an "important potential mediator of stress-related cardiovascular function" (p. 33) and related the effect to disproportionate arterial CO_2 reduction and myocardial O_2 reduction, one of its sequelae. Neill and Hattenhauer (1975), and many others, have cautioned about reduced myocardial O_2 in HV. Rasmussen, Jull, Bagger, and Henningsen (1987) classified their patients on the basis of their ECG S-T segment response to HV-challenge: 25% showed abnormal reactions and had a coronary arterial caliber (diameter) reduction of 54%, compared with 7% in those with a normal ECG response to HV. Some of the abnormal responders showed up to 100% constriction after HV. After 4 years, 32% of those with the abnormal response had died versus only 12% of the others.

Angelone and Coulter (1964) described system resonance between breathing and heart rate. Pinciroli, Rossi, Vergani, Carnevali, Mantero, and Parigi (1986) were able to reconstruct respiratory waveform from the ECG. Disturbances in RSA, other than those mentioned in connection with sympathetic arousal, have also been noted: Piggott et al. (1973) observed differences between respiration and heart rate patterns in psychotic children and normal controls.

Cardiac IBI has a number of intrinsic patterns not directly related to breathing (Sayers, 1973). Power-spectrum analysis of heart rate fluctuations by Akselrod, Gordon, Ubel, Shannon, Barger, and Cohen (1981) has yielded some revealing clues to the IBI-driving mechanisms, including peaks at low frequency (0.04 and 0.12 Hz). They conclude that the "tonic activity of the renin-angiotensin system normally damps the amplitude of these fluctuations" (p. 220). Wei and Chow (1985) and Lee and Wei (1983) conducted a study of pulse power spectral composition and found normal and abnormal pulse frequency clusters, and a connection to pulse power diagnosis of Chinese medicine—from which they distanced themselves with a disclaimer.

The Effects of Hyperventilation on Neurons and the Nervous System

Assessing the effects of HV on neuronal cells is typically accomplished by experimentally varying the concentration of CO_2 and hydrogen ions in their environmental milieu. It is concluded that the influence of

PCO_2 on neuronal cells is due to changes in extracellular pH. But Walker and Brown (1970) showed that different types of neurons respond in a unique way to varying CO_2 concentrations. In a study of the abdominal ganglion cells of *Aplisia californica*, they reported that, in the presence of 5% CO_2, some neurons are depolarized while others are hyperpolarized; others were unaffected. They concluded that extracellular pH changes result in changes in membrane chloride conductance in the "responsive" cells; and, in human cortical neuronal cells, that CO_2 may hyperpolarize some neurons while depressing the function of others (e.g., respiratory center neurons).

In 1932, Brody and Dusser de Barenne showed that HV gives rise to a distinct augmentation of the excitability of the cerebral cortex. Specifically, they referred to the motor cortex. Their article was entitled "Effect of hyperventilation on the excitability of the motor cortex in cats," and its publication preceded by five years that of Kerr, Dalton, and Gliebe (1937), who are usually, though clearly erroneously, credited with coining the term hyperventilation.

The effects of varying CO_2 concentration in the brain have led a number of investigators to hypothesize CO_2's role in pathophysiology. The effects of cerebral extracellular PCO_2 are typically thought to center on (a) hypocapnia and its cerebral arterial vasoconstrictive effect; (b) alkalosis, and its effect on OHb dissociation; and (c) the resultant tendency to hypoxia and vasospasm when PCO_2 is low for extended periods. Numerous investigators have suggested that HV is directly responsible for a number of pathophysiological conditions relating to chronic hypoxia and/ or to increased pH, which manifest themselves in the form of relatively well-known neurophysiological disorders including depression and other affective disorders (Katz, 1982) and epilepsy (Lennox, 1928; Lennox & Lennox, 1960; Meyer & Gotoh, 1960; Meyer & Waltz, 1961).

Hyperventilation and Brain Hypoxia

Although it has been shown that different neuronal cells in the brain have their own characteristic response to hypocapnia, the brain as a whole seems to respond to it in a manner suggesting that, irrespective of the final pathway, the net result is hypoxia. Siesjo, Berntman, and Rehncrona (1979) reported that even a moderate reduction in brain O_2 supply is accompanied by symptoms of neurological dysfunction. These include changes in acuity of the dark-adapted eye, impaired short-term memory, diminished vision, and light-headedness. Reduction in brain metabolism following HV has also been thoroughly documented (Gibbs, Williams, & Gibbs, 1949; Gotoh, Meyer, & Takagi, 1965; Gottstein et al., 1970; Granholm,

Lukjanova, & Siesjo, 1968; Lennox & Lennox, 1960; Meyers, 1979; Raichle & Plum, 1972; Withrow, 1972).

Siesjo, Berntman, and Rehncrona (1979) held that failure of brain neuron function is not due solely to deficient ATP in hypoxia. Hypoxia, it appears, reduces neurotransmitter synthesis (Blass & Gibson, 1979). HV contributes to an increase in the action of acetylcholinesterase (Darrow & Pathman, 1944). Furthermore, hypoxia increases brain lactic acid, leading to lactic acidosis and respiratory compensation. Granholm, Lukjanova, and Siesjo (1968) reported that hypocapnia ($PaCO_2$ below 20–25 mm Hg) is accompanied by a progressive increase in brain lactate level, altering both cellular and extra-cellular pH.

Brain hypoxia is typically evident in elevated mean *theta* in the EEG as well as in the typical ictal patterns. As hypoxia becomes more profound, the potential for syncope increases, and in some persons who are prone to it, there is an increased likelihood of seizure. Holmberg (1953) summarized it this way:

> . . . hypocapnia is probably the essential factor which produces slow waves in the EEG during hyperventilation. Hypoxia gives a strong support but is unable to produce any such effect without co-existing hypocapnia. (p. 376)

Hyperventilation and the Electroencephalograph

The relationship between $PaCO_2$ and the "fundamental" EEG frequency has been known for some time. Lennox, Gibbs, and Gibbs (1938) observed that the EEG changes with varying conditions that also influence seizure threshold. One of these conditions was HV in which the seizure sufferer, as they put it, "blows off" CO_2. They showed that there was a more or less linear relationship between the dominant frequency of the EEG and $PaCO_2$ (see Chapter 3). It was also very clear that HV resulted in a decrease in dominant frequency and in increased voltage of low-frequency activity in the *theta* range. Employing a bidirectional, pulsed, ultrasound blood velocimeter, Hauge, Thorensen, and Walloe (1980) found a linear relationship between brain arterial blood flow and $PaCO_2$ controlling end-tidal PCO_2 ($ETCO_2$) by voluntary HV. Previously, Darrow and Pathman (1944) showed a relationship between EEG slow waves and increase in heart rate, and Brill and Seidmann (1942), the occurrence of HV-potentiated EEG dysrhythmia as occurring separately from ictal activity. Engel, Ferris, and Logan (1947) reported that HV interacts with blood sugar level in determining the degree of EEG slowing. They also showed that changes in $PaCO_2$ and pH, following HV, occur for the most part in the first 30 to 60 seconds; one single deep inspiration and expiration is able to reduce CO_2 volume by 5% to 7% and CO_2 tension by 7 mm Hg to 16 mm Hg. Rubin and Turner (1942) had earlier shown that slow potential (defined as anything below 8 Hz), as *theta* was known, increases with HV and changes in blood sugar. Their data plotting blood sugar level and slow potential activity, over the course of 210 minutes after insulin administration, are mirror-image curves. They concluded that lowering blood sugar below 120mg% influences the EEG response to HV.

Engel, Romano, and McLin (1944) observed the EEG in HV while studying vasopressor and carotid-sinus syncope, and noted the same pattern of EEG slowing. In every case of syncope, slow waves appeared to the point of unconsciousness. Meyer and Gotoh (1960) reported that HV produces rapid reduction in alveolar CO_2 in the first 5 to 10 breaths; hypocapnia resulting in cerebral arteriolar vasoconstriction (vessel diameter reduced by as much as 50%); pH shift toward alkalinity; and EEG slowing. They attributed the EEG slowing to ischemic hypoxia. Subsequently, Meyer and Waltz (1961) showed that hypocapnia and anoxia may be produced independently and that they result in similar EEG changes.

Holmberg (1953) supported earlier investigators on the relationship between HV and seizures, most notably that of the Lennoxes and the Gibbses in the middle and late 1930s. He confirmed the fact that spontaneous spike-and-waves, and conspicuous idiopathic seizure patterns, can be increased threefold in the resting EEG by HV.

It is clear from these studies and countless others that appear in the literature, but which have not been cited here, that there is a direct relationship between breathing and the frequency/voltage (spectral) composition of the EEG. The evidence overwhelmingly suggests that breathing changes precede, and in fact cause, EEG changes.

Hyperventilation and Idiopathic Epilepsy

In a recent publication summarizing the behavioral methods that have shown promise in seizure control (Fried, 1993a), I included my own research indicating that the incidence and severity of idiopathic epileptic seizures can be decreased significantly in some persons by the self-regulation of breathing. This study was instituted on the basis of the fact that a strong causal relationship has been consistently shown between seizure activity, EEG dysrhythmia, and HV. The goal of the training was to normalize alveolar PCO_2, and thereby stabilize brain blood flow and metabolism. This work encountered a considerable amount of criticism and disbelief. But the connection goes back at least to 1928 when Lennox reported that HV is a common feature in seizure sufferers. In 1938, Cobb, Sargant, and Schwab instituted synchronous recording of respiration and EEG, and in 1941, Schwab, Grunwald, and Sargant attempted "regulation

of epilepsy by synchronized recording of respiration and brain waves."
Then, inexplicably, such efforts faded from view.

Historically, the predominant theories of seizure etiology center on
the model of cerebral neurons out of control, recruiting neighboring units
until a massive, synchronized discharge occurs. The aptly named Lord
Brain (1962) stated it this way:

> There seems no doubt, however, that whatever its immediate or remote cause, an
> epileptic attack is the manifestation of a paroxysmal discharge of abnormal electrical
> rhythms in some part of the brain. (p. 129)

This means that when brain neurons decide on paroxysmal electrical
rhythms they do so, and a seizure ensues—never mind why. And Penfield
(1939) wrote that "from a physiological point of view, epilepsy may be
defined as a tendency to periodic involuntary explosions." Or, epilepsy is a
tendency to unpredictable seizures. Physiologically speaking, of course!

Gowers (1907) held that seizures were migraine, which suggests a
metabolic and cerebrovascular etiology, in comparison to the neuron-gone-
bonkers (neurogenic) theory of Brain, cited above. Metabolic theories are
exemplified by that of Gibbs, Lennox, and Gibbs (1940), who stated that:

> . . . considering all those links between carbon dioxide and epilepsy, namely that (1)
> the influence of carbon dioxide on the EEG, and (2) the abnormal values of carbon
> dioxide in arterial and jugular blood of patients with petit mal and grand mal, and (3)
> the abnormal variation of carbon dioxide preceding grand mal seizures in such a way
> as to indicate a causal relationship, we may conclude that carbon dioxide plays a
> significant role in the etiology of epileptic convulsions. (p. 109)

Himwich (1951) likewise proposed that, in addition to exerting physiological effects, CO_2 may also be involved in epilepsy. Penfield and Jasper (1954)
later allowed the possibility that etiological factors in seizure conditions
might include a spectrum of events broader than just neuronal hyperexcitability:

> The possibility that there may be intermediary metabolic defects, or abnormal reac-
> tivity of certain cerebral vessels must be considered. It might be related to vascular
> instability such as migraine, or to some obscure metabolic defect. (p. 495)

Penfield and Jasper (1954), and Darrow and Graf (1945), reported the
"blanching" (ischemia) of vessels in the arteriolar bed of the brain, which
occurs with HV. Darrow and Graf (1945) produced it experimentally in
cats, by HV. The transient ischemia was said by them to have the appearance of sausage links. Earlier, Brody and Dusser de Barenne (1932) concluded that HV causes hyperexcitability of the motor cortex of the cat.
Grote, Zimmer, and Schubert (1981) likewise examined the effect of severe
hypocapnia on the brain of the cat. Their report is just as emphatic as that
of Darrow and Graf, though less graphic:

> During marked hyperventilation a pronounced increase of cerebrovascular resistance (CVR) and a subsequent decrease of total regional cerebral blood flow (CBF) . . . as well as alterations of brain metabolism . . . are typically observed. The metabolic changes, which are characterized by elevated cortical tissue levels of lactate, pyruvate and NADH and an increase in the lactate/pyruvate ratio and in the NADH/AND+ ratio, are explained as direct and indirect hypocapnic effects. (p. 195)

They report that when first lowering $PaCO_2$ to 25 mm Hg there was a homogeneous decrease of cerebral blood flow (rCBF) in corresponding areas of both hemispheres. I calculated that reduction from their published data to be a little over 20%. Severe hypocapnia (16 mm Hg) dropped rCBF about another 5%, with varied regional blood flow reactions. Severe hypocapnia, while it seemed to favor generalized cerebral arterial vaso-constriction, as previously noted, also induced hypoperfusion in some brain regions, and hyperperfusion in others. And among other things, there was a significant loss of extracellular potassium as HV induced further hydrogen expulsion. Numerous other investigators, including Schneider (1961), have reported electrolyte loss. But the disturbance in rCBF triggered by HV is of particular importance and will be discussed in greater detail below.

It is in many ways remarkable that these reports, and similar ones, did not initiate a major turning point in focusing investigators away from the hypothetical "neuronal instability" theory, to a metabolic dysfunction theory of the etiology of seizures. Some investigators, however, did pursue such a line of research, most notable among them, J.S. Meyer and colleagues (1960, 1961). Tarlau (1958), in a study of EEG changes in neurogenic chronic respiratory acidosis, reported that CO_2 tension is directly involved in the production of slow EEG waves and that this is the most important factor influencing the EEG spectrum. To support his position, he cited an early study by Lennox (1928), cited earlier, concluding that many epilep-tics show a marked irregularity in respiration rate and depth.

Mattson, Henniger, Gallagher, and Glaser (1970) proposed that there is a mechanism through which anxiety leads to HV which, in turn, lowers arterial blood CO_2, thus triggering seizures. They concluded this on the basis of polygraphic studies of HV and the EEG. In those patients who showed a marked tendency to HV unconsciously when anxious, there was no obvious overbreathing. Yet they observed a 50% fall in $ETCO_2$ and EEG when seizure activity increased, concluding that involuntary chronic HV increased EEG epileptiform activity and seizures. Swanson, Stavney, and Plum (1958) proposed two equally likely theories of seizure etiology: (a) that CO_2 has specific effects on neuronal activity, and (b) that CO_2-related change in acid-base balance is the relevant variable in seizure etiology.

A theory of neuronal hyperexcitability is deceptively appealing. In the first place, it may be observed indirectly as a "focus" on the EEG. This focus permits the hypothesis of a lesion lying below the point on the scalp where the signal is strongest. That there is a massive discharge during a seizure gives rise to the "recruitment" theory, and so on. In the case of idiopathic seizures of the most common kind, there is little hard evidence to support these hypotheses.

The metabolic theory is decidedly less esoteric than the neurogenic theory, but it is parsimonious. HV, for whatever reason, leads to hypocapnia and alkalosis which cause severe paroxysmal constriction in the arteriolar bed of the brain with regional differences in blood flow and perfusion. Regional brain metabolism is impaired resulting in a seizure. Gotoh, Meyer, and Takagi (1965) mapped out the process, adding that HV also lowers cerebral tissue O_2 concentration by the Bohr effect, compounding the anoxia resulting from cerebral vasoconstriction. They reported a decrease of from 30% to 40% in CBF in persons volunteering to hyperventilate, and found that EEG slowing appeared at a cerebral venous O_2 tension of 21 mm Hg. Gottstein, Berghoff, Held, Gabriel, Textor, and Zahn (1970) reported that after one to two minutes of HV, glucose arterial-venous (a-v) difference increased, PCO_2 dropped from 32 to 16 mm Hg (pH rose from 7.48 to 7.73), CBF was reduced, and there was a markedly augmented lactate level in cerebral venous blood. Under ordinary conditions, one would expect about 7% of glucose to be converted to lactate, but during HV it rose to 13%, indicating a significant increase in anaerobic glucose utilization.

The study by Grote et al. (1981) which so elegantly describes the effect of hypocapnia in the cat was preceded by a number of such studies on humans. Raichle and Plum (1972) reported in an equally elaborate study that:

> Acute hypocapnic-hyperventilation (HV) in healthy animals and man causes an immediate cerebral vasoconstriction with a consequent rise in cerebral vascular resistance (CV) and a fall in cerebral blood flow (CBF), changes that parallel the fall in carbon dioxide tension (PCO2). It is generally accepted that the effect of HV is mediated by this change in PCO2, for it is the most potent cerebral vasoconstrictive agent known. Acute changes in PCO2 between 20 and 60 torr [mm Hg] have been shown to change CBF 1 to 2 ml/min/100 gm of brain per 1 torr change in PCO2. (p. 566)

The decline in CBF translates to about 2% for each 1-torr (mm Hg) decrease in $PaCO_2$.

Detailing the physiology of CBF and rCBF in epilepsy is greatly benefited by the recent application of the Positron Emission Tomographic (PET) scanning technique. Engel (1984) reviewed its application in the study of rCBF, and cerebral regional glucose metabolism. The technique isolated "one or more zones of hypometabolism . . . that correlated with the site of epileptogenic lesions, determined by scalp and depth interictal and ictal EEG recordings . . . and with the location of determined pathological changes in the brain" (p. S181). Significantly, these "zones of interictal hypometabolism may become hypermetabolic during seizures." Stefan, Bauer, Feistel, Schulemann, Neubauer, Wenzel, Wolf, Neundorfer, and Huk (1990), using the PET scan technique, observed the ictal hyperperfusion during seizures of temporal and frontocentral onset—which they report inducing in their patients with HV. They report that, among other things, "during spontaneously occurring epileptic seizures, ictal [PET scan] measurements . . . disclosed a regional hyperperfusion that corresponded with the onset of the ictal EEG activity" (p. 163).

Why would hypocapnia result in cerebral hyperperfusion? The only answer consistent with the evidence is that since hypocapnia induces apnea, a common occurrence preceding seizures, a rapid buildup of CO_2 during the convulsion reverses vasoconstriction, restores CBF, and might act differentially on regional brain units with hypoperfusion. This explanation seems consistent with Meyers's (1979) theory of the causation of anoxic and hypoxic brain pathology, that O_2 deficiency injures brain tissue as a function of the accumulation of lactic acid during hypoxia. The factual basis of the theory is well documented and may be relevant to seizure disorders. At first, the blood flow stasis of the hypoperfused area obstructs the vessel. This is followed by local anoxia, edema, and rapid lactic acid accumulation. Lactic acid accumulation changes membrane permeability, breaking down the blood brain barrier, and if sustained, causes local tissue damage. Lauritzen et al. (1983) using the PET scan to study CBF in migraine observed mechanisms like those described by Stefan et al. (1990) in epilepsy, and concluded that "confinement of the regulation abnormalities to the area of oligemia [reduced blood volume] supports our contention that the blood flow changes are caused by a change in local metabolism" (p. 669).

During generalized idiopathic seizures, cerebral metabolism increases two- to fivefold, and the need for substrate rises. The increased metabolic demand is met by a rise in cerebral blood flow (reduced cerebrovascular resistance). But after 30 to 45 seconds of convulsions, the composition of arterial blood gases is about the same as it would be with an equivalent amount of breath holding (i.e., apnea) (Magnaes & Nornes, 1974).

Neurogenic theories lean on the postulation of hypothetical seizure-inhibiting processes. So far none with any power to do so reliably has emerged. But the metabolic theory needs no such thing. During the seizure, $PaCO_2$ rises sharply, because while breathing stops, metabolism increases, raising blood CO_2 levels and restoring local cerebral blood flow.

CO_2 inhalation is the most effective means known for suppressing seizures. It is unfortunate that its clinical use to control seizures is not practical because it is more effective than currently prescribed anticonvulsant medications, and it has virtually no known side effects. Brick (1958) observed over 50% seizure reduction with CO_2 inhalation. Others have also reported this (Caspers & Speckmann, 1972; Meduna, 1958; Pollock, 1949; Wang & Sonnenschein, 1955; Woodburry & Kemp, 1970). According to William of Ockham, sometimes the simplest theory may be the best one.

Chapter 7

Respiration, Hyperventilation, and Mental Disorders

Introduction

Most clinicians still cannot get over their doubts that hyperventilation causes organic and psychological symptoms, because they still tend erroneously to regard it as simply breathing too fast. The traditional view of HV as a symptom of hysteria is alive and well. But chronic HV, chronic respiratory alkalosis, is a physiological disorder of the acid-base balance of the blood taken seriously by the medical physiologists Krapf, Beeler, Hertner, and Hulter (1991), who first published confidence limits for expected changes in blood plasma bicarbonate concentration, and pH, as recently as 1991, in the *New England Journal of Medicine*.

Chronic respiratory alkalosis (chronic HV) is a renal compensated deficit of blood CO_2 ($PaCO_2$) (i.e., hypocarbia); the homeostatic juggling act of balancing blood pH is critical (within extremely narrow limits) to metabolism and, indeed, to life itself. As Krapf et al. (1991) point out, it may be primary (or uncomplicated) or secondary in response to metabolic acidosis. By simply observing breathing rate and mode, there is no way of knowing which of these prevails.

Whereas anxiety may cause primary HV, cardiovascular, heart, and renal disease, for instance, may cause secondary HV. The a priori assumption of primary HV is risky. Other factors being equal, Krapf et al. (1991) reiterated that hypokalemia resulting from chronic HV may be severe enough to upset cardiac electrolyte balance. Considering the common presence of chest symptoms, and ECG-trace abnormalities (arrhythmias) in hyperventilators, one cannot underestimate the need for medical evaluation in this client population.

Symptoms of the Hyperventilation Syndrome

In his classic description of the hyperventilation syndrome (HVS), Rosett (1924) used hyperpnea, essentially the HV-challenge, to study its effects (previously demonstrated by Haldane and Poulton in 1908). Although the protocol of his study is unclear, he apparently had patients "voluntarily overbreathe," noting that the procedure was safe except in epilepsy. He reported that:

(a) Very deep breathing, at 12 breaths per minute in a normal person, produces tetany in 15 to 30 minutes;

(b) Initially, there is a slight transient tremor of the eyelids and facial musculature—usually one side only (and typically the right side);

(c) Tremors are replaced by muscular rigidity in the face and hands—the lips form a circle, close against the teeth, thumb and fingers are extended; the width of the hand is reduced to the "obstetrician's hand" configuration;

(d) If hyperpnea is discontinued at this point no rigidity is noted in other parts of the body;

(e) Subjective sensations of slight dizziness and rigidity, numbness, and tingling in the affected parts are noted;

(f) Primary sensations of gross contact—pain, heat, and cold—are rendered more acute; reaction to stimuli is enhanced; on the other hand, the exercise of judgment is blunted, the power of attention is lessened, and consciousness is reduced. (pp. 332–333)

Normal persons react differently to hyperpnea than do those with organic conditions. Those afflicted with central nervous system abnormalities had a greater diversity of "abnormal states of consciousness," while persons suffering from pain demonstrated a lower threshold to the effects of HV. These findings have since been replicated repeatedly.

HV-challenge has been shown to produce an astonishing array of sensory, affective, and somatic symptoms, for example, dizziness, faintness, apprehension, anxiety, depression, panic, and phobia, and a considerable constellation of somatic sensations including chest pain and muscle spasms (Hill, 1979; Lewis, 1957; Lum, 1976). Kerr, Dalton, and Gliebe (1937) listed the following symptoms in 36 of 50 of their patients with the diagnosis of "psychoneurosis with anxiety neurosis" who also showed signs of hyperventilation: weakness and fatigability; numbness and paresthesia; palpitations and increased heart rate; dizziness; muscular contractions, twitching, trembling, convulsions, and tetany; difficulty in swallowing, talking, and breathing; precordial pain; dyspnea (diaphragm spasm); epigastric pain; and constipation.

Huey and Sechrest (1981) compiled the following list of symptoms from reports in the clinical literature (Ames, 1955; Christophers, 1961; Lowry, 1967; McKell & Sullivan, 1947; Pincus, 1978; Singer, 1958; Yu, Yim, & Stansfield, 1959): light-headedness, giddiness, dizziness, faintness; fainting, syncope; headache; blurred vision; tremors, twitching; numbness, tingling, prickling (paresthesia); chest pain, pressure, discomfort (usually precordial); nausea; vomiting; abdominal gas pain and abdominal extension; lump in the throat; dry mouth; dyspnea, difficulty breathing; weakness, exhaustion, fatigability; apprehension, and nervousness. These symptoms are unexplainable in conventional medical terms and have been said to "mimic" organic disease (Missri & Alexander, 1978; Pincus, 1978). Those who have them tend to make frequent and often fruitless visits to physicians and even to hospital emergency rooms. Lum (1975) calls them the clients with the "fat folder syndrome," referring, of course, to the sheer bulk of their medical charts. Much is troubling them. They are in pain or discomfort, but are typically told "it's all in your mind." Even when HV is suspected, they are told that it is "only hyperventilation," somehow disqualifying further serious consideration. HV is thought by many mental health professionals to be a manifestation of hysteria (Lowry, 1967).

Huey and Sechrest (1981), summarizing the work of Lewis (1957), noted that the original diagnosis of 150 persons with HV was one or more of the following:

(1) Cardiovascular
    coronary heart disease
    rheumatic heart disease
    hypertensive heart disease
    congenital heart disease
    acute rheumatic fever
    cor pulmonale
    paroxysmal auricular tachycardia
(2) Respiratory
    asthma
    emphysema
    "respiratory tract infection"
(3) Neurological
    epilepsy
    brain tumor
    poliomyelitis
    cerebrovascular accident
(4) Psychological
    "nerves"

"functional"
hyperventilation syndrome
(5) Gastrointestinal
    cardiospasm
    peptic ulcer
    cholecystitis
    cholelithiasis
(6) Musculoskeletal
    fibrosis
    myositis
    arthritis
(7) Endocrine
    islet cell tumors of the pancreas
    pheochromocytoma
    hyperthyroidism
    hypothyroidism
    insulin reaction
    "glands"
(8) "Allergic reaction"

It is clear that the hyperventilation syndrome may take any number of different forms and perhaps either cause or mimic organic disorders.

Psychological Manifestations of the Hyperventilation Syndrome

Because of the confusion of psychologists, psychiatrists, and other medical specialists attending the diagnosis and treatment of HV (Bass & Gardner, 1985a), it is common that it may go unrecognized in clinical practice. A client's complaint of breathing difficulty, common in stress and anxiety, is more often viewed as a symptom and ignored, rather than viewed as a potential etiological factor in other presenting problems. But despite the fact that clinicians may not readily identify HV, it has been recognized for some time. Haldane and Poulton demonstrated its effects in 1908, and Hofbauer (1921) classified it as hysteria and neurasthenia: "Diese 'hysterishe tachypnoe' ist seit lange bekannt." [This hysterical tachypnea has been known for the longest time.]

Remarkably, there is no reference to HV in the most recent edition of the Diagnostic and Statistical Manual of Mental Disorders (DSM-III-R, third edition, revised [1987], American Psychiatric Association) which is the standard reference book for all mental health professionals. It lists all the psychiatric syndromes and symptom categories currently used in assessing mental disorders, but contains no index entries for any of the terms commonly relating to breathing difficulty, such as hyperventilation, dyspnea, hypocapnia, or respiratory alkalosis. Yet, "dyspnea" is the first symptom listed for panic disorder, followed by dizziness; palpitations; chest pain or discomfort; choking or smothering sensation; vertigo or unsteady feeling; feeling of unreality; paresthesia (tingling in hands and feet); hot and cold flashes; sweating; faintness; trembling or shaking; fear of dying, going crazy, or doing something uncontrolled during an attack (p. 231). This is an incomplete but not incorrect set of criteria for the HVS. Lum (1976) would add fatigability, weakness, exhaustion, sleep disturbance, and nightmares to the list of psychic manifestations of the HVS. These symptoms clearly coincide with those of panic disorder in the DSM-III-R, and clinicians who work with HV patients would readily recognize the 12 criteria of panic disorders as sufficient evidence of HV to warrant the use of the challenge maneuver, were they so inclined.

None of the 12 criteria is excluded from any of the classical standard reports on HV symptomatology (Bass, 1981; Brashear, 1983; Brown, 1953; Burns, 1971; Carryer, 1943; Compernolle, Hoogduin, & Joele, 1979; Engel, Ferris, & Logan, 1947; Gliebe & Auerback, 1944; Hardonk & Beumer, 1979; Heim, Blaser, & Waidlich, 1972; Hill, 1979; Kerr, Dalton, & Gliebe, 1937; Lewis & Howell, 1986; Pincus, 1978; Singer, 1958; Waites, 1978). Is HVS synonymous with panic disorder? According to Clark, Salkovskis, and Chalkley (1985), perhaps it is. The illustrative case, "The Housewife," given in the DSM-III *Casebook* (Spitzer, 1981), underscored the dilemma:

A 28-year-old housewife presented with the complaint that she was afraid she would no longer be able to care for her three young children. Over the past year, she had recurrent episodes of "nervousness," light-headedness, rapid breathing, trembling, and dizziness, during which things around her suddenly feel strange and unreal. (case 172, p. 268)

The discussion of this case states:

Clearly this woman has had recurrent panic attacks, characterized by light-headedness, rapid breathing, trembling, dizziness, derealization [*sic*] (things around her feel unreal). (p. 269)

The DSM-III diagnosis is Axis I: 300.21, agoraphobia with panic attacks.

Rosenbaum (1982) listed HV as one of the physical signs and symptoms of anxiety and included "valvular disease" as a physical cause of anxiety-like symptoms; Liebowitz and Klein (1981) cited mitral valve prolapse (MVP) as a cardiovascular disorder linked to anxiety-panic syndromes. MVP has, very tentatively, been cited in connection with HVS, but its connection to it is unclear (Klein & Gorman, 1984). It is a silent, functional symptom, detected as a "murmur" or click, appearing as part of a constellation of cardiovascular disorders attributed to autonomic dysfunction, including extrasystole and tachycardia.

While fear of dying, frequent in both panic disorder and HVS, might have swung the pendulum, the data collected by Gorman, Klein, and Leibowitz, in their various reports in connection with the effects of lactate infusion (venous blood gases curiously showed a higher pH in patient groups than in controls), should have given the strongest impetus to the linking of panic disorder with HV. Shader, Goodman, and Gever (1982), commenting on this finding, pointed out the presence of chronic respiratory alkalosis in these panic sufferers. More about this later.

I have encountered HV in numerous clients, but I see no evidence for a distinct HV-personality type, though they share common features, such as anxiety manifest against a background of labile peripheral and cerebral vascular instability. Their physiological responses are very similar to persons with neurological symptoms of allergy (Beauchemin, 1936; Davidson, 1952; King, 1981). But some investigators postulate a type of life-style component that hyperventilating clients seem to share. Lum (1976), for one, described such persons this way:

> The majority of patients studied have shown obsessional and perfectionist characteristics; a personality type excessively vulnerable to the uncertainties and untidiness of life itself.
>
> The quiet overconscientious secretary with the always tidy desk and immaculate typescript; the houseproud mother or the gifted wife, who finds her own creativity frustrated by the chores of home and motherhood; the executive subject to pressure from directors above and workers below.
>
> Dislike of delegation, difficulty in decision making, dislike of compromise.
>
> Frequently hyperventilators, particularly men, are less tense at work and are most happy when driving themselves hard in their chosen career. It is not uncommon for them to get symptoms at weekends or on holidays and yet be asymptomatic at work. This fits well with the personality type familiar to cardiologists as most prone to cardiac infarction: the aggressive personality, with enhanced competitive drive, inability to relax, addicted to work and tension.
>
> Phobic traits, usually mild, are frequent, particularly claustrophobia.
>
> Hyperventilators, particularly women, are often quiet, undemonstrative and adverse to the public display of emotions, masking their own anxieties with an outward semblance of tranquility. (p. 217)

He further states that these examples underline his view that they are drawn commonly not from the ranks of the psychologically inadequate (which the label "anxiety neurosis" would tend to convey), but from the "gifted, the conscientious or the ambitious" (p. 217). I have also had such clients, but it would be misleading to suggest that this personality description, though often correct, is a criterion for establishing the likelihood of the HVS. I have seen numerous persons with severe chronic HV who were unmotivated, unsuccessful, untalented, and unpleasant. It should be noted that Lum seems to have described the so-called Type A client whose treatment, Benson (1975) suggested, should include breathing retraining.

Respiratory Patterns and Mental Disorders

In 1935, Christie reported the use of the spirometer to study breathing patterns in "neuroses." It had been well established that overventilation caused numerous organic and psychopathological conditions; its connection to "cardiac neurosis," or Da Costa's "effort syndrome," was accepted (White & Hahn, 1929), as was its relationship to epilepsy (Rosett, 1924) and to neuromuscular disorders. Christie concluded that spirometer tracings are of significant value in diagnosis and differentiation of certain types of "respiratory neuroses." His focus on anxiety and hysteria led him to conclude that they were respiratory in nature, and he called them "respiratory neuroses."

Clausen (1951) also studied respiratory movements in neurosis and psychosis, and summarized an extensive review of previous investigations which examined breathing patterns in persons with psychopathological conditions. He cited Finesinger (1943), Hattingberg (1931), Kohlrausch (1940), Romer (1931), and Sutherland, Wolf, and Kennedy (1938), among others. They reported the following breathing patterns in persons with "neurotic type" psychological disorders: sighing; increased respiration rate (tachypnea); irregularity of breathing (inhalation and exhalation)— disturbances of coordination; sharp transition between inhalation and exhalation; curtailed expiration and prolonged inspiration; respiration wholly or mainly thoracic; shallow respiration; inspiratory shift of median position. They also found respiratory disturbances in the psychoses, including lower rate (in catatonics); shallow abdominal amplitude; tachypnea in schizophrenics; greater incidence of regular breathing in schizophrenics than in normal persons; and smaller tidal volume in schizophrenics (Corwin & Barry, 1940; Finesinger, 1943; Kempf, 1930; Patterson, 1933; Thompson & Corwin, 1942; Thompson, Corwin, & Aster-Salazar, 1937; Wittkower, 1935; all cited in Clausen, 1951). And, in this connection, I would like to bring to your attention two most astonishing reports. Loevenhart, Lorenz, and Walters published an article in the *Journal of the American Medical Association (JAMA)*, March 16, 1929, titled "Cerebral stimulation," in which they report the pharmacological effects of the injection of (sublethal) doses of cyanide, and the inhalation of mixtures of O_2 and CO_2 on psychosis. It follows their previous report (Loevenhart, Lorenz, Martin, & Malone, 1918), "Stimulation of the respiration by sodium cyanid [*sic*] and its clinical application," which appeared in *Archives of Internal Medicine*, in 1918.

Loevenhart et al. (1918) summarized previous reports on the respiratory-stimulant effect of cyanide concluding that it is based on a response to tissue hypoxia: cyanide decreases O_2 absorption. But previous investigators held that its effects were transient and therefore had no practical value in medical pharmacotherapeutics. Loevenhart et al. disagreed, and thought its rejection was based, among other things, on blind fear of cyanide because it is a poison. In their laboratory tests of its effects on respiration, initially in dogs, they chose sodium cyanide over potassium cyanide because of the "depressing effects of potassium on the heart." They also tested caffeine, citrate, strychnine, sulfate, atropine, and lactic acid, discarding them as therapeutic agents for various reasons, but their conclusions regarding lactic acid might have foretold the outcome in more recent studies:

> . . . The effect of lactic acid when administered under the conditions stated varies remarkably in different animals. In some dogs no effect whatever was noted, while in others it proved to be quite an efficient stimulus to respiration. (p. 111)

In response to injection of cyanide, they concluded that:

(a) It causes stimulation of respiration (in increasing doses, up to the point of death);
(b) It works rapidly (6 to 9 sec);
(c) Intensity and duration of stimulation are dose-related; and
(d) Slow continuous intravenous injection causes continuous stimulation of respiration of almost any desired intensity. At this point in the report, they footnote that "The action of cyanid [*sic*] in these experiments reminds one of the stimulation of the respiration by carbon dioxid [*sic*]" (p. 112).

Constant stimulation can be maintained for several hours, even in the presence of increased intracranial pressure which normally paralyzes respiration. Naturally, they describe the doses and injection rate in detail. They then proceeded to test this procedure on 10 clinical cases chosen on the basis of putative intracranial pressure, respiratory depression due to other causes, paresis, "dementia paralytica," catatonic schizophrenia, and so on, and conclude that:

> The therapeutic use of sodium cyanid [*sic*] in these cases has fully confirmed the results of the animal experiments, in that we have never had experience with any drug whose administration calls forth *so exact a response* in functional [respiration] activity as is to be noted under the cyanid [*sic*]. (p. 123) (my italics)
> On the other hand, we have seen in addition to the stimulation of the respiration

observed during and immediately following the administration of the drug, a marked improvement in the general condition of many of these cases. (p. 124)

One patient who was expected to die had normal pulse and temperature the day after the treatment. But the message to us, embedded in this study, is that:

> Evidence of stimulation of the cerebrum as a whole, especially the psychic centers, was obtained in a number of cases. Thus, several patients, who had their eyes closed for a long time, opened their eyes and looked about. In two instances they yawned quite naturally as though they were awakening from a long sleep. The most interesting instance of psychic stimulation was observed in case 10. *This patient who had dementia praecox, entered the hospital June 27, 1917, and up to the time of the injection had not spoken a word, so that no history was obtainable except from the meager statements on his commitment papers. After receiving an injection of 102 cc of fiftieth-normal sodium cyanid [sic] within a period of sixty-four minutes, the patient conversed, answered questions and attempted to explain his prolonged silence.* (p. 128) (my italics)

The seizures of this 21-year-old man also stopped for the duration of the treatment effectiveness.

In 1929, Loevenhart, Lorenz, and Waters reported being encouraged by the effect of intravenous injection of a 0.1% (0.001) solution of sodium cyanide, "at the proper rate." Noting its similarity to the effects of CO_2, they undertook to test CO_2 inhalation and reported that with the proper gas mixture, administered by standard inhalation apparatus used in anesthesia, they were able to:

> [succeed] in producing what we term cerebral stimulation in cases of dementia praecox, manic depressive insanity, and involutional melancholia. Every case treated has shown a positive response; that is, evidence of increased psychic function. The degree and nature of the response has varied to a considerable extent. The most favorable and striking reactions occurred in those patients who had been mute and mentally inaccessible for long periods of time. (p. 880)

Among the responses to CO_2 were lifting of catatonia, expressing depressive and "hebephrenic" thoughts, reduced muscle tension, initial fear and apprehension, followed by calm; sudden seeming comprehension of the situation, and speech utterance in the otherwise mute. These effects lasted from 2 to 20 minutes, followed by retrograde changes:

> Gradually the voice becomes less audible; the response to questions becomes halting with long lapses; the facial expression becomes set; eye movements cease, and attention can no longer be obtained. The patient makes no effort to comply with commands. The muscular rigidity recurs and in the course of two or three minutes the patient lapses to his former condition of mutism, negativism, and complete inaccessibility. It is especially striking to note how completely the former muscular state is resumed. This reproduction is faithful to the minutest degree; the same posture, the same facial grimace, and apparently the same mental state. In some cases the lapse to the original state is remarkably sudden, so that a sentence begun is left unfinished. (p. 881)

Quite a story, wouldn't you say? Revolutionized psychiatry? No one paid any attention to it; they were tripping all over each other pursuing psychosurgery—for which Egas Moniz received the Nobel Prize in medicine, in 1936, and shortly thereafter, an assassin's bullet. And so it goes. How can you fail to follow up on the conclusions that:

> Sodium cyanide administered intravenously in proper dosage causes cerebral stimulation in the stuporous state of certain psychoses.
> By these simple chemical procedures, the mental processes in certain psychotic patients are restored toward normal for a period of from two to twenty-five minutes.
> The method of approach in certain stuporous or inaccessible psychotic patients here presented permits a period of contact with the individual which offers opportunities for further physiologic and psychologic investigations. (p. 883)

And all you have to do to produce this phenomenon is to stimulate respiration.

The Inspiration–Expiration Ratio

Clausen (1951) suggested an inspiration–expiration (I/E) ratio for the spirometric observations (i.e., for pneumographic recordings from the thorax and abdomen). His pattern variables consisted of duration; variation coefficient of duration for the thoracic curve; variation coefficient of duration for the abdominal curve; inspiration–expiration ratio for the thoracic curve; variation coefficient of the I/E ratio for the thoracic curve; I/E ratio for the abdominal curve; variation coefficient of I/E for the abdominal curve. He reported the following observations:

(a) Neurotic women use a smaller part of the respiration cycle for inspiration than do neurotic men;
(b) Neurotic men have a significantly more rapid respiration than do normal men (15.7 versus 10.9);
(c) In neurotic men and women, the I/E ratio is highest for the abdomen; this means that a larger part of the respiration cycle is employed for expiration in abdominal than in thoracic breathing;
(d) Psychotic men have a faster respiration than do normal men, as well as a higher I/E ratio for thoracic breathing.

Clausen (1951) concluded that normal men breathe more slowly than normal women; and that sex differences in breathing disappear among neurotic and psychotic subject groups. Furthermore, neurotic men and women have a lower I/E ratio than do a comparable group of normal men. Thoracic breathing is found more frequently in women (normal or abnormal), and I/E in abnormal respiration is distinctly sharper in neurotic men and women than in normal men and women. He explained these differences as due variously to sex differences, anatomy, and culture.

Finesinger (1943) reported a somewhat less elaborate scheme for describing and quantifying aspects of breathing patterns, employing 7 variables relating to spirometric tracings. He concluded that among groups of persons with anxiety, hysteria, reactive depression, and so forth, the highest abnormal spirogram scores were found for the anxiety group, and the lowest, among schizophrenics.

The Resting Breath Rate

Dudley, Martin, Masuda, Ripley, and Holmes (1969) reported the use of four respiratory variables that they found useful in detecting breathing pattern changes induced by changes in emotional state: rate; minute ventilation; $ETCO_2$; and anatomical dead space. They reported that specifiable breathing patterns accompany changes in emotion. The rate or depth of breathing may increase (sometimes both); sighing increases (mostly in anxiety but sometimes in anger or resentment); and the breathing rate decreases when subjects feel tension, or are "on their guard." Breathing became especially irregular when anger was suppressed.

Another index is the resting breath rate (RBR). Skarbek (1970) found that RBR may be a personality characteristic, proposing that it may be a measure of the initial level of excitation/inhibition present when a person is not engaged in speech. He reported a decrease of 3 to 4 breaths per minute in psychiatric patients when clinical improvement was noted. He also found that the therapeutic use of phenothyazines tends to result in a decrease of the RBR, while the use of electroconvulsive shock therapy and antidepressants tends to increase the RBR.

The Ventilatory Response to Carbon Dioxide

In 1970, Clark and Cochrane administered the Eysenck Personality Inventory (EPI) to 44 patients with chronic airway obstruction to see if personality affects alveolar ventilation. The EPI is used to assess "neuroticism" and "extraversion." They reported that extraversion appeared to be a significant factor but that neuroticism was not. And they concluded that the personality of a patient may play an important part in determining alveolar ventilation.

Subsequently, Saunders, Heilpern, and Rebuck (1972), Shershow, King, and Robinson (1973), and Singh (1984a, 1984b), addressed the issue of "alveolar ventilation," using the ventilatory response to carbon dioxide (VRCO₂). The VRCO₂ is based on the fact that, when breathing a gas mixture containing CO_2 in excess of the usual PCO_2 found at sea level, a healthy subject will show a degree of increase in breathing rate. The $VRCO_2$ tends to be consistent over time in any given individual; correlates positively with anxiety, extraversion, and aggression; correlates negatively with Minnesota Multiphasic Personality Inventory (MMPI) scales of depression, psychopathology, psychasthenia, and social introversion; and shows strong positive correlation with neurotic personality traits, but only in women. With the EPI also, Saunders, Heilpern, and Rebuck measured the extraversion/introversion versus neuroticism dimensions, and reported a significant correlation between extraversion scores and $VRCO_2$ in women. They found no correlation between the $VRCO_2$ and neuroticism in either sex.

Shershow, King, and Robinson (1973) reported elevated standard scales of the MMPI in low $VRCO_2$ subjects. Singh concurred with the conclusions of other investigators that the $VRCO_2$ is a constant measure over time for a given individual. High responders do not, apparently, become low responders. Is the $VRCO_2$ a trait, or "type" marker? In the general population, the range of $VRCO_2$ is estimated to be between 0.5 and 9.0 l/min/mm Hg PCO_2; and the distribution is approximately normal, with a standard deviation of 1.0 l/min/mm Hg PCO_2. The following ratio is proposed:

$$\frac{\text{ventilation}}{PCO_2}$$

A positive correlation between this ratio and anxiety, extraversion, and aggression and a negative correlation with depression have been reported. The $VRCO_2$ has also shown that transcendental meditation (TM) can lower $VRCO_2$ in the meditative state (Singh, 1984b).

Hyperventilation and Anxiety

Breathing changes are typically noted in anxiety. They may consist of irregularity (I/R ratio), shallow breathing (low Vt), increased breathing rate, and increased Vmin (Burns & Howell, 1969; Christie, 1935; Dudley et al., 1964; Finesinger, 1943, 1944; Finesinger & Mazick, 1940; Heim, Blaser, & Waidlich, 1972; Huey & Sechrest, 1981; Skarbek, 1970; Suess et al., 1980; Tobin et al., 1983). There are few exceptions to these observations, the most notable being in schizophrenia, where breathing abnormalities do not seem to be prominent (Damas-Mora et al., 1976, 1978; Goldberg, 1958; Hardonk & Beumer, 1979).

We are cautioned about the generalizability of these conclusions, however, because they seem contaminated by methodological problems. For instance, Huey and Sechrest (1981) pointed out that many of these studies were based on individual cases, that their design does not conform to modern standards, and that the literature is not recent. Furthermore, patient subgroups were frequently pooled within a given report, creating difficulty in the interpretation of the statistical summaries; and diagnostic criteria for assigning a given individual to a particular subgroup were frequently omitted from the report. Finally, operational definitions of the independent variable were seldom used, and it was seldom indicated who classified the patients. The necessity for operational definitions of anxiety is deemed crucial since that definition is frequently constructed from analogies derived from animal models. That is, our understanding of "anxiety" may be based on a composite of the behaviors cited in research reports on experimental anxiety, in the tradition of Hunt and Brady (1955), Masserman and Yum (1946), and Pavlov (1927).

These definitions contrast sharply with psychodynamic ones and often result in a strange amalgam of two opposing views. For instance, Kolb (1968), in a more-or-less traditional "dynamic" paradigm, stated that:

> . . . anxiety is generally considered now a state of tension signaling the potentiality of an impending disaster, a warning of danger from the pressure of unacceptable internal attitudes erupting into either consciousness or action, with the consequent responses of the individual personality or society to this eruption. (p. 62)

Davison and Neale (1982) defined anxiety as "physiological arousal accompanied by unpleasant sensations of fear and apprehension not related to an immediately hazardous situation"—in the tradition of Cannon (1927). These explanations of anxiety assert an internal state of arousal characterized by tension and apprehension noxious to the individual; furthermore, it is related to anticipation of some future event or events. Although some cognitive theorists (Ellis, 1962), for instance, related anxiety for the most part to the present clash of irrational ideas or beliefs, it is typically viewed as a response to the future. In a sense, arousal is preparatory to anticipated conditions requiring it. There are alternate ways of viewing the role of the future in present cognition. Conditioning addresses that role. Salter (1961), for instance, states that:

> . . . anxiety is thus basically anticipatory in nature and has great biological utility in that it adaptively motivates living organisms to deal with (prepare for or flee from) traumatic events in advance of their actual occurrence, thereby diminishing their harmful effects. (p. 221)

Here, the common element "anticipatory" proposes that anxiety is learned fear. Unfortunately, many publications dismiss the distinction between anxiety and conditioned fear, and previously cited studies have used conditioned fear as a model of "experimental anxiety." But the traditional use of "anxiety" and "neurosis," derived from the Pavlovians, was in connection with behavior resulting from the failure to visually discriminate and not from learned (conditioned) fear.

A synthesis of the research studies obliges us to differentiate anxiety from fear, conditioned or otherwise. But it may be said that (a) it is anticipatory of a nonspecific arousing situation; (b) the arousal is reported to be unpleasant, and attempts are made to avoid it; (c) it does not appear to be based on the elicitation of a specific conditional response; and (d) it is irrational insofar as the anticipated danger is not, by objective criteria, potentially physically harmful.

In the many studies where electric shock caused arousal, the probability of shock was real and painful, and potentially harmful. Such studies are misleading if they describe the outcome as neurosis or anxiety. Simply because therapeutic strategies may be used to control or reduce them does not prove that they are anxiety or neurosis. But practically, any explanation of anxiety that satisfied conditions a, b, c, and/or d, above, is satisfactory insofar as we typically perceive anxiety sufferers to be persons who are "sitting on the outside" and "running on the inside." Naturally, when one runs (in actuality or metaphorically), breathing will be different from that at rest.

For instance, anxiety is apparently accompanied by a state of arousal during which action is essentially inhibited—the "sitting on the outside, running on the inside" phenomenon. Breathing changes associated with anxiety seem to be related more closely to whether the emotional state is "action-oriented," as in anger, rather than "nonaction-oriented," as in depression (Dudley & Pitts-Poarch, 1980). These correlates give no hint as to causal relationship, and it is not clear whether inhibited action causes anxiety or results from it. The Pavlovians would say that inhibition of action is characteristic of the individual—a type-linked characteristic—thus making anxiety a trait. Therefore, the arousal pattern, including HV, is a trait characteristic.

Some speculate that anxiety causes HV, while others speculate the opposite. Goldberg (1958) thought that HV "is one aspect of the individual's anxiety reaction, and the mechanism whereby certain physical symptoms are produced in patients suffering from various psychiatric symptoms." Thus, one suffering from a psychiatric syndrome featuring anxiety will hyperventilate; and she or he who hyperventilates will have additional symptoms due to HV.

If this theory is correct, then it should be routine in all psychiatric conditions to determine which of the somatic complaints are the result of the HV. This modest proposal would, if implemented, yield some rather remarkable results, if the research literature is to be trusted. To Walker (1984), HV may be "a symptom of the panic disorder spectrum, a separate syndrome and a primary cause of panic attacks." He concluded that HV plays a significant role in all anxiety disorders and should be listed as a psychosomatic disorder.

Bonn, Readhead, and Timmons (1984) stipulated that HV should not be dismissed as secondary to fear, but that it may, per se, produce symptoms and imitate or aggravate panic. Huey and Sechrest (1981) suggested that persons who are anxiety-prone hyperventilate as part of their anxiety response to life stresses. Lum (1981) supported the position of Rice (1950), that anxiety is produced by the symptoms of HV, proposing that HV may, in many persons, simply be a bad habit. This is one of the very few of his assertions to which I take exception.

Hardonk and Beumer (1979) reported that emotions and tension can induce HV in the same way as physical exertion. But they are not certain whether the tension results from repeated HV attacks or whether it causes an attack. It is doubtful that there are many instances of HV due to physical exertion, since the body expels the increased CO_2 with increased metabolism.

Phillipson and Sullivan (1978), however, stated that arousal makes possible an appropriate integrated response to stimuli that includes behavioral as well as ventilatory, cardiovascular, and other adjustments. They point out that when we look at breathing we are seeing only a small part of the arousal system. The effects of HV infiltrate all aspects of physiological functioning.

In an article entitled "Agoraphobia, the panic attack and the hyperventilation syndrome," Ley (1985a) suggested that:

> The panic attack consists of a synergistic interaction between hyperventilation and anxiety, the nature of which is a positively accelerated loop: with excessive expiration of CO_2, moderate overbreathing produces relatively mild symptoms (e.g., slight dizziness) which can be tolerated for prolonged periods. If, however, respiration rate increased somewhat, the symptoms of hyperventilatory hypocapnia increase in both number and intensity *very rapidly* to the point where tolerance gives way to alarm and fear. When fear is elicited, heightened sympathetic nervous system activity contributes to an increase in respiration rate and thereby increases the intensity of the hyperventilation syndrome, which in turn increases fear, which in turn increases respiration rate and so on. The panic attack will in this way grow in intensity until the sufferer either falls into unconsciousness and thereby stops hyperventilating or engages in behavior which leads to a reduction in the amount of CO_2 dissipated. (p. 79)

This is essentially a type of fear-elicitation theory and is a plausible explanation of what one often encounters in clinical situations. I am inclined to endorse it, although it differs somewhat from my own beliefs in that it omits any mention of the organic/systemic variables that make a particular individual more or less anxiety prone. These variables include an inherited predisposition to the effects of hypocapnia due to, perhaps, morphological aspects of vascular structure and function, hemodynamic and O_2 transport mechanism, metabolic variables, and chemoreceptor threshold sensitivity.

I think that, for the most part, the chronic hyperventilator is prone to anxiety *and* other extended arousal-related somatic and psychological disorders, including panic, phobia, depression, and so forth. (Holt & Andrews [1989] found hypocapnia in agoraphobics [mean $PCO_2 = 35.0$ torr], panic disorder [35.2 torr], social phobics [34.7 torr], and generalized anxiety sufferers [36.0 torr], as compared to normal controls [37.3 torr]). Symptoms other than those elicited in nonprone persons (e.g., dizziness) may be essentially weak points in that person. If there are deficiencies in the vasculature and the O_2 transport system, further jeopardy by hypocapnia (Mathew & Wilson, 1990) may result in reasonably severe hypoxia and may manifest itself as the product of paroxysmal vasospasms, that is, migraine, Raynaud's disease, angina, or idiopathic epileptic seizures. If there are deficiencies in the striated musculature, fasciculation, cramping, and tetany may follow abnormalities in calcium metabolism. Other deficiencies may lead to irritable bowel syndrome.

In a recent study, Mathew and Wilson (1990) contend that:

> . . . anxiety is often accompanied by an increase in respiratory rate and reduced arterial levels of CO_2. . . . Hyperventilation is a common symptom of acute anxiety and panic, and hypocapnia has been held responsible for a number of somatic symptoms of acute anxiety. (p. 840)

According to these authors, acute anxiety, and panic, are hypoxic phenomena due to the reduced cerebral blood flow that accompanies HV. This seems a pretty straightforward description of a particular somatic type, and does not preclude the conditionability of the phenomena. We encounter essentially the same thing in another recent report (Gibbs, 1992), which also examines the relationship between HV and CBF. This "study was designed to test the hypothesis that panic disorder is associated with greater sensitivity of cerebral arteries to changes in arterial PCO_2 by measuring basilar artery flow with transcranial Doppler ultrasonography before and during hyperventilation" (p. 1589). Gibbs found that panic disorder patients have an exaggerated reduction in basilar artery flow during hyperventilation compared with control subjects.

Several things come to mind. First, this study by Gibbs is also clearly aligned with the somatic-type theory. Second, his hypothesis of "greater sensitivity" hardly does justice to his finding of an "exaggerated" reduction in blood flow in panic sufferers. Third, he inexplicably dismisses this exaggerated reduction in basilar artery blood flow as the cause of panic attack because it does not appear in all patients. There would be no validity in physiological research if that were the criterion. For instance, no conventional medication works in every case—anticonvulsants have, at best, a 60% to 80% *hit rate*, with complete seizure elimination in the neighborhood of 45% to 60%. Finally, the study is methodologically sound, but I question his reasoning, and fault his apparent disregard for previous research. As a professor of research methodology for many years, I would give him no more than a B− because of this glaring oversight—there are just 7 reference citations. He fails to cite Mathew and Wilson, who published in the same journal just two years earlier, and who find the relationship between acute anxiety and panic etiologically significant—and managed to find 117 relevant references. Is the Gibbs agnosia a coincidence, or just another example of the, unfortunately all too common, "Don't confuse me with the facts, my mind is made up"?

I contend that chronic hyperventilators are a somato-autonomic type, in the Pavlovian sense. And both their reactions to the world, stress, and HV and their reaction to the effects of HV form a more or less closed feedback loop where components of the system become indistinguishable once the cycle is set into motion.

Is There a Valid Hyperventilation Symptoms Scale?

Breathing modes and HV in particular correlate with various psychological and biological markers. But numerous investigators have listed all of the symptoms which they have observed in HV, or which they suspect to be etiological in HV, in the hope of showing the diversity of its effects. In contrast, some list a common core of symptoms which they believe identifies HV. To validate it, a high score on this list must show a high positive correlation to hypocapnia (alveolar PCO_2 below 38 torr). It would be better still if scores on this checklist were to vary linearly with PCO_2.

There are two major components to the impetus to find a common symptomatology. First, such a set of symptoms validates the existence of HVS as a diagnostic entity, a fact which, as you have seen in earlier chapters, is still in dispute in some quarters. Second, and perhaps somewhat less desirable, is that a set of symptoms becomes the criterion for differential diagnosis of HVS. Medical symptoms are the basis for differential diagnosis, but typically, they are validated by laboratory test procedures.

This test procedure is based on the fact that similar symptoms may come from entirely different disorders. For instance, hypertension may be a symptom of many diseases, including pheochromocytoma, an adrenaline-secreting tumor. Only blood tests can validate this diagnosis. Thus, treating someone for "stress" because of hypertension, and many of the other symptoms that accompany elevated blood levels of catecholamines, including HV, may prove hazardous.

Differential diagnosis by symptom is certainly better than having no criteria, especially when a client has been referred after thorough medical examination and blood tests have ruled out organic disease. Backing up this diagnosis with a psychophysiological respiratory profile, including capnography, is, in my opinion, evidence of the coming of age of our discipline.

Before there was HVS, there was DaCosta's Syndrome, effort syndrome, neurocirculatory asthenia, neurasthenia—Let's see, did I leave anything out?—Ah, yes: cardiac neurosis, anxiety neurosis, hysteria, and more recently, stress. You will recall that that controversy centered on whether these were not only the same thing, but were in fact HVS. For this reason, I am including here the list of Wheeler, White, Reed, and Cohen (1950) (see Table 1). It looks a whole lot like a list of HVS symptoms, doesn't it? (This list was published just 13 years after Kerr, Dalton, & Gliebe and there is, of course, no reference to them in the Wheeler et al. study.) What's more, the Kerr et al. (1937) report gives the laboratory values for each of their subjects. These include CO_2 before HV (vol %); CO_2 after HV (vol %); chlorides before HV (mg %); chlorides after HV (mg %); calcium (total); calcium (diff.); serum protein (total); serum albumin; serum globulin; blood sugar; serum magnesium; RBC magnesium; hematocrit; urine pH before HV; urine pH after HV; urine ammonium total before HV; urine ammonium total after HV; urine ammonium per cc before HV; urine ammonium per cc after HV; urine acetone before HV; and urine acetone after HV. It is clear from the comprehensive and specific nature of these tests that they understood the physiology of HV. For their list of symptoms, see Table 2.

They also reported that 14 of their patients experienced diaphragmatic spasm which was, parenthetically, attributed by Harris, Hoff, and Wise (1954) to hysteria. Soderstrom (1950), on the other hand, related this "clonic spasm of the diaphragm" to cardiac systole in two patients, and its correspondence to cardiac systole in the others to coincidence. I think that he was wrong in the latter case. Diaphragmatic "spasm" as indicated by high frequency, apparently clonic, spasms is not uncommon in certain individuals, and is related to the beating of the heart against the diaphragm, forcing air out with each beat. There is no evidence that it is

Table 1. Symptoms of Neurocirculatory Asthenia
Percentage of Each Symptom in 60 Patients and 102
Healthy Controls*

Symptoms	Patients	Controls
palpitation	96.7%	8.8%
tires easily	95.0	18.6
breathlessness	90.0	12.7
nervousness	87.6	26.5
chest pain	85.0	9.8
sighing	79.3	15.7
dizziness	78.3	15.7
faintness	70.0	11.8
apprehension	60.7	2.9
headache	58.3	25.5
paresthesias	58.2	7.2
weakness	56.0	3.0
trembling	53.5	16.7
breath unsatisfactory	52.7	3.9
insomnia	52.7	4.0
unhappiness	50.0	2.1
shakiness	46.5	15.7
fatigued all the time	45.1	5.9
sweating	44.9	38.0
fear of death	41.8	2.0
smothering	39.7	3.9
syncope	36.7	10.8
flushes	36.2	—
yawning	34.6	14.0
pain radiating to left arm	30.0	2.0
vascular throbbing	29.0	1.1
dry mouth	25.1	1.1
nervous chill	24.4	—
frequency	18.6	2.1
nightmares	18.3	9.2
vomiting and diarrhea	14.0	0.0
anorexia	12.3	3.0
panting	7.9	—

*Reprinted with permission from E. O. Wheeler, P. D. White, E. W.
Reed, and M. E. Cohen (1950): Neurocirculatory asthenia (anxiety
neurosis, effort syndrome, neurasthenia). *JAMA*, 142:878–889.

pathophysiological and it is certainly not hysteria. The capnogram tracing, from a 35-year-old man suffering anxiety, illustrates the phenomenon (see Figure 1).

Grossman and DeSwart (1984) list the symptoms of HV, as well as their relative frequency, observed in their patient population (see Table 3).

Table 2. *Some Physical Phenomena Associated with Anxiety States and Their Relationship to Hyperventilation**

Since 1928, fifty patients have been admitted to the University of California Hospital whose conditions have been diagnosed as psychoneurosis with anxiety neurosis.

Number of patients with symptoms similar to the ones now described as associated with hyperventilation	36
Number of patients without these symptoms	14
Number of patients with the following symptoms:	
Weakness and fatigability	18
Numbness and paresthesia	14
Palpitation and increased cardiac rate	12
Dizziness	10
Nausea and vomiting	4
Muscular contractions:	
Twitching, trembling, convulsive states	14
Tetany (not on basis of hypoparathyroidism)	9
Difficulty in swallowing, talking, breathing (pharyngeal-laryngeal spasm)	8
Precordial pain (intercostal muscle and diaphragmatic spasm)	4
Dyspnea (diaphragmatic spasm)	14
Epigastric pain (diaphragmatic spasm)	2
Constipation (spastic colon)	5

The figures given above are compiled from the descriptions of the symptoms and signs that are given, and not from the results of formal experimentation.

*Reprinted with permission from W. J. Kerr, J. W. Dalton, and P. A. Gliebe (1937): Some physical phenomena associated with anxiety states and their relationship to hyperventilation. *Annals of Internal Medicine*, 11:961–992.

Notice once again that breathing is at the top of these lists. More recently, van Dixhoorn and Duivenvoorden (1985) reported on the "Efficacy of [the] Nijmegen Questionnaire [NQ] in recognition of the hyperventilation syndrome" (after Nijmegen University, The Netherlands). Sixteen items are thus scaled:

never	rarely	sometimes	often	very often

......I...............I...............I...............I..............I......

The questionnaire was administered to 75 patients with the clinical diagnosis of HVS, and it shows a high degree of differentiation between HVS and non-HVS patients. The list, clustered into one of three components, is shown in Table 4; the Nijmegen Questionnaire is shown in Table 5.

Initially tested on 263 patients, the NQ differentiated well (around 80%) between those who reported symptoms on provocation, and those who did not. The NQ was intended to "[provide] empirical support for the possibility of a circumscribed definition of HVS" (p. 199). I assume this

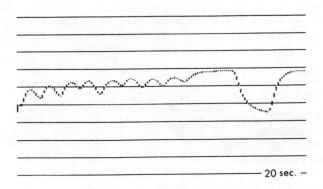

20 sec. –

TIME=11/10/87 13;36;54 22 UPDATE #18 PEAK CO2=5.58 AVG. CO2=5.08%

Figure 1. Cardiac oscillation in end-tidal breath ($PETCO_2$) tracing: Wave pattern is produced when the heart, beating against the lungs, mechanically forces small additional amounts of air out during expiration in deep-diaphragmatic breathing.

to mean that it was hoped that the NQ could be a reasonable alternative to the capnogram and the HV-challenge. It certainly makes sense since the NQ poses no health hazard, unlike the "challenge," and capnography is not yet routine.

Statistical analysis revealed that the NQ has three components: (a) the subjectively experienced difficulty in breathing; (b) peripheral sensations, including Chvostek's sign (tightening around the mouth); and (c) central tetany (i.e., neurological signs plus chest and abdominal sensations). The number of false-positives was smaller than the false-negatives, encouraging its use as a screening instrument. The authors refer to hypocapnia, hypocarbia, and alkalosis, but there are, unfortunately, no alveolar PCO_2 data to corroborate their conclusions. Perhaps that is the next step.

Hyperventilation and Panic Attacks

A systematic review of the research and clinical reports that relate HV to panic disorder may be summarized by citing examples of the contemporary view of this relationship. For instance, Clark, Salkovskis, and Chalkley (1983) and Salkovskis et al. (1986) reported that the sensations in panic attacks are similar to those in HV. They contended that stress causes an increase in ventilation (increasing pH and decreasing PCO_2), resulting in unpleasant sensations to which the person responds with apprehension. Carr and Sheehan (1984) hold that panic attacks differ from anxiety in response to stress in normal (nonpanic-prone) persons. They cited charac-

Table 3. Frequency of Positive Responses to Complaint Items among HVS and Non-HVS Subjects*

Item	Percent positive responses		Significance level
	HVS Ss	non-HVS Ss	
Fits of crying	14.5	6.5	0.01
Unable to breathe deeply enough	44.5	33.5	0.03
Suffocating feeling	54.5	41.0	0.009
Rapid heartbeat	41.5	27.0	0.003
Feeling of unrest, panic	54.5	38.5	0.002
Tingling in feet	20.0	17.0	
Nausea	38.0	31.5	
Confused or dream-like feeling	35.0	27.5	
Feeling of heat	42.0	34.0	
Pounding heart	50.0	27.0	0.0000
Stomach cramps	19.0	18.0	
Toe or leg cramps	10.5	12.5	
Shivering	25.5	16.5	
Irregular heartbeat	18.5	11.5	0.07
Tingling in legs	16.0	11.5	
Feeling anxious	30.0	21.0	0.05
Chest pains around heart region	40.0	37.5	
Stiffness in fingers or arms	18.5	13.0	
Cold hands or feet	20.5	20.5	
Feeling of head warmth	29.0	20.0	0.05
Stiffness about mouth	6.5	4.5	
Stomach feels blown up	21.5	18.0	
Pressure or knot in throat	23.0	13.5	0.02
Tingling in arms	20.5	14.0	
Faster or deeper breathing than normal	42.5	18.5	0.0000
Hands tremble	38.5	25.0	0.005
Dizziness	69.0	50.5	0.0002
Stiffness in legs	7.5	5.0	
Blacking out	45.5	35.5	0.05
Tingling in body	5.0	4.0	
Tenseness	51.5	36.5	0.003
Need of air	27.5	16.0	0.008
Fainting	15.0	15.5	
Tingling in fingers	26.5	17.5	0.04
Tiredness	64.0	55.5	0.10
Headaches	47.0	51.0	
Tingling in face	10.0	4.0	0.03

*From P. Grossman and J. C. G. DeSwart (1984): Diagnosis of hyperventilation symptoms on the basis of reported complaints. *Journal of Psychosomatic Research,* 28:97–104. Reprinted with permission.

Table 4. Dimensional Structure of Hyperventilation Complaints

	Components		
	I	II	III
	Shortness of breath	Peripheral tetany	Central tetany
		*	
8 Constricted chest	0.81	0.16	−0.23
7 Shortness of breath	0.81	0.28	−0.12
6 Accelerated or deepened breathing	0.81	0.15	−0.01
11 Unable to breathe deeply	0.76	0.16	0.04
1 Chest pain	0.53	−0.13	−0.52
2 Feeling tense	0.48	−0.13	0.15
15 Palpitations	0.41	−0.22	0.29
13 Tightness around the mouth	0.02	−0.73	−0.07
12 Stiffness of fingers or arms	0.06	−0.72	−0.15
14 Cold hands and feet	0.10	−0.58	0.08
10 Tingling fingers	0.16	−0.57	−0.16
9 Bloated abdominal sensation	0.13	−0.03	−0.67
4 Dizzy spells	0.25	−0.06	0.62
3 Blurred vision	0.04	−0.11	0.55
5 To be confused, losing touch with environment	0.47	−0.08	0.54

*Figures represent loadings, correlations of the items with the components.
Note: Reprinted with permission from J. van Dixhoorn and H. J. Duivenvoorden (1985): Efficacy of Nijmegen Questionnaire in recognition of the hyperventilation syndrome. Journal of Psychosomatic Research, 29:199–206.

teristic age of onset and sex distribution data as evidence for the specificity of the panic response as well as the fact that panic attacks respond to different therapeutic strategies than those used to control nonpanic anxiety. Their suggestion that HV and panic share a common pathogenesis is yet another support of the type, or trait, theory. I have alluded to this, in the previous section, in connection with the reports by Mathew and Wilson (1990) and Gibbs (1992) that support the contention that HV-related changes in CBF in acute anxiety and panic disorder may be etiological.

Hibbert (1984) titled his research article "Hyperventilation as a cause of panic attack," leaving no doubt about his theory. Because beta-adrenergic agonists induce panic while beta-adrenergic antagonists tend to control it, he contended that panic of sudden onset may represent an endogenous form of anxiety. This is also important to the "type" theory since, without the endogenous predisposition, panic will not occur even in the face of considerable anxiety. Endogenous predisposition to panic attacks, in connection with HV, has been suggested. One of the most prominent predisposing factors is lactic acidosis.

Table 5. Adaptation of the Nijmegen Hyperventilation Symptoms List (NHSL)*

Name: _____   Date _____

A number of complaints are listed below that may possibly apply to you. Will you please circle one of the vertical strokes after each complaint?

	Never	Rarely	Sometimes	Often	Very often
1. Sharp pain in chest	—|____	____|	____|	____|	____|____
2. Tension	—|____	____|	____|	____|	____|____
3. Blurred, hazy vision	—|____	____|	____|	____|	____|____
4. Dizziness	—|____	____|	____|	____|	____|____
5. Confusion or a sense of losing normal contact with surroundings	—|____	____|	____|	____|	____|____
6. More rapid or deeper breathing	—|____	____|	____|	____|	____|____
7. Shortness of breath, difficulty breathing	—|____	____|	____|	____|	____|____
8. Tightness in chest	—|____	____|	____|	____|	____|____
9. Bloated abdomen	—|____	____|	____|	____|	____|____
10. Tingling in fingers	—|____	____|	____|	____|	____|____
11. Unable to breathe deeply	—|____	____|	____|	____|	____|____
12. Stiffness of fingers and arms	—|____	____|	____|	____|	____|____
13. Tightness around the mouth	—|____	____|	____|	____|	____|____
14. Cold hands or feet	—|____	____|	____|	____|	____|____
15. Heart palpitations	—|____	____|	____|	____|	____|____
16. Feeling of anxiety	—|____	____|	____|	____|	____|____

Sex: _____ Age: _____   Medication: _____

PCO_2: _____   Main complaints: _____

*The NHSL is reprinted with permission from P. van Doorn, P. Colla, and H. Folgering (1982): Control of end-tidal PCO_2 in the hypervenilation syndrome: Effects of biofeedback and breathing instructions compared. *Bulletin of European Physiopathology and Respiration.* 18:829–836.

The scenario for the manifestations of lactic acidosis predisposition goes something like this: The chronic arousal that accompanies stress and anxiety, including an increase in ventilatory drive, results in jeopardy of the body's O_2 transport system caused by the effects of hypocapnia. Consequently, there is a graded hypoxia that shifts the system to increased anaerobic metabolism. This shift results in the increased production of lactic acid and the tendency toward lactic acidosis. There follows a further increase in ventilatory drive to correct acidosis. These homeostatic adjustments are costly to the body and vacillate, causing change in metabolism and blood gas composition. Chemoreceptors are activated by these vacillations in metabolism and end-product metabolites and send afferent signals to the brain (Blass & Gibbson, 1979; Carr & Sheehan, 1984; Katz, 1982; Lowry, 1967; Lum, 1981). Panic is the result of these afferent impulses, for which the individual has no adequate labels. Thus, panic becomes the basis for *attribution*.

A number of studies have been conducted on the role of lactic acidosis in panic disorders. Most notable are those of Pitts and McClure (1967) and of Klein and his colleagues (Gorman et al., 1981; Klein & Gorman, 1984). In these studies, there is considerable evidence of HV in the client population and dyspnea is prominently mentioned, but curiously, there is no mention of the HVS or of the role that it might play in the metabolism of client populations manifesting lactate sensitivity.

In evaluating the role of HV in panic disorders, it is important to remember that investigators align themselves with one of two possible theories: (a) panic is a more severe form of anxiety, and (b) panic is the result of an endogenous process, including the arousal that occurs with anxiety and stress but is, in a sense, separate categorically from the anxiety continuum that is based on conditional fear. It is relatively simple to relate the arousal that accompanies anxiety with HV. But if panic disorder is not on a continuum with anxiety, how does HV contribute to it? I propose the following model.

In those who are morphologically and physiologically predisposed, the chronic arousal of an anxiety or stress reaction results in HVS. Initially, HV may have adaptive value, but when it is chronic, it depletes the stress-coping mechanisms of the body. For instance, the homeostatic adjustments necessary to compensate for respiratory alkalosis during chronic hypocapnia are costly to the body. And, as previously noted, there are numerous other changes in the body (in circulation, hemodynamics, and metabolism) that must be compensated for the body to achieve physiological synchrony. In these persons, chronic HV gradually produces chronic graded hypoxia, and especially cerebral hypoxia (Darrow & Graf, 1945; Fried, 1993b; Fried et al., 1984b; Penfield & Jasper, 1954).

Graded hypoxia results in depressed oxidative metabolism, decreased cerebral blood flow (by as much as 30%), and many other changes (i.e., cardiac, vascular, hemodynamic, and so forth). Thus, the first stage of chronic graded hypoxia, which has repeatedly been shown to be the case in chronic HV, is depression (of mood and activity). If the hypoxia becomes more severe, that is, if it exceeds some internal systemic/physiological criterion, there will be a second stage, a quantum leap to the endogenous conditions that give rise to panic attacks. Individuals will be responding to afferent as well as central signals of anoxia for which they have no adequate labels. They may attribute the sensations to ongoing activity, actual or cognitive, perhaps related to the stress exacerbating the graded hypoxia.

Internal conditions such as increase in catecholamines, typical in such situations, further exacerbate the anoxia by their demonstrated effects on

OHb affinity (Mairlbaurl & Humpeler, 1981). The third and final stage is asphyxia, where the panic subsides with the release of endogenous opioids, which have been shown to accompany (if not cause) ventilatory collapse (Denavit-Saubie, Champagnat, & Zieglgansberger, 1978; Moss & Scarpelli, 1981).

If this model is correct, it explains the interrelationship between HV, graded hypoxia, and mood depression (Katz, 1982) as covariates of metabolic activity and perhaps in response to anaerobic and metabolic end-products. Respiratory changes in depression have been well documented (Burns, 1971; Damas-Mora et al., 1978; Shershow, Kanarek, & Kazemi, 1976). This model applies only to endogenous depression, although breathing changes have also been noted in depression associated with grief (Jellinek, Goldenheim, & Jenike, 1985). Thus, it is not surprising that the panic stage of this chronic arousal syndrome may be accompanied by the fear of death so frequently encountered in connection with panic disorder (Lazarus & Kostan, 1969). The individual is responding to the signals of asphyxia.

Pincus and Tucker (1974) suggested that HV is a universal reaction to anxiety, but panic is not. Panic may be viewed as the result of a chronic endogenous process of gradually increasing proximity to anoxia, typical of persons who are predisposed to compensate for chronic sympathetic arousal and the attendant graded hypoxia with respiratory alkalosis and hypocapnia.

A note on the concept of "proximity to anoxia" is warranted in the light of a recent description by Klein (1992) of the extrapolation of a hypothetical *suffocation detector* from his CO_2 sensitivity studies. According to Klein, a physiological suffocation monitor misfires in response to CO_2 hypersensitivity. The response of the suffocation detector leads to sudden respiratory distress followed by HV, panic, and the urge to flee. The fact notwithstanding, that I have found fault with some of the research methods and conclusions drawn by Klein, and his colleagues, I rather find this theory elegant. It fits many of the things we know about the physiology of panic. Gibbs (1992), and Mathew and Wilson (1992), recently demonstrated HV and reduced CBF in panic attacks. Basilar artery ischemia is an excellent mechanism for depriving the brain of its blood supply. The vertebral arteries join the basilar artery, which enters the Circle of Willis from the posterior, while the carotid arteries join it from the anterior. Reduced CBF causes a rapid brain lactic acid build-up (Meyers, 1979) which will cause HV. If HV follows cerebral ischemia, other factors being equal, what sets off sensor hypersensitivity to CO_2? This sequence suggests that the same sensors, presumably chemoreceptors, misbehave. On the other hand, it is perhaps more likely that HV causes constriction of the basilar artery setting off the sequence. This in no way reduces the merit of a putative suffocation detector. I alluded to such a mechanism in *The Hyperventilation Syndrome* (1987).

Hyperventilation and Agoraphobia

Leitenberg (1976) reported that the incidence of phobias is about 77 per thousand capita. About two per thousand phobias are disabling, the most common of these being agoraphobia, the fear of open places. Agoraphobics usually have great difficulty leaving their home and traveling. Leitenberg said of them: "anxiety with somatic and autonomic components is a major feature of this disorder. In addition, agoraphobics often have a fear of fainting, and losing control in public due to anticipated recurrent panic attacks. Approximately 50% to 60% of patients suffering from phobia have this syndrome" (p. 127).

The DSM-III-R lists agoraphobia with panic attacks (300.21) and agoraphobia without panic attacks (300.22). The disorder may feature avoidance of crowds, stores, tunnels, bridges, streets, elevators, and similar locations. The initial phase of the disorder consists frequently of recurrent panic attacks. But panic disorder is specifically indicated as not being associated with agoraphobia. Thus, panic attacks may or may not be a feature of agoraphobia, but agoraphobia is not a feature of panic attacks. What is the role of HV in agoraphobia?

According to Lowenstein (1968), agoraphobia has its origin in an episode of HV. Lum (1981) stated that of over 2000 persons with HV treated in his clinic, one quarter displayed phobic symptoms. Bonn, Readhead, and Timmons (1984) strongly supported the contention that HV plays a singularly crucial role in agoraphobia. They compared the effects of treatment in their agoraphobic clients by "real-life exposure," with and without breathing retraining. They concluded that improvement in the control of panic attacks increased in the group receiving the breathing retraining consisting of diaphragmatic breathing training at 8 to 10 breaths per minute. This is a standard method of training clients to correct HV, although it is not the most efficient.

Garssen, van Veenendaal, and Bloemink (1983) contended that there is a striking similarity between the panic attacks in agoraphobia and the attacks of the HVS. Despite evidence suggesting endogenous mechanisms, they explained HV as a "learned response to stressful life events." This makes little sense since HV is maladaptive, results in discomfort, and may jeopardize physiological adjustment to life stresses. I know of no conditioning model that such "learning" might fit. Bonn, Readhead, and

Timmons quite correctly admonished us for continuing to employ learning theory in assessing the etiology of agoraphobia. That HV might be a "learned response to stressful life events" fits neither a classical nor an instrumental conditioning model, nor does it fit a cognitive learning model. Even worse, it overlooks vast amounts of physiological data that clearly support the endogenous nature of this phenomenon (Carr & Sheehan, 1984).

Ley (1985a, 1985b) asked whether symptoms of HV-hypocapnia precede the fear expressed in panic, and if agoraphobics show HV breathing patterns. The answer to both of these questions is "yes." It is, therefore, reasonable to conclude that panic disorder, agoraphobia, and HVS share the same pathophysiology; and it is not unreasonable to suppose that HV may trigger panic attacks and/or agoraphobia. This hypothesis is bolstered because (a) HV is usually reported in panic attacks and in agoraphobia; (b) HV has been shown to precede these events; and (c) breathing retraining has a salutory effect on these disorders.

The Search for Traits

The psychophysiological symptoms of HVS seem to be consistently typical in particular individuals, and they seem to run in families. There is a consistency to the label "headache sufferer," just as there was to "anxiety neurotic" and "hysteric." We treat that consistency as though it were a trait, or type, and for good reason. When a client recently told me that tension "causes" his migraine, I explained to him that it is only because he is so predisposed. He argued that everyone knows that tension causes symptoms. I replied that it may well be true, but the symptoms do not vary at random. Furthermore, if he did not believe me, I proposed that as a homework assignment he convert his headaches to an ulcer, which is far less disruptive in the short run.

Consistent with the belief that there are "types," behavioral physiology, just like traditional psychometrics, depends on basic assumptions about which parameters it is important to observe and what the quantitative variations in observations represent. Many efforts in that direction have been published, ranging from the Pavlovian typology (Pavlov, 1928, 1950), to that of Eysenck (1970), Davis (1987), and more recently, the Type A personality (Friedman & Rosenman, 1969; Jenkins, 1971). But assessment in clinical psychophysiology should serve to determine both present physiological status and the likelihood of success of a given course of treatment.

A physiological profile is made up of simultaneous observations on a number of variables which singly, and in combination, establish and verify some aspect of local dysfunction or general arousal level. Such a profile is a functional evaluation and is the basis for diagnosis, treatment, and outcome prediction. Let's look at a subset of variables in this example. Suppose that a client is being treated for frequent moderate to severe panic attacks. $ETCO_2$ is 3.6% (27 torr); arterial blood O_2 saturation, SaO_2, is 99%; breathing is rapid and shallow, about 27 b/min; hand temperature is 78°F and head-apex temperature is 87°F, in a room at 80°F; pulse rate is 112 per minute, with no RSA evident.

Wouldn't you say that this is a fairly typical psychophysiological profile? It features all of the concomitants of compensated lactic acidosis: rapid breathing, hypocapnia, tachycardia, left-shifted ODC; peripheral vasoconstriction, and so on. Wouldn't you consider it a safe bet to predict that an EEG power spectrum with elevated *alpha* probably came from someone else? But the same information leads different clinicians to postulate different types. To some, this is a hysterical type with somatization, previously known as "conversion" disorder.

To me, this seems to be a person with severe chronic hypoxia and secondary anxiety and panic. Tachypnea (rapid breathing) and HV produce respiratory alkalosis to compensate for lactic acidosis. Cold hands indicate impaired peripheral circulation consistent with the vasoconstrictive effects of low arterial CO_2 ($PaCO_2$). Pulse is concomitantly rapid. No wonder this client is anxious. I like to think of this conclusion as *rational attribution* (RAT). If your body is "out of synch," you may feel anxious. How do you feel when you have the flu? Miserable and depressed, right? In fact, it often seems that you will never get well again.

In the case of the flu, however, you know the cause of your misery. But if you don't even know that you have a disorder (e.g., anemia, thyroid dysfunction, hypoglycemia, etc.), you may attribute the way you feel to prevailing stressors: emotional or other psychological problems. That may be an *irrational attribution* (IRAT), based on correlation, and may not be valid. It is often helpful in therapy to identify IRATs (Fried & Golden, 1989).

In most persons, HV is not readily detectable without a CO_2 detector (capnometer): The classic "hysterical" overventilator puffing into a paper bag is a textbook fantasy, rare as the *emmetropic eye*. Isn't that why some practitioners employ the HV-challenge? They wouldn't need it if they had a capnometer. That is also why symptom assessment figures so mightily in the effort to identify persons whose symptoms may be HV-related (Freeman, Conway, & Nixon, 1986; Grossman & DeSwart, 1984; Huey & West, 1983; Nixon & Freeman, 1988; van Dixhoorn & Duivenvoorden, 1985, 1986).

Paradoxically, it is precisely those investigators who are equipped for capnometry to measure alveolar PCO_2 who have been foremost in developing HV symptom rating scales. These investigators are most aware of the need to clearly identify HV where an otherwise disparate set of symptoms has led to controversy over diagnosis. Though perhaps the most common, HV is only one of the reasons why a capnometer is essential in psychophysiology—not just respiratory psychophysiology. Idiopathic HV typically entails only a relatively small decrease in alveolar CO_2 (PCO_2), as observed in end-tidal CO_2 ($ETCO_2$). Commonly encountered organic disorders such as hypertension, diabetes, and kidney and heart disease, where metabolic acidosis may play a role, typically present with far lower $ETCO_2$.

Another client who sought my help had heart disease that soon proved fatal. The client was very agitated, nervous, and engaged in much sighing and chest heaving. The capnograph indicated severe hypocapnia, (i.e., $ETCO_2$ as low as 18 torr). I declined to teach her to relax because to do so might, in my opinion, have jeopardized acid-base homeostasis. I don't believe that one is likely to encounter Kussmaul breathing (see the following section), a symptom of metabolic acidosis (such as keto acidosis, or lactic acidosis) in psychogenic HV.

Metabolic Acidosis in HV and Panic Attacks

Another client was recently referred to me with severe and frequent panic disorder with agoraphobia. Resting breathing rate was 27 to 31 b/min, $ETCO_2$ was frequently below 24 torr, and SaO_2, measured by earlobe transducer, ranged between 89% and 93%. Breathing was of the Kussmaul type: exaggerated chest-heaving often called hyperpnea, or total HV (Shapiro, Harrison, & Walton, 1982). The client was cyanotic (bluish), with spasmophilic tremors (alkalotic muscular hypercalcemia [Durlach, 1969]). There was agitation and, in the vernacular, hysteria. Although he was quite clearly a fairly typical severe panic sufferer, there was an additional clue to the etiology of the complaints which no one seemed to consider relevant: severe anorexia. The little food the client ate consisted almost exclusively of milk products.

Breathing was, clearly, compensatory for fasting ketoacidosis. A referral to a physician was made, and hospitalization for observation followed. Routine blood tests, none that would have revealed the condition, were performed in the hospital and the client was discharged in the care of a psychiatrist for treatment of emotional hysteria. From there, the client slid between the cracks, as they say.

More commonly, lactic acidosis is the culprit in so-called psychogenic idiopathic HV; one doesn't hyperventilate to that degree without organic basis—as in a "bad breathing habit," or "hysteria." The connection between HV and hysteria is based on the encrusted presumption of typology. The hysterical type, usually thought to be a woman, hyperventilates when anxious: "They are just like that, don't you know," or are the "neurotic type." This is the basis for the concept of psychogenic HV, an armchair concept for which there is not a shred of scientific evidence.

Lactic acidosis is actually quite a common occurrence. Lactic acid is produced in the muscles and the brain, and production in muscle is drastically accelerated whenever there is an O_2 deficit (i.e., less O_2 is available than is required to supply energy needs). Lactic acidosis is, therefore, a hypoxic phenomenon (Katz, 1982) and can be, in the extreme case, the final pathway in any disorder that results in respiratory and circulatory collapse.

When blood flow to peripheral tissues is so diminished that O_2 delivery is not sufficient to meet metabolic demand, mitochondrial activity is impaired and ATP concentrations fall. The enzyme *phosphofructokinase* (PKF) is activated to speed up glycogen breakdown and glucose oxidation. This accelerated glycolysis leads to overproduction of pyruvic acid which reduces to lactic acid (Cohen & Woods, 1976; Huckabee, 1961; Kreisberg, 1980; Park & Arief, 1980). In the absence of hypoxia, lactate is transported in the bloodstream to the liver, where it is converted to glucose.

Huckabee (1961) proposes two subtypes of lactic acidosis: (a) non-hypoxic, with proportionate increase in lactate and pyruvate; and (b) hypoxic, with lactate disproportionately elevated in comparison to pyruvate. But Cohen and Woods (1976) prefer classification of excess lactate by symptoms, rather than by lactate/pyruvate levels, because blood pyruvate levels are unusually low and unstable. Cohen and Woods (1976) distinguish type A, with poor tissue O_2 perfusion and oxygenation from type B, with elevated blood lactate level in the absence of diminished tissue O_2 perfusion, and acidosis ranging from mild to severe. Type B includes that resulting from thiamine deficiency, and metabolic or respiratory alkalosis.

The average biofeedback practitioner, psychotherapist, or "breathing trainer" cannot be expected to evaluate type and degree of metabolic acidosis in a client. But by understanding the physiology of respiratory drive, she or he may strike such ludicrous concepts as hysterical overbreathing from the vocabulary and go on with the practice of clinical psychophysiology.

The Controversy over Lactate versus CO_2 Sensitivity in Panic Disorder: A Squabble over Types?

Here is a brief overview of the lactate/CO_2-panic-disorder debacle intended to expose the fits and starts of the search for a type that integrates physiology and psychology. In 1967, Pitts and McClure wrote that "excessive lactate production in standard exercise in patients with anxiety neurosis" was reported in four studies world-wide. In fact, under the names "effort syndrome," "neurasthenia," "circulatory asthenia," "cardiac neurosis," and "DaCosta's syndrome," as well as "anxiety neurosis," this phenomenon was reported in several hundred publications, in which many argued that these diagnostic categories were all actually the same thing, that is, HVS. But maintaining that they are different permitted the theory of an organic-type as opposed to a mental-type. A physiological basis for effort syndrome would point to an organic etiology for anxiety neurosis, making it a medical type, whereas, if classified a hysterical symptom, it would be a mental or psychological trait. Pitts and McClure's article in the *New England Journal of Medicine* is also notable for its selective myopia. Of the countless references relevant to this study, they cited just 11, including two on "circulatory asthenia." One was a statistics text I once assigned to my college undergraduates! There is not one single reference to hyperventilation in that Pitts and McClure article. Is it possible that they never heard of it? Not likely. Kerr, Dalton, and Gliebe published their classic study in 1937; Brown, in 1953; Engel, Ferris, and Logan, in 1947; Gliebe and Auerback, in 1944; Lewis, in 1957; and Meyer and Gotoh, in 1960. It may also be noted that "dyspnea," "smothering," "sighing," and "choking," appear in the list of symptoms in the Pitts and McClure article—4 out of 21 symptoms are directly breathing-related.

Was HV omitted because Pitts and McClure simply didn't believe it existed? Perhaps they were geared up to give the symptoms of anxiety an organic etiology, and HV and anxiety are symptoms of "hysteria" (Lowry, 1967), a psychiatric entity. Paradoxically, they cite Cohen and White (1950) who coauthored a number of excellent studies which do refer to effort syndrome and neurocirculatory asthenia. Effort syndrome had already been attributed to excess lactate well before Pitts and McClure published in 1967 (DeJours, 1964).

If you look at an article by Wheeler, White, Reed, and Cohen (1950) ("Neurocirculatory asthenia [anxiety neurosis, effort syndrome, neurasthenia]," *JAMA*, 142:878–889), you will find on the bottom of the first page (albeit in very small print):

Cohen, M.E., Consolazio, F.C., & Johnson, R.E. (1947) Blood lactate response during moderate exercise in neurocirculatory asthenia, anxiety neurosis or effort syndrome. *Journal of Clinical Investigation*, 26:339. (p. 878)

No reference is made by Pitts and McClure to this publication in one of the most highly respected journals; and despite the title it is obviously not one of the four studies they managed to find. The breathing-related symptoms might have been an impetus to look at another reference just below the one just cited:

Cohen, M.E., Johnson, R.E., Consolazio, F.C., & White (1946) Low oxygen consumption and low ventilatory efficiency during exhausting work in patients with neurocirculatory asthenia, effort syndrome, anxiety neurosis. *Journal of Clinical Investigation*, 25:292. (p. 878)

From the title alone, you would surmise that persons with this disorder have impaired metabolism. Isn't that what causes excessive lactate? But so narrow is their focus that they show no recognition of the connection.

Then, in 1974, Ackerman and Sachar criticized Pitts and McClure on methodological grounds and concluded that:

. . . alterations in acid-base balance and/or endogenous lactate elevation and/or a fall in serum calcium are not themselves necessary or sufficient conditions for the development of anxiety states. (p. 72)

It's not medical; it's not hysteria; it's conditioning! Ackerman and Sachar proposed an alternate hypothesis:

The anxiety neurotic, relieved of his physical symptoms, quickly extinguishes such learned secondary behavioral manifestations as phobic avoidance of crowded places with the aid of supportive psychotherapy. (p. 75) (their italics)

After some time pondering the meaning of "extinguish with the aid of," I gave up. Then, along came Gorman et al. (1984): Yes, it is excess lactate (as evidenced by the reaction to its increase by infusion) that causes panic after all—it is medical. It has the same physiology as HV, but it is not HV:

The role of hyperventilation in the pathogenesis of anxiety disorder is much speculated on but poorly understood. A familiar sight in the emergency room is a patient furiously breathing into a brown paper bag to abort an episode of psychogenic hyperventilation. (p. 857)

Now, if everyone is aware of the controversy centering on "the role of hyperventilation in the pathogenesis of anxiety disorder," how come it is so rarely cited? In 42 citations, Ackerman and Sacher (1974) cite only one report directly concerned with the connection between HV and lactate (Edwards, R.H.T. & Clode, M. [1970] The effect of hyperventilation on lactic acedemia of muscular exercise. *Clinical Science*, 8:269–276). Gorman et al. (1984) do not even cite that one. If, according to Gorman et al., endogenous lactate sensitivity leading to panic attacks is not of the hypoxia type, as evidenced by HV, what is it due to? Their answer: sensitivity of the *locus ceruleus*—yet a new type. But now, in 1986, they state in the last paragraph of their report that:

The weight of evidence provided herein indicates that hyperventilation is an integral part of an acute panic attack and that respiratory alkalosis dominates metabolic acidosis during lactate infusion and lactate-induced panic. Further work aimed at defining the nature of ventilatory physiology is warranted. (p. 1071)

So it is HV after all? That same old HV, symptomatic of hysteria? Oh no! A new, improved HV; not hysteria at all, but a physiological phenomenon of the acid-base balance. So, excess endogenous or exogenous lactate causes panic, according to these investigators, and HV is secondary . . . to what? Why would HV be thought to be secondary to a condition—lactic acidemia—known to cause it. In any case, the only condition that HV could be secondary to is hypoxia, a concomitant of lactic acidemia. This would have been a good time for them to fill in the gaps in the "false suffocation alarms" theory. Cerebral lactic acidemia is certainly an early step in the path that leads to reduced CBF by HV-induced brain vascular ischemia. They did not take that step.

Margraf et al. (1986) do not exactly see the matter resolved either, and the ubiquitous methodological problems crop up again. This time, it is not conditioning, but cognitive factors that interact with lactate sensitivity. And to further confuse the picture, Woods, Charney, Loke, et al. (1986) claim that panic is due to none of the above, but to CO_2 sensitivity. An interesting construct—in fact, a conundrum.

We infer that a person is more sensitive to one stimulus than another by response magnitude (i.e., latency, duration, amplitude, and frequency). We've abandoned perceptual traits in favor of physiological response types, from classifying the perceiver to classifying the responder (Albright, Andreassi, & Steiner, 1988; Braithwaite, 1987; Friedman & Rosenman, 1969; Jenkins, 1978; Juszczak & Andreassi, 1987; King, Bayon, Clark, & Taylor, 1988; Kopp & Koranyi, 1982; Lobel, 1988a,b; Schalling, Asberg, Edman, & Orland, 1987; Singh, 1984). And this is central to contemporary concepts of types or traits in clinical psychophysiology and in behavioral medicine.

Then in 1988, Gorman et al. published "Ventilatory physiology of patients with panic disorder," cited in Chapter 2 in connection with its "methodological problems." The last statement of their abstract merits special attention:

> Patients with panic disorder may have hypersensitive CO_2 receptors that, when triggered, evoke a subjective panic associated with an exaggerated ventilatory response and consequent hypocapnic alkalosis. (p. 31)

If not HV, then what is "exaggerated ventilatory response and consequent hypocapnic alkalosis?" As Shakespeare put it:

> What's in a name? That which we call a rose
> By any other name would smell as sweet. . . .
> (Romeo & Juliet, act II, scene II)

One possible explanation is that "hyperventilation" is still not entirely *kosher*, whereas "CO_2 sensitivity" is so scientific, so organic. This report seems to be a turning point in their thinking, for here, if I am not mistaken, is the germination of the "hypersensitive CO_2" component of their false suffocation alarm theory. By 1989, every effort to link HV to panic attacks was abandoned in favor of "CO_2 hypersensitivity." They unwittingly reinvented the wheel (see Meduna [1958], *Carbon Dioxide Therapy* [Charles C. Thomas]). There is nothing new under the sun, as they say; this is a most remarkable book, way ahead of its time. I can't be the only one who's read it.

The most amazing thing about this last publication by Papp, Goetz, Cole, Klein, Jordan, Liebowitz, Fyer, Hollander, and Gorman (1989) is its numerous disclaimers: Referring to previous studies, especially the "ventilatory physiology" study, which I reviewed in Chapter 2, they state that: "These studies, however, were confounded by inherent and technical and design problems. . . . we did not control for a number of psychological factors . . . known to affect CO_2 sensitivity." Never mind, it got published anyway!

Types of Physiological Assessment

Strong precedent in introductory psychology textbooks virtually mandates at least a passing reference to Kretchmer, Lombroso, and Sheldon's somatotypes. More advanced texts detail Pavlov, Eysenck, and now Jenkins. Typology has an illustrious past, and it deserves a bright future. Valid typology reduces predictive error; and in psychophysiology, it clarifies reasonable expectations of treatment outcome.

Pavlov: Excitation and Inhibition. According to Pavlov (1928) (Koshtoyants, 1950), behavior has "boundless variety." But because of its control by the nervous system, variety reduces to basic properties with "combinations and gradations." Using the method of conditioned reflexes, it was determined that the properties include (a) the strength of nervous system processes (i.e., excitation and inhibition which constitute the sum-total of nervous activity); (b) the equilibrium of these processes; and (c) their mobility. In addition, behavior has plasticity which means that various combinations of the properties are modified by conditioning (learning).

But it was evident from the start that dogs on whom the conditioning experiments were carried out differed. Some were "bold," others "cowardly." The bold ate at once when fed, while the others required days, in some cases weeks, to become accustomed to the procedure. In the bold dogs, conditioned reflexes developed rapidly, remaining constant across procedures, whereas in the cowardly, they formed slowly, requiring many repetitions, and remaining unstable.

It seemed that in the bold dogs, excitation is strong, while in the cowardly, it is weak. Strong excitation resists minor influences; weak excitation cannot overcome less important prevailing conditions. The result is external inhibition. It was initially thought that these dogs with weak excitation (i.e., strong inhibition) had a "weak type of nervous system." But by split/litter method (one half raised in a kennel, the other half given complete freedom), it was determined that in the more hazardous environment, natural caution and results of exploration increase inhibitory action to *any* new stimulus.

Another property of the central nervous system subdivided the dogs into two groups in accordance with excitation and "higher active cortical inhibition," by which is meant internal inhibition. In dogs with a strong excitatory process, positive conditioned reflexes are formed rapidly; inhibitory reflexes elaborate slowly and with obvious difficulty:

> When we subject the cortical inhibition in such animals to severe strain by means of very delicate differentiation, or by a frequent or protracted application of difficult inhibitors, their nervous system becomes fully, or almost fully, deprived of the inhibitory function; real neuroses set in, typical and chronic nervous diseases, which must be treated either by . . . a long rest . . . complete discontinuance . . . or by giving bromide. (p. 321)

Since the first property of the nervous system is excitation, animals are divided into strong and weak types. Another property is the preponderance of excitation and inhibition, with strong animals subdivided into equilibrated and unequilibrated. There exist a number of elaborations of the conditioning typology of Pavlov, integrating cortical excitation and inhibition with personality theory, with the object of determining the physiological basis of personality as well as therapy outcome in clinical populations.

If there are types based on conditionability, which differ in the rapidity of ANS and other learning, the stability, or retention, of the learning may depend on selecting the appropriate reinforcement strategy. This is a matter of considerable practical importance in predicting biofeedback/self-regulation treatment outcome. One such trait approach is that of H. J. Eysenck in which introversion–extraversion, a horizontal (X) dimension, is bisected by hysteria-anxiety, a vertical (Y) coordinate, to form quadrants in which one locates diagnostic categories.

Extraversion, neuroticism, and conditionability. Typically, the extravert (E), as opposed to the introvert (I), is outgoing, uninhibited, impulsive, and sociable, whereas neuroticism (N) is general emotional overresponsiveness and liability to neurotic breakdown under stress (Eysenck & Eysenck, 1968). Persons with high N-scores tend to have vague somatic complaints.

A high positive correlation was found between the Maudsley Personality Inventory (MPI), and the Eysenck Personality Inventory, which preceded it. It was found that dysthymic neurotics (i.e., those with anxiety, reactive depression, obsessive-compulsive behavior, phobias, etc.) tend to score high on E and low on N (neurotic introverts); and psychopaths score high on N and high on E (neurotic extraverts).

According to Eysenck and Eysenck (1968), neurotic introverts are oversocialized, while neurotic extraverts are undersocialized. The significance of these personality traits in the context of a behavioral clinical approach to treatment is that since introverts (anxiety neurotics) are said to have strong excitation and weak inhibition, while extraverts (psychopaths) have weak excitation and strong inhibition, introverts can be expected to be conditioned better than extraverts (Franks, 1957; Fried, Welch, & Friedman, 1967; Vogel, 1961). Better adjustment is not associated with high conditionability (N), but with above-average extraversion.

Type A Personality, the Jenkins Activity Survey, Braithwaite's Scale of Emotional Arousability, and $ETCO_2$. Another morphological approach to type and prediction was taken by Jenkins (1979) on the basis of Friedman and Rosenman's "Type A Personality" (1969). The Jenkins Activity Survey (JAS) is intended to assess coronary-prone behavior in terms of life-style activities which include extremes of competitiveness, striving to achieve, aggressiveness, impatience, haste, restlessness, and a feeling of time-pressure.

The Type A, coronary-prone individual differs from other persons who suffer anxiety depression and stress (Zyzanski, Jenkins, Ryan, Flessas, & Everist, 1976). For instance, Williams, Lane, Kuhn, Melosh, White, and Schanberg (1982) reported that compared to Type B, Type A male college students show "qualitatively distinct patterns of neuroendocrine responses" during mental work and sensory intake tasks. They were observed to have greater muscle vasodilation and enhanced secretion of norepinephrine, epinephrine, and cortisol; Albright, Andreassi, and Steiner (1988) also report cardiovascular differentiation of Type A persons. But the idea that Type A and B may be subsets of those who suffer stress and/or anxiety may be more apparent than real. If we interpret the research literature on the spirogram in mental disorders, we might conclude that Type A is a coronary type, while the "anxiety neurotic" is a ventilatory type. In Type A persons, stress-related increased blood levels of catecholamines reduce systemic blood flow and the resultant ischemic hypoxia corrodes the heart and coronary arteries. In the neurotic anxiety sufferers, the same process reduces cerebral blood flow and alters neurotransmitter biosynthesis.

Braithwaite (1987) developed the *Scale of Emotional Arousability* (SEA) to focus more specifically on physiological arousal than either the EPI or the JAS. Braithwaite's scale aims to measure neuroticism and is, therefore, more consistent with Eysenck's trait theory. It would be interesting to see if Type A's fall to the right or the left of the neuroticism intercept on the introversion–extraversion scale of the EPI. The average American college student did circa 1960 (Bendig, 1960).

Is there a direct connection to breathing? If higher breathing rate has a psychological or anxiety/stress component, one would certainly expect that it would show up as lower $ETCO_2$ in persons with increased anxiety or arousal. That is exactly what Fox (1991) found. As predicted, high scores on the JAS, which is not specific to stress or anxiety, did not identify persons with lower $ETCO_2$, while EPI and SEA scores showed significant negative correlation with $ETCO_2$.

Anxiety neurotics seem to have the lion's share of HV. As a practical matter, they are the mainstay of clinical practice. They are numerous, condition readily, adjust poorly, and have disordered breathing of a type that heightens their symptoms.

Chapter 8

Behavioral Treatment and Control of Breathing in Physiotherapeutic, Yogic, and Relaxation Methods

Introduction

Assessment and treatment methods in this chapter are those common in rehabilitation medicine and relaxation techniques, and are frequently used in the control of chronic, irreversible breathing problems. They are, in many instances, similar to yogic breathing practices, from which many have been derived. Chapter 9 details recently developed self-regulatory (biofeedback) methods.

Physiotherapeutic Breathing Techniques

Rehabilitation medicine and pulmonary physiology have had a considerable impact on the knowledge of the effects of HV and its treatment. L.C. Lum (1975, 1976, 1978–1979, 1981, 1983), a noted British thoracic surgeon and pulmonary physiologist, has reported the treatment of several thousand persons with HV and HV-related symptoms. In 1981, he recommended abdominal breathing retraining and reported that his clients were typically trained by professional respiratory physiotherapists (personal communication, 1983).

This is entirely appropriate, since physiatry is typically concerned with chest disease and physiology but not necessarily with "hands-on" treatment. The professionals who train patients in rehabilitation institutions are nurses, physical therapists (physiotherapists), and respiratory therapists, who most often work with clients who suffer from chronic obstructive pulmonary disease (COPD), including emphysema and cystic fibrosis. A variety of exercises were developed for these patients which include medication, relaxation exercises, inhalation therapy, and in many cases diaphragmatic breathing, as an important adjunct to other interventions and therapy (Haas, Pineda, Haas, & Axen, 1979).

Sinclair (cited in Basmajian, 1978) suggested the following:

Diaphragmatic respiration. We now come to the most controversial aspect of breathing exercises, the teaching of voluntary control of diaphragmatic or abdominal respiration. This is regarded as important in virtually all clinics, though with some differences in emphasis.

The patient is shown that the outline of his abdomen barely changes during respiration because of the abnormal mechanics of his movements, while his upper thoracic movement is accentuated.

Exercise to overcome this abnormal breathing pattern is best begun with the patient lying down, with bent knees supported by pillows, his hands resting on his lower front ribs. Attention is given first to the upper rib movement; he practices suppression of this until in quiet breathing it subsides toward a normal level. He then concentrates on abdominal movements, until his abdomen relaxes and distends in inspiration and tenses and retracts during expiration, which is usually taught to last up to twice as long as inspiration [presumably to conserve CO_2]. He practices prolonging expiration until he can exhale for ten to fifteen seconds without losing control of his next inspiration, which should not be associated with gasping or with upper chest movement.

Diaphragmatic expiration is encouraged during other body maneuvers. The patient may sit on a stool or chair, his feet apart and his arms relaxed. He leans forward as he expires, until his head is near or between his knees; at the same time he firmly contracts his abdominal muscles. He slowly uncoils during inspiration.

Next, the patient lies on his back with knees drawn up, draws one knee up to his chin during expiration and lowers it again during inspiration. This is repeated first with the other knee, then with both knees being lifted together. The shoulders and arms are relaxed.

By this stage, the patient should appear to control his breathing in relaxed positions so that there is much more normal abdominal movement and much less upper thoracic movement. He is now taught to maintain this breathing pattern while sitting or standing and during some of the bending swinging exercises practiced previously for relaxation. (pp. 581–582)

Haas, Pineda, Haas, and Axen (1979) suggested the following:

The basic exercise is done initially in the supine position and the right and left fetal positions. The patient is instructed to place his left hand on the thoracic cage just below the clavicle as a guide to limit excursion of the rib cage, thus emphasizing diaphragmatic breathing. His right hand is placed on the abdomen over the umbilicus. The patient is then instructed to inhale deeply through the nose, making an effort to push and distend his anterior abdominal wall outward, and then to exhale slowly and steadily through pursed lips while pushing his abdomen inward and upward. The movement of his hands will tell him if he is doing the exercise properly or not. If the hand on his abdomen moves up during inspiration, he is working correctly; if the hand on his chest moves, then he is inspiring using thoracic muscles instead of the diaphragm. Prolonged (pursed lip) expiration, optimally twice the inspiration duration, should be emphasized. (p. 129)

With some differences in emphasis, such as nasal breathing, most diaphragmatic breathing exercises are similar. They may be tailored to different body positions and activity levels, but they generally emphasize awareness of both abdominal and thoracic movement (excursions) and a deliberate control of the muscles affecting those motions.

Yogic Breathing Methods

Many methods describing the control of muscle tension and other discomfort accompanying chronic ANS arousal center on altering the degree of muscle tone by various means include breathing control methods invariably derived from yogic exercises, such as transcendental meditation (TM) or Zen (Zazen). These methods were incorporated into "behavioral medicine" or, more aptly, "behavioral physiology."

The origin of TM and other yogic methods of meditation may be traced to ancient Eastern cultural and religious practice (Lysebeth, 1979; Mahesh, 1963; Ramacharaka, 1905; Tohei, 1976). They teach breathing through the nose, rather than through the mouth, and abdominal breathing in a slow and rhythmic pattern, rather than chest breathing. The yogi follower believes that this form of breathing will facilitate the flow of an exogenous energy, called *prana* in India and *Qi* (pronounced chee) in China. But incorporation of TM as well as other yogic techniques into modern relaxation exercises is a matter of pragmatism, totally unrelated to the perception of benefits from this hypothetical energy flow.

In the West, we believe that these methods have empirically verified effects on hypertension, anxiety, and stress, especially in persons in whom these conditions are chronic. Consequently, they are included in many programs recommended by conventional medical practitioners as adjuncts to pharmacological and psychiatric therapeutics (Benson, 1975; Glueck & Stroebel, 1975; Stroebel, 1982). These methods also facilitate deep muscle relaxation, which inhibits anxiety (Jacobson, 1934, 1935; Wolpe, 1958, 1969; Wolpe & Lazarus, 1966).

TM came into vogue in psychotherapy and stress-management strategies of the 1960s because it was found to have salutary effects on a variety of disorders, including hypertension, migraine, Raynaud's disease, irritable bowel syndrome, colitis, and asthma (Badawi, Wallace, Orme-Johnson, & Rouzere, 1984; Beary, Benson, & Klemchuk, 1974; Benson, Beary, & Carol, 1974; Benson, Rosner, Marzetta, & Klemchuck, 1974; Blackwell, Bloomfield, Gartside, Robinson, Hanenson, Magenheim, Nidich, & Zigler, 1976; Carrington, 1984; Datey, Deshmukh, Dalvi, & Vinekar, 1969; Dudley, Holmes, Martin, & Ripley, 1964; Elson, Hauri, & Cunis, 1977; Glueck & Stroebel, 1975; Kanellakos & Lukas, 1974; Orme-Johnson & Farrows, 1977; Ornstein, 1972; Pelletier, 1977; Schwartz & Beatty, 1977; Shapiro, 1982, 1985; Stone & Deleo, 1976; Stroebel & Glueck, 1977; Wallace, 1970, 1972; Wallace, Benson & Wilson, 1971; West, 1979; Wolkove, Kreisman, Darragh, Cohen, & Frank, 1984; Woolfolk, 1975). But some clinicians who studied the benefits of TM held that it was not significantly better than resting (Holmes, 1984), or deep muscle relaxation as taught by Jacobson (1935) and by Wolpe (1969) (Lehrer, Woolfolk, Rooney, McCann, & Carrington, 1983; Morse, Martin, Furst, & Dubin, 1977; Travis, Kondo, & Knott, 1976).

TM differs from other passive meditative techniques. The meditator focuses his/her thoughts on a mantra; no other instructions are given. In *Shavasan*, the meditator is supine, lower limbs at a 30° angle, arms at a 45° angle to the trunk; the forearms are in midprone position, and the fingers are semiflexed; eyes are closed, with the lids drooping. Slow diaphragmatic breathing is taught, with a short pause after each inspiration and a longer pause at the end of each expiration. The meditator is then instructed to focus on the sensations at the nostrils (the coolness of the inspired air and the warmth of the expired air). Finally, she or he is instructed to feel the heaviness of different parts of the body (Datey et al., 1969).

Zen is another form of meditation. It is practiced in the *lotus* or *semilotus* position, with attention focused on breathing. When the meditator has mastered attention to aspects of breathing, she or he is given a "riddle" on which to meditate (Woolfolk, 1975). Benson and colleagues (1974a) extracted many elements from these techniques and developed a method that is said to produce a "relaxation response."

All yogic techniques have certain outcomes, including reduction of O_2 consumption; reduction of CO_2 expulsion; no change in respiratory quotient (ratio of O_2 in to CO_2 out); reduction in respiration rate; reduction in Vmin; change in power spectral composition of the EEG (decreased mean *theta* and *beta*, increased and coherent *alpha*); and change in state of arousal and awareness. It is because of its effects on breathing that these techniques are useful in the control of HV.

Transcendental Meditation

In 1957, Das and Gastaut undertook the study of the effects of meditation. Their equivocal findings have been attributed to the primitive conditions under which their studies were, of necessity, conducted. But their report of EEG, ECG, and muscle tension in meditation opened up the study of the physiological correlates of states of consciousness. The psychology paradigm for the study of "states" is to compare unknown and uncharted states with relatively unknown and uncharted states. For instance, take the phrase "Hypnosis is like sleep." It is, of course not like sleep (Evans, 1977), but it looks more like sleep than a waking state. Then we have "meditation is like deep muscle relaxation," which it is also nothing like. For one thing, meditation can result in suspension of breathing (Badawi et al., 1984; Farrow & Hebert, 1982).

What is TM? It is the process of focusing on a thought or word (mantra) until attention transcends its common meaning, and its subtler and deeper meanings emerge. It is predicated on a belief that, when the subtler meanings of thought are perceived, one then experiences the subtler aspects of life itself (Mahesh, 1963). In TM, it is held that *prana*, the cosmic vibratory energy of the universe, connects the votary to transcendental existence, where all subtle meanings of thoughts and being exist; and that this is established through the adoption of a "state" during which slow, rhythmic nasal and abdominal breathing (*pranayama*) prevails. TM, unlike other yogic methods, does not teach breathing, which changes due to meditation. In TM, breathing is not guided. One should do nothing to interfere with breathing, but simply allow it to reach *prana* through the process of meditation on the mantra.

A number of psychophysiological changes have been noted in TM, including slower breathing; lower ventilation volume (Vmin), heart rate, and blood pressure; and change in the EEG power spectrum, with an increase in the *alpha* band and transient *theta* (4 to 7 Hz) (Badawi et al., 1984; Elson, Hauri, & Cunis, 1977; Shapiro, 1982; Woolfolk, 1975). Benson, Beary, and Carol (1974) report a hypometabolic state.

But TM does, indeed, change breathing. Allison (1970) reported that breathing becomes slow and shallow during TM, with the rate dropping to about half of normal (i.e., six breaths per minute). Davidson and Schwartz (1976) highlighted breathing change during TM, as well as muscle tension, concluding on the basis of a number of studies (in particular, Timmons, 1982) that:

> . . . it appears that the amplitude of the abdominal and thoracic respiratory movements can covary with shifts in arousal and level of muscle tension. It should be noted

that the above measures do not, in fact, reflect respiratory rate, but rather indicate the relative contribution of abdominal and thoracic components. (p. 406)

It is not clear whether the deep muscle relaxation observed in TM accompanies, precedes, or follows a change in respiration to a primarily abdominal mode. I have observed that *simply slowing* chest breathing to about 10 to 12 breaths per minute can be uncomfortable for most trainees.

It is not surprising that slowing breathing coincides with a shift to abdominal breathing. I have observed this spontaneous shift repeatedly and I am at a loss to explain it. But, being practical, I would not permit this ambiguity to prevent the adoption of TM as a method of effecting breathing control in chronic HV, especially where monitoring of alveolar ventilation is not available. It still remains to be seen whether TM offers more than deep muscle relaxation.

How does TM compare with other methods, such as Jacobson's progressive relaxation? Lehrer et al. (1983) reported comparing their psychophysiological and therapeutic outcomes, and concluded that progressive relaxation seems to be a more effective therapeutic tool than TM. But their conclusion does not emphasize the special role of breathing in TM:

Because the experience in our laboratory has shown that Ss often spontaneously link their mantras with breathing, an attempt was made to restrict awareness of breathing to its effects to a limited facial area. Thus, during the fourth weekly meeting, rather than saying their mantras to themselves, the Ss were instructed to count their breaths (on exhalation) from 1 to 10, while focusing on air movement sensations at the tip of the nose. The instructions specifically did not, however, advise or train the Ss to alter their breathing in any way, as is commonly done in various "controlled-breathing meditative exercises." (p. 645)

Instruction to do anything other than repeat the mantra violates TM procedure, and the effect of changing the instructions to subjects concerning their breathing is not known.

Although there is considerable evidence that TM affects breathing in a way that would be beneficial in chronic HV, I have not adopted it in my treatment program. First, it does not appeal to many clients; and second, it is a fairly lengthy process requiring a level of patience that many "stress" clients do not have. Finally, generalization of TM to a level of activity not characterized by "focus on the subtler aspect of thought" (Mahesh, 1963) has not been established.

I prefer to help clients adopt a state of alert and wakeful relaxation unless sleeping is their main problem. Many fear that relaxation will make them less effective in their daily routine and occupation.

Modified Yogic Breathing Methods

TM alters breathing without direct instructions. There are other forms of yogic exercise, and some of these do control or guide breathing, often by developing self-awareness of the breathing process and modifying it in specific ways. In the next sections, I present breathing exercises without particular reference to the philosophies which they embody. They constitute, in composite, that body of techniques from which a set was chosen for use in connection with biofeedback of the percentage of end-tidal CO_2 ($PETCO_2$), as described in the next chapter. They share self-awareness of breathing and its attendant sensations; nasal breathing (as compared with oral); and rhythmic, slow abdominal (as compared with thoracic) breathing.

Many of the *nouveau* deep muscle relaxation exercises now incorporate some kind of breathing instructions. For instance, Fair (1983) proposed the following modification of Bernstein and Borkovec's (1973) instructions for home practice:

> Now take a deep breath and hold it—just notice that for a moment. Notice the pressure. Feel the sensation in your chest. And, now gradually relax and let the air flow out. Allow your whole body to begin to relax as you breathe out. Allow your breathing to become relaxed and rhythmical. (p. 187)

It may be useful to specify that a moment is a count of two, as in "Just hold it. One, two. Good." And it is assumed that the person has been instructed in abdominal breathing. But basically, this is a distillation of the genre of meditation-derived breathing instructions. It is important to teach the client that rhythm means timing. The hectic inner state of the chronically aroused is not amenable to smooth, rhythmic, slow breathing activity, as shown by van Dixhoorn and Duivenvoorden (1986).

Breathing through the Nose

Ballentine (1979) summarized much of what is known of the nasal cycle. There is a consistent shift in laterality in nasal breathing; as the tissues in one nostril swell, those in the other nostril recede (Keuning, 1968). This cycle alternates about every one and three-quarter hours. This is the infradian cycle where air flow increases in the nostril in which the mucosa is least swollen.

There is a complex set of physiological and cognitive changes that is said to accompany the predominance of right or left nostril breathing, including cerebral lateral dominance (Beubel & Shannahoff-Khalsa, 1987; Klein, Pilton, Prossner, & Shannahoff-Khalsa, 1986; Prohovnik & Risberg, 1979; Werntz, Bickford, & Shannahoff-Khalsa, 1987). We need to be aware of this cycle as we train clients to breathe through the nose. Training someone in nasal breathing typically consists of directing him or her to focus on the sensations created by air flowing through the nostrils and of determining which nostril is dominant and open at any given moment. It would go something like this:

> Place your left index finger lightly over your left nostril—press with enough force to close it, but not more. Breathe through your right nostril. Now repeat this with your right index finger on your right nostril: Press and breathe through your left nostril. Notice that air flows more smoothly through one nostril than the other. Which one? That one is your dominant nostril.

This alternating right and left nostril breathing is called a round. Each yoga master has a favorite number of rounds (between three and five) to recommend. The process of alternate nasal breathing is called *Nadi Shodhanam*. It should be performed slowly and gently, with no strain in its performance; breath should make no sound. There are variations, some relatively complex, but its main feature is to make the trainee aware of the sensations of nasal breathing. It also gives the clinician the chance to determine whether the client can actually breathe through the nose—some have obstruction, swelling, and, rarely, serious deviation of the septum. But most important, it illustrates for the client that, typically, one cannot easily hyperventilate when breathing through the nose.

Abdominal Breathing

In abdominal breathing, the abdomen is pushed outward with inspiration and the abdominal muscles contract during expiration. The object of this form of breathing is to lower the diaphragm, by contracting it, during inspiration so that the lungs are pressurized through this action rather than through the action of the intercostal (rib cage) muscles. Extension of the abdomen during expiration and contraction during inspiration is called reverse-breathing, and it is not uncommonly observed in chest breathers.

Chest breathing tends to be shallow, with minimal tidal volume, rapid and irregular, providing inadequate ventilation to the lower lobes of the lungs (Hughes, 1975). Abdominal breathing tends to normalize the blood flow in the lower lobes of the lungs and, if there is no pulmonary pathology, it ensures proper alveolar ventilation. Diaphragmatic breathing appears to increase negative pressure in the lower thoracic cavity, thus improving venous return of the blood to the heart (Ballentine, 1979).

Determining whether a person breathes with the chest or with the abdomen is relatively simple, though in some cases it may not be obvious; the chest movement may be subtle. The trainee is asked to place his or her hand on the abdomen and note motion with breathing; alternately, a light object may be placed on the abdomen, with the person in a reclining position.

Another method for determining breathing mode is to have the person straddle the middle and index fingers of the left hand over the rib located a few inches below the left nipple. (This may, of course, also be done with the right hand, on the right side of the body.) The motion of the chest may be gauged by noting the extent to which the fingers spread apart with inspiration.

The yogic system of classification denotes four categories or types of breathing. High breathing involves the clavicles, or collar bones. The chest rises and the collar bones are elevated; the abdomen is drawn in, and the diaphragm is raised. Pulmonary ventilation is minimal, despite the fact that maximum effort is employed. It has been said to promote mouth breathing because it requires maximum air intake. Middle breathing is rib, or intercostal, breathing. The diaphragm is pushed upward, and the abdomen is drawn in. The ribs are slightly raised and the chest somewhat expanded. Low breathing is abdominal or diaphragmatic (i.e., deep breathing). In low breathing, there is greater ventilation of the lungs than in high or middle breathing. It is the preferred breathing to correct HV.

In yogic complete breathing, elements of all three forms are employed in such a way, it is believed, as to fill the lungs completely with each inspiration. Ramacharaka yogi (1905) taught the following:

> Sit erect. Breathing through the nostrils, inhale steadily, first filling the lower part of the lungs, which can be accomplished by bringing into play the diaphragm, which descending exerts a gentle pressure on the abdominal organs, pushing forward the front walls of the abdomen.
>
> Then fill the middle part of the lungs, pushing out the lower ribs, breast bone and chest. Then fill the higher portion of the lungs, protruding the upper chest, including the upper six or seven pairs of ribs.
>
> In the final movement, the lower part of the abdomen will be slightly drawn in, which movement gives the lungs a support and also helps to fill the highest part of the lungs. (p. 40)

This is the first part of the exercise, and it is to be carried out as continuously and smoothly as possible—in one motion. He continued,

> Exhale quite slowly, holding the chest in a firm position, and drawing the abdomen in a little and lifting it upward slowly as the air leaves the lungs. When the air is entirely exhaled, relax the chest and abdomen. (p. 41)

These methods are the most commonly used. It is not intended that this be a thorough review of them, but rather an indication of their salient features. In general, all methods have the following in common:

(a) The trainee is made aware of the nasal function and of nasal breathing and is encouraged to breathe through the nose;

(b) The trainee is made aware of the rate and rhythm of his/her breathing and is encouraged to practice slowing his/her breathing;

(c) The trainee is taught to become aware of the difference between thoracic and abdominal breathing and is encouraged to breathe by contracting the diaphragm rather than by expanding the chest;

(d) The success of these methods depends on the ability of the trainee to gain awareness of the different sensations in breathing and to learn the proper movements in correct breathing.

The Relaxation Response

The recognition that meditative methods may lead to a particular hypometabolic state, with evidence of reduced somatic arousal, led Benson and colleagues (1974) to the development of a relaxation response. In a study of the effects of the regular elicitation of the relaxation response, in pharmacologically treated hypertensive patients, they indicated the following psychophysiological indices of that state: decreased O_2 consumption; decreased CO_2 elimination; decreased respiration rate; and decreased minute ventilation. And, of particular interest in connection with HV, were a marked decrease in blood lactate level and a slight decrease in blood pH. This state appeared to them to be an "integrated hypometabolic response" that may serve to counteract the effects of the "fight and flight" arousal response. Their assignment of this response to the hypothalamus was evidently based on the description by Hess (1957) of the tropotrophic and ergotrophic centers (Pelletier, 1977). Parenthetically, little has been made of the remarkable observation that blood lactate levels decrease markedly in this hypometabolic state. In fact, Garssen, de Ruiter, and van Dyck (1992) seem to have missed the point entirely. In the abstract of their report, titled "Breathing retraining: A rational placebo?" they state that an alternative to breathing retraining is "the induction of a relaxation response," and the presentation of an explanation for the threatening symptoms. They assert that this is intended to give the patient a distracting task to practice when panic occurs, and to promote a feeling of control. If they do indeed induce a relaxation response, panic ceases *because* blood lactate levels drop, according to current research. But they cite no references to the research on the psychophysiology of the relaxation response and, with few, mostly ancient exceptions, seem not to have access to research reports published in the United States.

The methods used to elicit this response were derived from yogic meditation, and TM in particular. They consist of:

(1) *Mental device.* There should be a constant stimulus, such as a sound, word, or phrase repeated silently or audibly, or fixed gazing at an object. The purpose of these procedures is to shift away from logical, externally oriented thought.

(2) *Passive attitude.* If distracting thoughts do occur during the repetition or gazing, they should be disregarded, and attention should be redirected to the technique. One should not worry about how well he or she is performing the technique.

(3) *Decreased muscle tension.* The subject should be in a comfortable posture so that minimal muscular work is required.

(4) *Quiet environment.* A quiet environment with decreased environmental stimuli should be chosen. Most techniques instruct the practitioner to close his eyes. A place of worship is often suitable, as is a quiet room.

Benson and colleagues reported that most trainees learn this easily in about one hour (Beary, Benson, & Klemchuck, 1974; Benson, Beary, & Carol, 1974; Benson, Rosner, Marzetta, & Klemchuck, 1974; Wallace, Benson, & Wilson, 1971). It appears to be the case that:

> . . . the physiologic changes during meditation differ from those during sleep, hypnosis, and autosuggestion and characterize a wakeful hypometabolic physiologic state. (Wallace, Benson, & Wilson, 1971, p. 795)

This relaxation response is a combination of relaxation, Zen, TM, Eastern meditation, and counterconditioning. The specific instructions to the subject are as follows:

(1) Sit quietly in a comfortable position.

(2) Close your eyes.

(3) Deeply relax all your muscles, beginning at your feet and progressing up to your face. Keep them deeply relaxed.

(4) Breathe through your nose. Become aware of your breathing. As you breathe out, say the word "one" silently to yourself—e.g., in . . . out, "one"; in . . . out, "one"; and so on.

(5) Continue for 20 minutes. Occasionally open your eyes to check the time. When you finish, sit quietly for several minutes at first with closed eyes and later with open eyes.

(6) Do not worry about whether you are successfully achieving a deep level of relaxation. Maintain a passive attitude and permit relaxation to occur at its own pace. When distracting thoughts occur, ignore them and continue repeating "one." With practice, the response should come with little effort. Practice the technique once or twice daily, and not within 2 hours after any meal, since

digestive processes seem to interfere with the elicitations of anticipated changes. (Benson et al., 1974, p. 291)

Many other techniques consider the role of breathing in both stress and
stress reduction. Stroebel's *Quieting Response* (1982) is another excellent
example.

The Quieting Response (QR)

The QR is a set of exercises available on eight tape-recorder cassettes.
Designed to help people to cope with stress, it teaches a tension reduction
skill which can be used in most places where one can find solitude such as
the home and the workplace. Its aim is to "minimize the negative effects of
annoying or stressful situation whenever and wherever they occur."

The first cassette teaches about fight or flight and compares it to the
QR. It encourages you to take responsibility for your health by practicing
the exercises daily for at least six months. The second cassette teaches slow,
deep, diaphragmatic breathing, and the simultaneous cultivation of a
passive attitude. The third one teaches muscle tensing and relaxing and
integrates it with your breathing, suggesting also increased awareness of
posture and muscle tension. In the fourth, you are taught to relax smooth
muscles (i.e., those over which you do not exert control). (For instance,
arteries may constrict or dilate, depending on the level of tension in your
body. The diameter of arteries may determine blood flow to extremities
and internal organs.) In the fifth cassette, skeletal and smooth muscle
relaxation are integrated using self-suggestions and images. The sixth
reviews and consolidates the first five, using a nine-step procedure. The
seventh reviews the procedure in the sixth, and adds a tenth procedure.
The eighth cassette teaches using the QR in daily life. The ten QR
summary exercises are listed below:

(1) Sit or lie down in a comfortable position with your eyes closed.
(2) Carry out quiet, easy breathing for 30 to 40 seconds.
(3) Lift your arms slowly, high above your head, and take a deep,
    deep breath. Hold your breath and then slowly lower your arms
    and hands, and when your arms and hands touch your sides or
    your chair, breathe out and go completely limp.

    Hold your arms in front of you as if you were praying. Take a
    deep breath, and, holding it, press your hands together until you
    feel your arm muscles begin to tremble. Maintain that tremble as
    long as you can, and then breathe out and go completely limp.

    Take a deep breath and hold it, slowly drawing your hands
    toward your face. When your hands touch your face, breathe out

and let yourself go completely limp, letting your hands fall to your sides.

Again bring your hands to a prayer position, holding them about 3 inches apart. Notice a feeling of warmth between your hands, as you continue breathing deeper and deeper. Then relax and bring your hands to your sides in a comfortable position.

(4) Imagine a spot of warm sunlight on the top of your head.

(5) While doing this, imagine your body as a hollow vessel.

(6) Now let the warm sunlight shining on your head slowly flow into the vessel, filling it, beginning with your toes, moving on up through your legs, your abdomen, and your chest.

(7) Feel the warmth reach your shoulders, where it spills over and flows into your arms and fingers, filling your arms until your body begins to have a warm and heavy feeling.

(8) Continue to pay attention to quiet breathing.

(9) With your eyelids closed, gently focus your eyes on an imaginary point just in front of the tip of your nose. Imagine that spot is a ball of warm sunlight which now changes to the misty, cool, white-blue light of a winter room, filling your mind like a blank screen. Float in this state for several minutes.

(10) Conduct your daily review, making your mind like a blank movie screen, and playing the activities of your day backwards on that screen, observing objectively and passively, reacting neither positively nor negatively to events during your day.

(The cassettes are distributed by Willow Heart Publications, P.O. Box 284, Columbia, Conn. 06237.) Every exercise, no matter how harmless it may seem to be, should be done with caution and consideration for the possibility that a particular client should not engage in it by virtue of a contraindication. For instance, a given client may have a preexisting condition making the exercise hazardous. She or he may have sustained an injury to muscle or bone, or there may have been recent surgery. Great care must be taken to ensure that the exercise is safe for a given person. More about that in the next chapter.

Chapter 9

Behavioral Assessment and Breathing Training in the Treatment of Hyperventilation, Asthma, and Other Conditions
Integrating Guided Visual Imagery, Music, and Physiological Feedback

Introduction

The modalities of the psychophysiological profile detailed in Chapter 5 are respiration rate (breath/minute); respiration mode and pattern (chest versus abdominal, inspiration–expiration ([I/E] ratio); alveolar CO_2 ($ETCO_2$, or $PETCO_2$); arterial blood oxihemoglobin (OHb) saturation (SaO_2); pulse rate; cardiorespiratory synchrony (RSA); blood pressure; electroencephalograph (*alpha* versus *theta*); and peripheral vasotonus (hand, scalp apex temperature). These parameters monitor target behaviors in biofeedback training. In any combination, or subsets, they may also be dependent or independent variables in any controlled approach to the treatment of breathing disorders.

Respiration Rate

Reports of normal breathing rate in a person at rest vary from 12 and 14 b/min (Clausen, 1951; Comroe, 1974) to as high as 18 b/min (Bell, Davidson,

245

& Scarborough, 1968; Nakamura, 1981). I would take exception to the higher value and propose that a respiration rate of 15 is pretty much at the upper limit of normal for both men and women. In a normal, healthy person at rest, an objective of breathing retraining is the self-regulation of respiration rate at no more than 9 to 12 b/min, assuming normal Vt and PCO_2.

Figure 1 shows that there are two ranges in the relationship between (a) ventilation and breathing rate, and (b) breathing rate and inspiratory volume. First, inspiration is drive dependent; but above a certain point, it becomes volume dependent.

Respiration Mode and Pattern

Unusual and idiosyncratic breathing patterns are common in persons with HV, and in those with asthma, emphysema, and other breathing disorders. One may observe chest-breathing; and not uncommonly, the pattern and rhythm of breathing are halting, with numerous hesitations, deep sighs, and other spasms and irregularities. In retraining, abdominal (diaphragmatic) breathing is usually regarded as superior to chest (thoracic) breathing during normal, nonstrenuous activity (Basmajian, 1978; Egan, 1973; Haas et al., 1979): An objective of breathing retraining is the adoption of a predominantly abdominal breathing mode to effect greater tidal-volume (Vt), with more or less normal minute volume (Vmin).

In Figure 2, the capnographs illustrate breathing patterns in five clients and one control subject (Fried et al., 1984a). Ventilatory difficulty is indicated in the fifth client, with emphysema, by the slight apnea, followed by CO_2 retention and gradual return to expulsion. This maneuver may serve to conserve CO_2, thereby increasing respiratory drive.

End-Tidal Carbon Dioxide

Depending on how it is measured, one may observe alveolar CO_2 concentration as partial pressure (PCO_2) in torr, or as percentage of end-tidal CO_2 ($PETCO_2$). The normal limits range around 5% (38 torr) (Ruch & Fulton, 1961; Shapiro, Harrison, & Walton, 1982). An objective of training is self-regulation of $PETCO_2$ at 4.75 to 5.0% (36 and 38 torr) for women, and 4.75 to 5.25% (36 and 40 torr) in men, with normal rate, Vt, and Vmin.

Cardiorespiratory Synchrony

The synergistic action of the heart and lungs, presumably under the modulating effect of vagal tone, appears as a cyclical increase with inspiration, and decrease with expiration of the heart rate, that is, respiratory

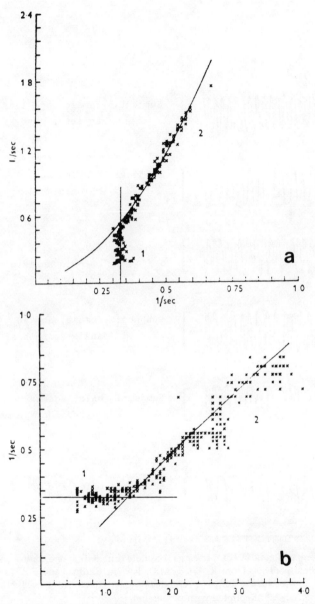

Figure 1. (a) Relation between ventilation and breathing rate, and (b) relation between breathing rate and inspiratory volume in a human subject. Reprinted with permission from F. J. Clark and C. von Euler (1972): On the regulation of depth and rate of breathing. *Journal of Physiology*, 222:267–295.

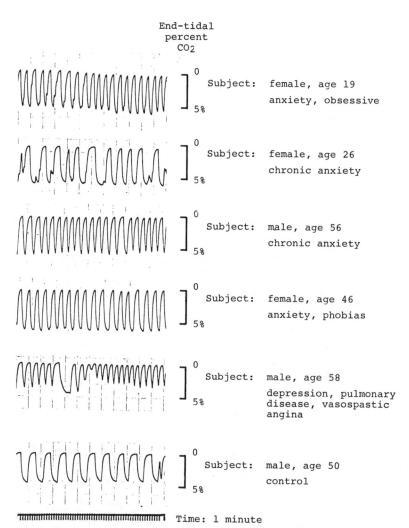

Figure 2. Comparison of PETCO$_2$ tracings (1-minute duration) in one control and 5 hyperventilation clinic patients. From R. Fried, M.C. Fox, R. Carlton, and S.R. Rubin (1984): Method and protocols for assessing hyperventilation and its treatment. *Journal of Drug Therapy and Research*, 9:280–288. Reprinted with permission.

sinus arrhythmia (RSA). It is typically absent in HV and is usually restored with normal breathing (Cacioppo & Petty, 1982; Fried, 1987a). In a person at rest, doing deep-diaphragmatic breathing at around 3 to 5 b/min, with $ETCO_2$ at about 5%, and an I/E ratio of about 1.0, RSA may show a highest-to-lowest pulse rate difference of over 10 b/min. However, 5 to 8 b/min is more typical (Fried, 1987b).

Figure 3 shows the RSA as the change in the cardiac interbeat interval (IBI) in a young woman undergoing deep-diaphragmatic breathing training (see Chapter 5). The seven very long lines in session 1 are trace disruptions due to sighs. RSA shows a sort of "scallopping" and is barely evident in session 1; by session 3, it is becoming evident and occurs over a 7 to 8 beat cycle, though sighing is still prominent. By session 5, sighing has disappeared; and by session 19, RSA is becoming more profound: Although average pulse rate changes little, the difference between the faster and slower IBIs is greater.

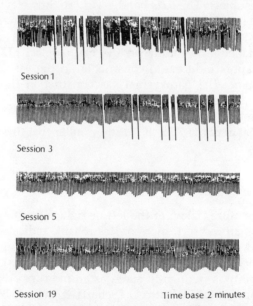

Session 1

Session 3

Session 5

Session 19   Time base 2 minutes

Figure 3.   Changes in respiratory sinus arrhythmia (RSA) after 19 breathing training sessions in a 34-year-old client with idiopathic seizures. In session 1, the tachometer is frequently interrupted by sighs, and no RSA is evident. By session 3, sighing is less frequent, and RSA is evident; by the 5th, sighing is eliminated, but the shorter downward stroke of the tachometer indicates that the heart rate is somewhat rapid; and by the 19th, the heart rate has slowed considerably, and the RSA is quite evident. Reprinted by permission from R. Fried, S. R. Rubin, R. M. Carlton, and C. M. Fox (1984a): Behavioral control of intractable idiopathic seizures: I, Self-regulation of end-tidal carbon dioxide. *Psychosomatic Medicine*, 46:315–332.

The Electroencephalograph

An abnormal brain wave pattern, with elevation in *theta* (4 to 7 Hz), and depressed *alpha* (8 to 13 Hz), is a signature of HV (Blinn & Noell, 1949; Brill & Seidmann, 1942; Holmberg, 1953; Lowry, 1967; Meyer & Gotoh, 1960). It has also been reported to follow hyperpnea in normal persons, and is common in vasopressor and carotid sinus syncope in migraineurs and idiopathic seizure sufferers (Engel, Romano, & McLin, 1944; Fried et al., 1984; Gibbs, Lennox, & Gibbs, 1940; Holmberg, 1953; Swanson, Stavney, & Plum, 1958). An objective of breathing retraining is the normalization of the EEG power spectrum.

Figure 4a shows the capnograph of a young woman who suffers from migraine. Her IBIs show virtually no RSA, the capnograph is erratic, and the EEG shows peaks at 5 and 7 Hz, in the *theta* band, and an *alpha* elevation at 14 Hz. By comparison, Figure 4b shows marked RSA, normal capnograph, and EEG power spectral composition in a 22-year-old asymptomatic control subject. The *theta* band is very slightly elevated between 4 and 6 Hz, but it is well below *alpha* which shows a prominent peak at 12 to 13 Hz.

The HV-challenge is routine in the neurological EEG examination because hypocapnia induces (a) constriction in the vascular bed of the brain; (b) in some, the paroxysmal vasoconstriction that leads to the spike-and-wave; (c) and in others, to seizures. Figure 5 illustrates the decrease in cerebral blood flow with alkalosis: When pH is 7.5, CBF is about half of that at pH = 7.38. It is little wonder that this maneuver can trigger seizures.

Finger Temperature

Skin temperature, taken at the left or right index finger, is conventionally used as an indirect, more-or-less reliable indicator of peripheral blood flow and muscle tension (Hersen, Eisler, & Miller, 1977; King & Montgomery, 1980). Low finger temperature (85°F or less) or erratic temperature variability is frequently taken as an index of ANS-sympathetic arousal (Blanchard, Morrill, Wittrock, Scharff, & Jaccard, 1989; Danskin & Crow, 1981; Engel & Chism, 1967; Fox & Simpson, 1973; Hertzman & Dillon, 1939; Ziegler & Cash, 1938).

You may find it useful to gauge temperature at the first handshake with your client. It may be a good indicator of sympathetic ANS arousal. But it is not reliable. HV causes peripheral, as well as cerebral, vasoconstriction. Restoration of peripheral blood flow, as indicated by an increase in finger temperature, suggests a criterion for the effectiveness of

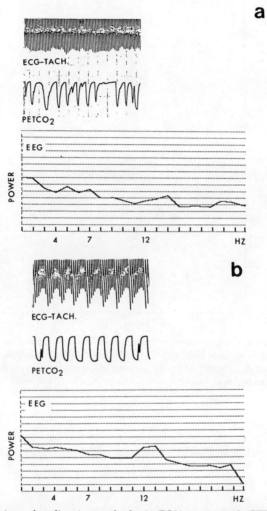

Figure 4. Comparison of cardiac sinus arrhythmia (RSA), capnograph (PETCO$_2$), and EEG power spectrum in an idiopathic seizure sufferer. Before training (a), there is no RSA, breathing is irregular, and the EEG shows *theta* elevation at 5 and 7 Hz. After deep-diaphragmatic breathing training (b), *theta* is depressed, and there is *alpha* elevation at 12 and 13 Hz. From Fried, R. & Rubin, S. R. (1984). Efecto de la biorretroalimentacion del dioxido de carbono del volumen respiratorio final sobre la hiperventilacion cronica y la epilepsia idiopatica. *Revista Latinoamericana de Psicologia*, 16:421–433.

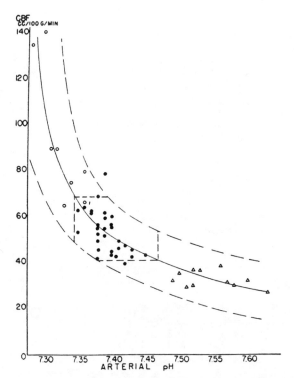

Figure 5. The relationship between cerebral blood flow and arterial blood pH. Reprinted with permission from S. S. Kety and C. F. Schmidt (1948): The effects of altered arterial tensions of carbon dioxide and oxygen on cerebral blood flow and cerebral oxygen consumption of normal young men. *Journal of Clinical Investigation,* 27:484–492.

breathing retraining (Bacon & Poppen, 1985; Fried, 1987a, 1987b, 1989, 1990a, 1993b).

Physiological Volumetric and CO_2 Feedback Methods in Breathing Retraining

Physiological feedback methods often rely on transducers or other means, and inform the trainee about behavior outcome; but the simplest maneuver involves the "hands-on-the-chest-and-abdomen" technique, where the trainee watches excursion of the hands with breathing.

Monitoring Thoracic and Abdominal Mechanics:
Impedance and Pneumographic and Other Changes

Observing chest movement in psychiatric disorders is well documented. Finesinger (1943) reported significant differences between controls and individuals said to suffer hysteria, reactive depression, and schizophrenia, in the incidence of "sighing respiration," citing earlier studies in which a spirometer was used to observe breathing in mental patients—one, by White and Hahn, dated to 1929 (see Dyspnea, Chapter 4).

According to Mead (1960), for any given level of alveolar ventilation, there is a particular respiratory frequency that is least work-costly. Furthermore, at the breathing rate commonly observed in transcendental meditation (3 to 5 b/min), there appears to be a sort of "resonance" to cardiac functioning, evident in phase correspondence between respiration rate and the cardiac IBI (Angelone & Coulter, 1964). Thus, there is a compelling correlation between inefficient mental functioning and breathing that also has been observed in numerous other ways.

Timmons et al. (1982), using strain gauges, reported that chest breathing tends to predominate in sleep and corresponds to changes in the EEG. Lum (personal communication, 1983), monitoring $ETCO_2$, as well as thoracic impedance, found a high degree of agreement among thoracic impedance measurement, tidal volume, and ventilation, replicating numerous previous studies. Hamilton, Beard, and Kory (1965), in an excellent study of the relationships among chest impedance change, tidal volume, and ventilation, reported that although the placement of electrodes affected the reliability of measurement, a high (positive) correlation was obtained between transthoracic resistance, or capacitance changes, and ventilation (special electrodes were used).

What is more important is that a linear relationship was demonstrated between lung volume change and impedance change in subjects in the standing, sitting, or supine positions, whether the breathing pattern was normal, predominantly thoracic, or predominantly abdominal, demonstrating clearly that monitoring impedance may offer a highly reliable method of monitoring lung ventilation.

More recently, the work of Tobin et al. (1983) amply validated thoracic impedance monitoring. Other noninvasive methods were described by Allison, Holmes, and Nyboer (1964); Cohn, Rao, Broudy, Birch, Watson, Atkins, Davis, Stott, and Sackner (1982); Cohn, Rao, Davis, Watson, Broudy, Sackner, and Sackner (1979); Goldensohn and Zablow (1959); and Sackner, Broudy, Davis, Cohn, and Sackner (1979). Inspiration and expiration are measured as changes in electrical resistive impedance, matching closely corresponding volumetric values obtained with a Collins spirometer.

These studies were preceded by those of Geddes, Hoff, Hickman, and Moore (1962); additional calibration methods were proposed by Kubicek, Kinnen, and Edin (1964), and by Chadha, Watson, Birch, Jenouri, Schneider, Cohen, and Sackner (1982), among others. Some investigators have cautioned about the inherent propensity of measuring devices to alter breathing so as to make it unlikely that one can observe true volumetric changes (i.e., "true" meaning as one breathes naturally). But they are unquestionably superior to those spirometers which use face masks, and sometimes nose clips (Askanazi, Silverberg, Foster, Hyman, Milic-Emili, & Kinney, 1980; Gilbert, Auchincloss, Brodsky, & Boden, 1972). They cautioned about decreased respiratory frequency, with concomitant and variable increase in tidal volume, and the irritating effects of these devices. Weissman, Askanazi, Milic-Emili, and Kinney (1984) reported that the use of a mouthpiece and nose clips increased minute ventilation (Vmin), tidal volume (Vt), and mean inspiratory flow (Vt/Vi)—though not frequency. Nose clips alone resulted in decreased frequency, and increased Vt, but Vmin and Vt/Vi were unchanged. Maxwell, Cover, and Hughes (1985) report that the dead space in tube-breathing affects Vt, though not frequency, and that a face mask with a high flow of air did not significantly alter breathing pattern. But external devices such as nose clips and mouthpiece, by themselves, significantly raised Vt and slightly lowered frequency.

Consequently, I opted not to employ such methods to monitor ventilation in most of my clients; for the same reason, I do not typically employ "myofeedback" (thoracic muscle feedback) for breathing retraining in HV. But it has considerable merit in the treatment of asthma where tension in the scalene muscles of the neck has been shown to constitute an important impairment. Peper (1988) prompted my application of this technique, as well as the use of the incentive inspirometer following publication of his notable results in this area (described in greater detail later in this chapter).

Typically, monitoring ventilation and thoracic and abdominal muscle activity, despite claims to the contrary, is to a degree sufficiently disruptive to change breathing even though it is claimed to be noninvasive. "Invasive" is usually interpreted to mean entering the body in some manner; therefore, these methods which use electrodes, strain gauges, or other sensors which encircle the body are not, strictly speaking, invasive. And I do use these techniques when I train some persons with asthma, or with other forms of intransigent resistance to abdominal outward excursion.

Most of my clients have "functional" breathing disorders with hypocapnia. This is not to say that tidal volume (Vt) is not affected. Their breathing behavior, bracing, and what not cause low PCO_2. I suspect that this client population predominates in the practice of clinical psycho-physiology. There are, of course, other cases, when the primary problem is organic, or trauma, or another disability of the thoracic and abdominal musculature impairing the mechanics of motion. Then, these devices are indispensable. In most cases, I focus mostly on training the breathing behavior, monitoring alveolar PCO_2 to make sure that they do not inadvertently hyperventilate.

Physiology is in many ways analogous to electronic circuit design, that is, everything is predictable pretty much within the tolerance of the components. You just simply can't lose *pieces*: If PCO_2 is correct, and if breathing is slow and rhythmic, and the client appears comfortable, volume has to be at least near normal. This is borne out by the standard nomographs which reflect a sort of human physiological circuit design.

I learned from many years of experience that the best criterion for proper breathing, in my client population, is $ETCO_2$. It can be trusted to be an accurate measurement of alveolar CO_2 (Comroe, 1974; Hughes, 1975). Furthermore, in private practice, as compared to a research laboratory, volumetric monitoring is cumbersome and distracts the trainee; elaborate calibration procedures before training are time-consuming.

On the other hand, since change in impedance is also embedded in the ECG baseline, baseline shifts give a rough estimate of chest excursion (Angelone & Coulter, 1964). The shift in the overall baseline from which the ECG traces "drop" is the reflection of the changes in chest impedance that correspond with chest excursion. Because of its rather extensive deviation, it can readily be calibrated to reflect volume change.

Monitoring End-Tidal Carbon Dioxide

I have reported elsewhere (Fried et al., 1984b; 1990; 1993a,b) the procedures for the control of HV in idiopathic seizure sufferers. HV control is used to reduce hypocapnia and alkalosis in that patient population. Several self-regulation methods had been developed to control idiopathic seizures. The most prominent among these involved one or another form of EEG conditioning (Bowersox & Sterman, 1981; Finley, 1976; Kuhlman, 1979–1980; Kuhlman & Allison, 1977; Lubar & Bahler, 1976; Lubar et al., 1981; Qui, Hutt, & Forrest, 1979; Sterman, 1977a, 1977b; Sterman & Friar, 1972; Sterman, Macdonald, & Bernstein, 1977; Wyrwicka & Sterman, 1968). I chose to pursue the two methods that resulted in explicit concomitant breathing changes (Chase & Harper, 1971; Harper & Sterman, 1972).

Several investigators had reported breathing training methods in which they observed alveolar gas composition. Brigo et al. (1968) at-

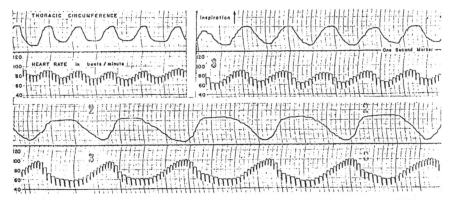

Figure 6. Comparison of phase between breathing and heart rate fluctuations for different rates and styles of breathing. Reprinted with permission from A. Angelone and N.A. Coulter (1964): Respiratory sinus arrhythmia: A frequency dependent phenomenon. *Journal of Applied Physiology,* 3:479–482.

tempted to rehabilitate emphysematous patients by regulating breathing with a metronome. They conceded that their breathing retraining showed little CO_2 modification, and no pH change, though PO_2 increased. I would question any breathing training procedure in which no change in PCO_2 is observed, but in emphysematous patients, alkalosis is not typically the problem.

Because of the pathological condition of the alveoli in emphysematous lungs, it would be a mistake to generalize these findings to persons who do not have chronic obstructive pulmonary disease, especially emphysema, but who show hyperpnea, as did the patients in these findings.

Khan (1977) reported training persons with bronchial asthma with biofeedback using a (Monaghan) pulmonary function analyzer. The feedback signal varied with the degree of airway resistance. But the problem in hyperventilators, for the most part, is not airways resistance but hyperpnea and uneven pulmonary ventilation. In the context of uneven pulmonary ventilation, Johnston and Lee (1976) monitored the upper rectus abdominis, the lower rectus abdominis, and the external oblique muscles, combining EMG with spirometric measures. This method, effective in teaching abdominal versus thoracic breathing, unfortunately gives no indication of gas composition in the lungs during the training procedure.

Breslav, Shmeleva, and Normatov (1986) reported alveolar CO_2 biofeedback during administration of a "respiratory mixture" intended to produce hypoxia. They wished to train pilots to stabilize $PaCO_2$ and avoid detrimental effects of hypocapnia and hypoxia. The feedback signal was an oscilloscope trace analog of PCO_2. van Doorn, Folgering, and Colla (1982) and Naifeh, Kamyia, and Sweet (1982) also used "instrument" biofeedback, the former using a polygraph trace of PCO_2, and the latter, a pitch modulated tone. All these studies used face masks.

The van Doorn et al. (1982) study compared "breathing instructions" to biofeedback:

> The ten subjects in the breathing instruction group received a stenciled training schedule containing breathing instructions to be used at home twice a day for 10 min. The essence of this program was that patients should learn to breathe slowly and not too deeply, thereby gaining control over their breathing pattern. Abdominal ventilation and counting for the duration of the inspiration and expiration served as a way to accomplish this. Introduction of this program and first exercises were done in presence of the therapist. . . . (p. 832)

These instructions are exceptionally naive. Furthermore, we are left in the dark about what they mean by "deeply," what the therapist contributed, or what the "count" was. Not surprisingly, we are given no data on breathing rate or rate change. It was studies like these that gave impetus to my determination to devise successful training methods which achieved both physiologically consistent and replicable breathing rate reduction with PCO_2 normalization.

The Initial Intake Interview

Before training begins, it is essential to establish that there is no determinable organic basis for the HV or tachypnea and that there is no extant condition that contraindicates biofeedback or breathing training. Two conditions that would immediately be red flags are low blood pressure and diabetes. Breathing training has an astonishingly rapid effect on blood pressure; it may plummet after a few minutes of sustained slow diaphragmatic respiration. It has also been shown that relaxation training reduces insulin dependence; one possible reason for this is that stress reduction reduces blood glucose (Guthrie, Moeller, & Guthrie, 1983).

When the client first comes into the office, I always shake his or her hand. I note whether it feels warm, cold, moist, or dry (these indicate arousal); then I note the breathing pattern. Is it rapid or slow? Shallow or deep? Does she or he sigh or exhibit reverse breathing, thoracic or abdominal motion? Are his or her clothes tight at the belt? When I ask the first question on the intake form, "How do you spell your name?", does the chest heave before answering? This is an indication of dyspnea (air hunger), and is common in chronic HV; such persons have to catch their breath before they can speak.

The intake form first covers personal and family data: spouse, children, parents, siblings. I try to determine the health of the family to determine if there is any pattern of chronic illness; if any family member died, what was the cause of death? If any family member has a major or chronic illness, what is it? How is it treated? Next, the head and neck region. Does the client have any of the following: migraine; dizziness; blurred vision; vertigo; bruxism (at night); jaw clenching; faintness; itching around the eyes; nasal swelling (chronic) or obstruction; deviation of the septum; moments of fading consciousness; tightness of the neck muscles; tightness of the throat; difficulty swallowing; dryness of the throat or excessive salivation; tinnitus; dermatitis of the scalp or neck; seizures (epileptic); syncope.

Next, it covers the trunk and abdomen. Is there pain or tension of the shoulder muscles; chest pain; frequent sighing and chest heaving; pain in rib cage muscles or sharp shooting pain "that makes you want to keep your chest expanded and not breathe" (diaphragmatic spasm); palpitations (heart pounding); asthma; bronchitis (morning smoker's cough); heartburn; stomach gas; indigestion not relieved by antacids; irritable bowel (diarrhea associated with tension); indigestion with nausea and vomiting associated with tension (abdominal migraine); frequent urination; irregular or painful menstrual periods; frequent bladder infection; vaginal yeast; hypoglycemia; diabetes; hyper- or hypotension; dermatitis; excessive sweating; flatulence.

Next, the arms and legs: coldness of the fingers and toes; spasms of the fingers and toes; spasms of the arm, thigh, or calf muscles; tingling sensations in the fingers; dermatitis.

Does she or he, or a blood relative, have chronic pulmonary lung disease; stroke; heart disease (angina, etc.); diabetes; high blood pressure; epileptic seizures; allergies, "food sensitivities."

Then, these questions are asked:

(a) "Are you currently being treated for a medical condition? What condition? How are you being treated? What medication do you take?"
(b) "Do you have any allergies?"
(c) "Do you have any food sensitivity? Are there any foods that you crave? That you must have? That make you feel better or worse when you eat them?"
(d) "Do you use alcohol or any controlled substance (marijuana, cocaine)? Do you smoke? How much?"

The psychological assessment centers on symptoms:

(a) "Do you feel that you are under constant and great stress?"
(b) "Do you experience anxiety? Under what circumstances?"
(c) "Do you experience panic attacks? Agoraphobia?"
(d) "Are you depressed?"
(e) "Do you have mood swings?"
(f) "Do you suffer from "PMS" or menstrual pain?"
(g) "Do you tire easily?"
(h) "Is it an effort to get through the day?"
(i) "Do you have difficulty concentrating on what you do?"
(j) "Do you have obsessive thoughts? Compulsions? Rituals?"
(k) "Do you have phobias? Fears?"
(l) "Do you think that you have a serious physical condition (that is incurable) that no doctor has been able to diagnose?"

She or he may be referred by a professional who can verify that there is no psychosis. Thus, the intake interview is meant to elicit the somatized and psychological symptoms that are most frequently encountered in persons with HVS: tension; fatigue; inability to concentrate; a sense that things are unreal; depression; anxiety; panic attacks; phobias; dyspnea, tachypnea, air hunger; headaches; migraine; Raynaud's syndrome; irritable bowel syndrome; gastritis; indigestion; chest pain; stress, family, and other coping problems; as well as evidence of graded hypoxia; impaired immune system reaction such as frequent colds, tonsillitis, or ear infections; aggravated or frequent allergy symptoms; bronchitis; vaginal yeast (chronic or recurring); or flareup of otherwise "curable" diseases; and so on. I also look for any factors that are known to potentiate HV, chronic autonomic arousal, or the effects of these two factors. For instance, I look for ways that clients potentiate vasopressor or vasotonic change, such as consumption of foods rich in tyramine (a sympathomimetic that augments catecholamine release (Fried, 1990a); hypoglycemia; thyroid dysfunction; evidence of anemia, or variant hemoglobin; evidence of hystamine reaction such as dermographia.

The Hyperventilation Provocation Test and the Think Test

Grossman and DeSwart (1984) recommended detecting HVS by symptoms; and van Dixhoorn and Duivenvoorden (1985) recommend the *Nijmegen Questionnaire* to assess it (see Chapter 8). I think that in the long run such instruments may contribute to the validity of HVS, still contested in some quarters, as capnometry becomes more popular and supports symptom observations. Correlation of the questionnaire with PCO_2 should help to settle that issue in the future.

Although the capnometer is obviously the only really accurate means of establishing HV, which is, after all, a ventilation phenomenon, the use of symptoms lists is unquestionably more desirable than the HV challenge, or provocation test. It is a common procedure in medicine to validate clinical symptoms by routine laboratory procedures and there is no reason why we cannot do likewise where such procedures exist.

The use of hyperpnea to elicit symptoms dates back to Rosett (1924); but its present form is typically attributed to Beumer and Hardonk (1971). A number of investigators are beginning to opt for other methods, and rightly so. If you consider the potentially dangerous consequences of HV to coronary and brain circulation, you may be less likely to employ it frivolously, but history records that, with notable exceptions, medical physiology has little regard for the HVS. That may be why it more or less discounts its hazards.

In 1941, Wood reported on Da Costa's Syndrome. He attributed the dull persistent type of precordial pain reported in neurocirculatory asthenia to respiratory malfunction. Though he thought, as did others (Kerr, Dalton, & Gliebe, 1937; Soley & Shock, 1938), that HV may be responsible, he ultimately aligned himself with Guttman and Jones (1940), and later White (1942), who concluded that the respiratory symptoms were of cardiac origin. I do not think it a coincidence that White, a noted cardiologist, should have come to that conclusion. Friedman reviewed this research in the *American Heart Journal*, in 1945, and reported that ". . . we were unable to detect any basic cardiovascular abnormality in patients with this syndrome" (p. 558).

Subsequently, Wheeler, White, Reed, and Cohen (1950) cited Soley and Shock (1938) (and Freud!), but not Friedman (1945), in their report on neurocirculatory asthenia—in which there is, of course, no mention of the HV hypothesis. They apparently just plain ignored a report which contradicted their point of view, published just four years earlier in their own journal. However, in 1943, Finesinger summarized his conclusions about the "spirogram" in psychiatric disorders. He noted irregularities in breathing tracings and found that their incidence was greatest in anxiety groups, and least in schizophrenics. The Loevenhart et al. (1929) studies, detailed in Chapter 7, employing cyanide as a respiratory stimulant to awareness in psychotics, would certainly have predicted this observation.

Apparently spurred by evidence that anxiety affects breathing, Finesinger followed an earlier study (Finesinger & Mazick, 1940) with a report entitled, "The effect of pleasant and unpleasant ideas on the respiratory pattern (Spirogram) in psychoneurotic patients" (1944). These studies may be the major historical antecedents to Nixon's "Think Test" (1986, Nixon & Freeman, 1988). Finesinger (Finesinger & Mazick, 1940) concluded that:

The respiration pattern of the anxiety groups is characterized by the highest spirogram scores, with high values for sighing respiration, upper and lower major fluctuations [in the I & E phase of the tracings], upper minor fluctuations and upper points off the line. The group of hysterias and reactive depressions has a moderately high spirogram score, a high percentage of sighers, moderately high values for sighing respiration, high values for upper major fluctuations, the lowest values for points off the line. (p. 166)

It is this frequency of breathing irregularities noted previously by Christie (1935) that led him to the term "respiratory neurosis." I think that history may bear witness to the fact that this may have been a poor choice of words: "Neurosis" is mental (Freud is cited in some studies of neurocirculatory asthenia by Wheeler et al., 1960). Medicine then zeroed in on the heart as a possible cause of this alleged "neurosis."

In the later study, Finesinger had patients and controls "state what ideas came to mind on being asked to think of pleasant ideas and unpleasant ideas" (p. 660). After a preliminary period of spirometric observations lasting from 3 to 6 minutes, the subjects were instructed to think of pleasant ideas, and after another period of spirometric observations, to think of unpleasant ideas. This was followed by another spirometric observation period; then they were told to relax and were disconnected from the apparatus.

First, unpleasant ideational stimuli increased sighing respiration and irregularity in other aspects of the spirogram. Second, patients with "hysteria," "anxiety neurosis," and "reactive depression" reacted to unpleasant ideational stimuli with excessive respiratory lability as gauged by greater irregularity of the respiratory pattern. Those with compulsions, hypochondriasis, and schizophrenia were less reactive.

More recently, Nixon (Nixon & Freeman, 1988) questioned the usefulness of the HV-provocation test because, among other things, it lacks the "component of emotional arousal required to provoke a hyperventilation response in many subjects" (p. 277). He initially undertook to evoke that response with hypnosis (1986), and in patients thought to have HVS on the basis of medical history and symptoms, $PETCO_2$ decreased three times as much as in the controls. This particular report also cites 19 primary sources of information on respiratory response to psychological "challenge" and in some instances, *mean fall* and *lowest mean* $PaCO_2$. These averaged 7.1 and 28.96 torr, respectively. If psychological stress can cause an average drop in $PaCO_2$ of 7 torr (18%), that would be a profound alkalotic challenge to acid-base homeostasis, and to the ODC. Such findings are consistent with my observation that symptoms begin to emerge below 30 torr.

Nixon (Nixon & Freeman, 1988) proposed the *Think Test* to screen for HV, and validated it in over 90 patients with cardiovascular symptoms.

Resting $ETCO_2$ was obtained; then they were asked to perform the forced HV-provocation test (FHVPT) with $ETCO_2$ monitoring, with FHVPT, in the manner of Hardonk and Beumer (1979), that is, 60 breaths per minute, for 3 minutes, with PCO_2 dropping below 19 torr. The rate of return to resting $ETCO_2$ is plotted for 3 minutes following FHVPT. If the ratio

$$\frac{PETCO_2 \text{ at rest}}{PETCO_2, \text{ 3 minutes after FHVPT}}$$

is greater than 1.5, chronic HV is considered to be likely. The *Think Test* was as follows:

> . . . patients were instructed to close their eyes and recreate in their minds a time or place when they had experienced their typical symptoms: They were invited to think back and remember all the feelings and sensations which were present at that time. The pattern of their breathing was specifically not mentioned. After this, topics that had appeared to have an important emotional content during history taking were reintroduced and the patient was invited to remember the effect that this feeling had on them. A fall in $PCO_2 > 10$ mm Hg which was maintained spontaneously for more than 1 min was considered significant. (p. 277)

The fascinating thing about these studies is that they do not settle the question of "type" or "trait." Individuals with HVS report chest symptoms with virtually no exception. Does this mean that these "high anxiety" individuals hyperventilate, and in so doing drive their chest symptoms; or are they anxious because they are a cardiac type, which leads to HV? Or is HVS a psychological anxiety disorder with physical symptoms, or a cardiac or respiratory disorder with concomitant psychological symptoms?

General Training Procedure

In most instances, training proceeds by steps:

(1) Breathing training: The client is taught deep-diaphragmatic breathing with physiological monitoring, and biofeedback, where appropriate, from session to session until she or he can sustain about 10 consecutive deep-diaphragmatic breaths with comfort and normocapnia.
(2) Relaxation training: A modified systematic muscle relaxation program, the RAR(TH), is taught and the breathing is integrated into it.
(3) Advanced maneuvers: "Complete" respiration is combined with imagery.

First Test of "Receptivity."   The client is asked to sit up and lean back in the chair, head resting comfortably against the back of the chair. Then, she or he is asked to close the eyes. If a slight decrease in breathing rate occurs now, lasting perhaps one or two breaths, sometimes accompanied by a slight increase in finger temperature, it strongly predicts that she or he will have little difficulty learning deep-diaphragmatic breathing.

Second Test of "Receptivity."   The client is told, "Now when you inhale, please hold your breath and count to two. As you exhale, hold it and count to two."

If she or he cannot do this simple task, it may be that there are problems with the mechanics of breathing, perhaps an inability to control respiratory muscles. In asthma clients especially, there may be what appears to be a reluctance to exhale. This restriction of end-tidal volume impairs inspiration since there is still more air left in the lungs than one would normally expect. I have noted in many cases that PCO_2 is near-normal in asthma clients and often even elevated because this increase in the volume of *dead air space* favors CO_2 retention. Such a mechanism has adaptive value since it tends to keep the ODC near normal. However, if there is even a slight elevation in PCO_2, there will also be an increase in respiratory drive causing diaphragmatic fatigue.

Biofeedback

Physiological (bio-)feedback is, with some exceptions, principally an open-loop system, where feedback typically provides "knowledge of results" for performance correction. We recognize this empirically when, in thermal biofeedback, we ascribe initial drop in hand temperature to performance anxiety.

The Profile

A modified psychophysiological profile is obtained before training begins and a decision is made about which modalities will be monitored. The modified profile in Figure 7a is the initial psychophysiological profile of a professional woman in her early forties, who sought help for tension, anxiety, and headaches. Breathing rate is approximately 18 b/min (30-second screen duration); $PETCO_2$, 4.6 (as read directly from the capnome-ter) (33 torr); arterial O_2 saturation (SaO_2), 97.9%; pulse rate, about 68; hand temperature, 79.5°F; and scalp apex temperature, 92.8°F (room temperature is 76°F). Breathing rate is elevated with low CO_2 (hypocap-

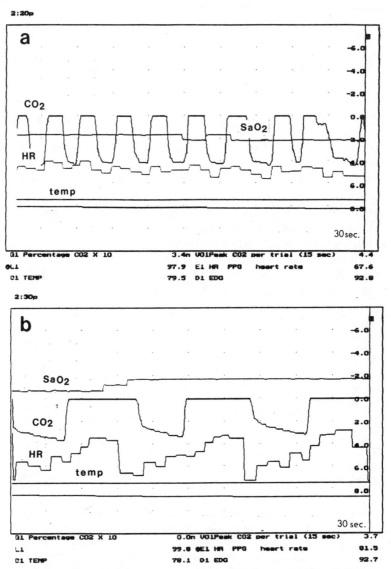

Figure 7. Psychophysiological respiration profile (PRP) showing $PETCO_2$, SaO_2, heart rate, and hand and scalp temperature before (a) and during two sessions (b and c) of deep-diaphragmatic breathing training. Screen duration is 30 seconds. Breathing drops from 18 breaths/minute to 3 breaths/minute.

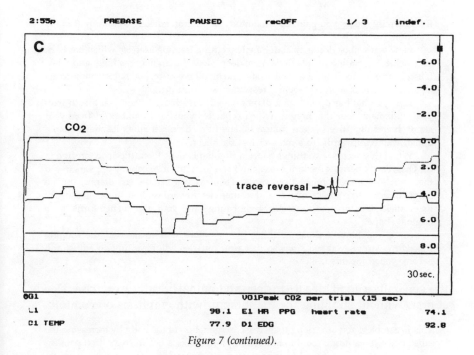

Figure 7 (continued).

nia). Peripheral vasoconstriction is likely. But because she is a runner, pulse rate is relatively low. SaO_2 is elevated above normal (95% to 98%), suggesting a left-shifted ODC, consistent with hypocapnic alkalosis.

Breathing Training (Day 1)

The client is coupled to the physiological interface by the electrodes, sensors, and cables, and the general training is explained. The traces on the video monitor are explained to the client who is then instructed as follows:

> Please put this book flat on your abdomen, spine up, and please push it out as far as you can. That's good. Now relax. Thank you. Did you feel any pain or discomfort? No. Good.

The degree of outward excursion is noted, and the monitor trace changes are discussed. A note of caution to therapist and client: Most persons are unused to deep abdominal/diaphragmatic excursion. It may be strenuous. If training proceeds too quickly, she or he may experience painful diaphragmatic cramps; should these occur, stop the exercise immediately:

If an exercise causes you pain, or discomfort, stop it immediately, and bring it to my attention.

Now you will be doing an abdominal breathing training exercise which has been very helpful in getting people to do more deep, slow abdominal breathing, and relax. It helps reduce muscle tension, pulse rate, and blood pressure, and helps people to get a general sense of alert well-being, relaxation and comfort.

Here is what happens during diaphragmatic breathing—when you breath with your abdomen. Your diaphragm, which separates your lungs and heart from your stomach and digestive system, contracts; and in so doing, it alters its shape from a dome, vaulted upwards, to a more or less flat sheet.

When this occurs, two things happen simultaneously: First, the space created in the chest cavity permits the lungs to expand and fill with air. Second, it appears to you that your abdomen is pushed outwards. Then, as you exhale, the diaphragm, no longer directed to contract, relaxes and resumes its upward vaulted shape. Because of its elasticity, the air is pushed out of your lungs and your abdomen returns to its original shape.

Since you haven't done anything like it before, I have divided the training procedures over several sessions so that your muscles will have time to adjust and become toned for this task.

It is generally a good idea to do deep abdominal breathing exercises slowly at first, without straining the diaphragm, with emphasis on comfort.

This is aerobics. You are trying to increase oxygenation of the body by increasing the efficiency of breathing. You do not need to plunge, like a health freak, into pain-as-a-measure-of-success. If you experience pain and discomfort, you are doing it *wrong*.

Do you feel dizzy? If not, good. If you feel dizzy, you are overbreathing—hyperventilating. You are putting too much effort into it, too early in the game. Make the motions a little more subtle: not so far out on inhale and not so far in on exhale. If you feel dizzy, stop and rest a little while until it passes, which it usually does quickly.

Close your mouth. Breathe in and out only through your nose. Breathing through your mouth tends to promote hyperventilation. Look at your hands.

As you inhale, keep your chest down. Let the hand on your abdomen rise as the air fills your abdomen.

Now let's look at the screen and see how you're doing.

If there is difficulty in compliance, try:

Place this book on your lap (spine up, so that it won't slide off). Now, without coordinating it with your breath at all, push the book out as far as you can with your abdomen.

When you inhale, your abdomen should move out about as far as it did when you pushed the book. If it did not move out much, don't worry; you may be tense, that's to be expected. It will improve with practice.

On exhale: Slowly—but never so slowly that it creates discomfort—pull your abdomen back as far as it will go, but do not let it raise your chest. Good. Now don't stop. Don't pause; repeat the inhale and exhale procedure once more. Rest for a moment.

Now let's look at the screen and see how you are doing.

Now, once again: Inhale . . . fill up. And, exhale . . . pull all the way back.

Repeat this procedure three times, then stop.

> Let's see how you are doing. Here is what's happened to your breathing; . . . and to
> your oxygen and carbon dioxide; . . . your hand and head temperature now are. . . .
>   That's all for today.

Doing much more than this may be counterproductive, possibly causing cramps or dizziness. There may be a slight tendency to hyperventilate at first. Many of my clients do. It will pass and, with practice, it will disappear.

Second Training Session (Day 2)

The client is prepared for the exercise in the same way as day 1:

> Please sit back in your chair. Place your hands on your knees for a moment. Let
> yourself relax. Close your mouth.
>   Place your hands on your chest and abdomen as you did yesterday. Once you get
> the knack, you can do it without your hands.
>   Now, looking at your hands, inhale, holding down your chest, and letting your
> abdomen fill up. Then, exhale slowly, and pull your abdomen all the way back.
>   Now let's look at the traces on the monitor.

Then the procedure is repeated several times and the performance explained and discussed.

> That's enough for today.
>   Did you find it to be any easier? Did your abdomen move further out when you
> inhaled? Did the hand on your chest remain more or less motionless? Can you pull
> your abdomen a little further in?

I recommend only very short exercise sessions the first few days. Diaphragm and abdominal muscles need time to tone up.

Third Training Session (Day 3)

> Let's see you do the exercise without your hands. Prepare yourself in your chair, as you
> did yesterday. Try it.

After three consecutive deep breaths, performance is explained and discussed.

> Does your chest remain more still as you inhale, and is your abdomen moving
> outward? If it is, good. If not, go back to using your hands. But, if you can, proceed
> breathing in and out four times in a row—close your eyes.
>   If you still need to use your hands, then proceed, eyes closed, and imagine what
> your hands are doing. Good.
>   That's it for today.

I usually make it a practice to review the pre- and posttraining profile, and to review signs and symptom frequency and severity after a session. As soon as the client can sustain deep-diaphragmatic breathing for at least 10 to 15 consecutive breaths without hypocapnia, the breathing exercise can be integrated with a modified form of muscle relaxation, imagery, and music. See also *The Breath Connection* (Fried, 1990a, Insight/Plenum).

Diaphragmatic Fatigue

Figures 7b and 7c show consecutive screens during the training procedure. Figure 7b shows a good breathing configuration at about 6 breaths per minute, and the RSA is prominent and synchronized with breathing. Figure 7c shows 2 to 3 breaths per minute, and trace reversal due to fatigue at the beginning of the last inspiration in the capnogram.

The physiological traces on the monitor are the best means for making sure that you, the practitioner, are in control of what your client is learning. She or he can't get good practice with a fatigued diaphragm. I have often criticized studies in which the instructions to the client are wrong, vague, or absent. You must take responsibility for training and guiding your client so that the resultant behavior is the best that technology, plus all that you know, can produce. Think about what is required to produce deep-diaphragmatic breathing behavior and mechanics—you are teaching it. The computer monitors breathing, PCO_2, SaO_2, and so on. You can stop the screen and then discuss the traces and the data with the trainee, after short training segments of a few consecutive breaths, allowing a brief rest period. When the trainee improves, training segments may be lengthened. Occasionally, she or he may have difficulty with abdominal breathing. Instructions then include:

> As you inhale, fill up your abdomen as much as you can. That's it. Good, keep going. You've got lots of room. Keep going. Keep filling. Good.
> Now see how the trace has changed.

Guided Imagery, PETCO$_2$ Biofeedback, and EEG: Rapid Induction Hypoarousal (RAR™)

The procedure described above has been published elsewhere (Fried, 1987a, 1990a). It is adapted for the treatment of HV in a variety of clinical subpopulations, and is an integral program for devising a strategy of biofeedback centering on breathing training. Keeping in mind the link between HV and panic disorder, it would seem best to do breathing retraining so as to produce rapid inhibition of sympathetic ANS arousal. If, as research suggests, panic is a reaction to brain hypoxia and elevated lactate levels then, to be effective, breathing must correct these conditions.

Meditation (especially TM), yoga, modified versions of yoga, and the relaxation response (Benson et al., 1974) tend to promote a hypometabolic state with many of the components that seem desirable to counter HV. But they do not provide it quickly. Many clients would benefit from retraining but become discouraged or impatient. The more rapid and profound the change, the more she or he will be motivated to practice the training procedure.

The most effective of the yoga-derived techniques, in achieving diaphragmatic breathing, is probably TM. But clients are not equally adept at it, and there is no immediate knowledge of results—an absolutely essential component of self-regulation strategies.

A review of the available biofeedback techniques by Glueck and Stroebel (1975) confirmed that EEG biofeedback, for one thing, is difficult for the average practitioner to implement. Although *alpha* training has been shown to be associated with states that entail deep, rhythmic, diaphragmatic breathing, Glueck and Stroebel nevertheless recommended the "mantra-type passive meditation" of TM. Many of the previous findings on breathing alterations in TM were also confirmed by Wolkove et al. (1984), who stated that "these observations suggest an alteration in wakefulness, more subtle than sleep or the unconscious state, can significantly affect chemical and neural regulation of breathing."

Thus, I decided to teach the client to induce a wakeful relaxed state in which she or he is breathing in synchrony with a natural physiological rhythm, using biofeedback, not to self-monitor but as an adjunct to finetune the induction of this state. That is, I would monitor the effect of the induction and adjust the instructions to clients in accordance with the outcome of their efforts to engage in a hypoaroused activity.

I acquired a frequency spectrum analyzer to monitor the EEG online and used an X-Y recorder to "dump" the momentary power-spectral composition of the EEG on to "hard copy." Electrode placement is described in Chapter 5. The client and I can watch breathing pattern and mode, end-tidal CO_2 and rhythm, the composition of the EEG changing with breathing, and the finger temperature at the beginning and end of each session. Occasionally, I may check the client's blood pressure.

Inducing a response inhibiting sympathetic ANS arousal by the induction of hypoarousal requires the client to acquire both a different "mind-set," and a change in muscle tension pattern. This is accomplished by instructions to imagine the following:

Do you like the beach? Good.

> I will give you instructions to imagine that you are on your favorite beach. Are you comfortable? Good.
>
> During the time that you are imagining the scene that I will suggest to you, I will be watching these instruments, and I will be giving you information about what they tell me that you are doing and what is happening to you. Periodically, I will ask you to open your eyes and to look at these instruments also so that you can see for yourself how you are doing.
>
> O.K.? Let's begin.

If there is evidence of exceptional tension, I instruct the client in a modified form of Jacobsonian relaxation (e.g., alternately squeezing or contracting and relaxing the brow, nose, and cheeks; shrugging the head into the shoulders; squeezing and relaxing the shoulders, upper arms, fists, chest muscles, stomach, and thighs; and stretching the calves). Then, I proceed:

> Now, please close your eyes and imagine that you are on your favorite beach. Look around you. You are standing on the beach. There are a few people about. You can just make out some people out of the corner of your eyes, but you can't see them clearly and you can't hear them talk.
>
> The sun is shining. It is midmorning. It is warm but not hot. Feel the sun warming your shoulders and your arms. Let the warmth flow right into your body. Feel the relaxation of being on this pleasant warm beach, and let it flow right through your body. Good.
>
> Now then, look at the ocean before you. Feel the sun? See the beach? Look at the ocean again: it is calm. Look at the surf now: it is gently coming up on the beach and receding. See it gently coming up on the beach? And receding? Nod your head if the answer is "yes." Good.
>
> When the surf comes up on the beach next, take a breath and let it out slowly as the surf is receding from the beach. Good.
>
> You are relaxed, alert, awake.

The next action is coordinated with the $PETCO_2$ trace on the video monitor. As the trace indicates that inspiration is beginning, I say:

> Now, the surf is coming up on the beach.

And as expiration begins:

> Now the surf is receding from the beach.

Thus, the motion of the surf is synchronous with the inspiration and expiration phases of breathing. Feedback is given during the first few breaths:

> That's good. Very good. Here is the surf coming in now. Good. And now, going out. Good.

When the client is breathing slowly, as almost invariably happens, about 3 to 5 breaths per minute, or less, $ETCO_2$ initially rises slightly. The instructions are now altered:

> You are doing well. Your breathing is rhythmic and slow, and your lung gas-composition is adjusting well. I will now stop the action on the screen so that you can see this for yourself. Now please open your eyes.

The screen is "frozen" and I can then discuss the pattern with the client:

> Here is where you were breathing in, and here is where you are exhaling. You can see how nice and smooth the pattern is. Good.
> Let's begin again. It is mid-morning. You are on the beach, and the sun is shining. The sun is warm but not hot. Feel the warmth on your shoulders, relaxing your body.
> Let it flow through your arms . . . and to your hands. Look at the ocean in front of you. It is calm. You are relaxed, comfortable, alert. Alert—not at all sleepy. Awake and alert.
> Look at the surf gently coming up on the beach. Good. And now receding. Good.

At this point, she or he is usually synchronizing breathing with the imaginary action of the surf as it rapidly returns to the slow, rhythmic pattern. In some cases, I have noted that the breathing automatically shifts to the abdominal mode, but this is not frequent. In persons in whom thoracic breathing prevails, I add:

> As you are breathing in with the tide, push out your belly. Breathe by pushing out your belly as far as it will go when you breathe in. Good. Now, pull back your belly to breathe out. Good.
> As you are standing on the beach and breathing with the surf, put your right hand on your belly and push your hand out as you breathe in. Good. And pull your belly in as you breathe out with the receding tide.

Each session consists of three to four such image-related exercises, lasting from 2 to 3 minutes each. At the end of the session, a "hard copy" of the capnograph, and other details, including EEG, finger, and head temperature changes, are discussed. On subsequent sessions, the previous record is discussed before training begins, and some goals of the training are established.

I have found this procedure to be exceptionally rapid in inducing a slow, deep breathing, and the concomitant EEG is astonishingly similar to that reported in TM. Some, though not all, clients have produced the pattern on the first training session in as little as 3 to 5 minutes. For instance, the client whose breathing is shown in the pretraining capnograph (Figure 8a) slowed from 30 breaths per minute after only 3 minutes of training (Figure 8b). The evaluation began at 1:32 P.M., and the imagery instructions were given at 1:35 P.M.. The capnograph shows that the recording was made at 1:38 P.M.

I will also stop the client and freeze the spectrum analyzer screen when there is a substantial elevation in *alpha*, and discuss the meaning and implication of *alpha* elevation. When clients show that they understand

TIME=06/14/85 13;32;30 52 UPDATE #1 PEAK CO2=3.96 AVG. CO2=3.96%

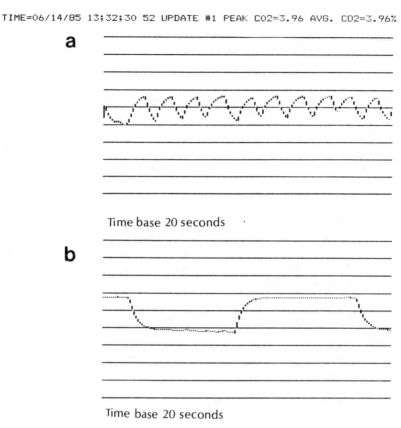

Figure 8. Capnographs of a 20-year-old woman with severe anxiety. Before training (a) breathing rate is 30 breaths/minute. After 5 minutes of deep-diaphragmatic breathing training (b), breathing rate is a little over 3 breaths/minute.

what *alpha* elevation, mean *theta* decrease, and transient *theta* mean, I also inform them of those occurrences:

> Good. And now you are showing a strong *alpha* response and there is no *theta*. How do you feel?

When she or he shows a good breathing configuration, and there is *alpha* elevation and mean *theta* reduction, and end-tidal CO_2 is decreasing, the instructions are changed again:

> Now you are doing very well. You are relaxed and alert. Why don't you go ahead and set the pace yourself? And as you are breathing in with the surf and out as the surf

recedes from the beach, tell yourself "I am relaxed and alert, warm and comfortable and alert."

I have found it important to use the words "alert" and/or "awake and not at all sleepy" on the inspiration phase of breathing. And I use "relaxed, warm, comfortable," on the expiration phase. I consider it important for the client to associate the proper words with the energizing and the passive phases of breathing, as contraction of the diaphragm is active, and breathing out is passive.

Second, at no time do I set a respiration rate for the client. I give no indication that there is a desired breathing rate. Yet, she or he typically tends to adjust automatically to the 3 to 5 b/min rate of TM and Zen. It is also common that after several minutes of this breathing, using surf imagery as the "metronome," as it were, there will be a decrease in $PETCO_2$, signifying a decrease in metabolism. When this does not occur, the client is probably not relaxing.

I do not generally permit $PETCO_2$ to decrease beyond a certain point without checking the client's blood pressure. That is, if it drops below 4%, I will ask the client if she or he experiences dizziness, faintness, or any discomfort. Lower PCO_2 can be taken to mean hypoarousal, but it can also signify hypocapnia. It is important to differentiate between the two.

Hypocapnia will be accompanied by elevated *theta* and symptoms of HVS, whereas hypoarousal is an asymptomatic state of reported well-being and alert comfort. If the client reports feeling good, relaxed, and alert, I will usually continue the training for another 30 seconds, always watching for sudden changes in breathing rate, rhythm, and percentage of end-tidal CO_2, as well as *theta* EEG. In extreme cases, syncope is usually preceded by a sharp drop in blood pressure and a significant increase in *theta* (Engel, Romano, & McLin, 1944). None of my clients has had syncope with this training procedure, probably because hypotensives are excluded from training; but breathing training has been shown to have a profound effect on blood pressure (Benson et al., 1974; Blackwell et al., 1976; Datey et al., 1969; Stone & DeLeo, 1976).

Superficially, the method described above appears to produce a pattern that looks like the one in the hypometabolic state of TM, Zen meditation, and Benson's relaxation response. It is characterized by a state of alert relaxation and comfort, a sense of well-being, decreased PCO_2, increased finger temperature, and an EEG in which *alpha* is coherent and predominant and *theta* is depressed with the exception of "transients."

The psychophysiology of the meditative state has been described in detail by numerous investigators since its initial study by Das and Gastaut (1957). (See also Chapter 8.) Its effectiveness compares favorably with relaxation and biofeedback for lowering blood pressure (Patel, 1973, 1975a, 1975b). Its other dimensions have also been examined and compared with biofeedback and relaxation, including the hypometabolic and hypoarousal states, and systematic changes in hemodynamics, cardiac function, acid-base homeostasis, cerebral function, and EEG (Badawi et al., 1984; Elson, Hauri, & Cunis, 1977; Farrow & Hebert, 1982; Fenwick et al., 1977; Jevning et al., 1978; Orme-Johnson & Farrows, 1977; Shapiro, 1982; Wallace, 1970a,b; Wallace, Benson, & Wilson, 1971; West, 1979; Wolkove et al., 1984; Woolfolk, 1975).

Three main aspects of the meditative state induced by TM, Zen, or other yogic methods, even Benson's, distinguish it from relaxation, biofeedback, and hypnosis: (a) altered metabolism, (b) respiratory suspension, and (c) a characteristic EEG pattern. Consonant with these three dimensions, the method described above, with imagery and biofeedback for the rapid induction of a hypoarousal state, is most like meditation. I call it the Rapid Alert Relaxation (RAR)™ exercise; and I included it with a stress reduction program, called *The ARTSystem™*, which I developed for The Prudential Life Insurance Company, in 1989.

Altered Metabolism

It is a basic tenet of physiology that respiration determines metabolism at any given instant. Consequently, numerous investigators have asked why meditation, unlike relaxation, most forms of biofeedback, and hypnosis, produces a hypoaroused, hypometabolic state. Fenwick et al. (1977) reported a decrease of about 16% in CO_2 output with TM. Wallace (1970a, 1970b) reported about 20% reduction in O_2 consumption after about 5 minutes of TM, and there are many other similar reports. These observations have not been reported in connection with most forms of biofeedback, relaxation, or hypnosis. In the rapid-induction method (i.e., RAR™), using biofeedback and imagery, as described above, there was no direct measure of O_2 consumption, but if the evidence from the TM studies is to be believed, there was no change in the respiratory quotient (QR) when O_2 consumption decreased.

This means that if respiration rate in my clients decreased and PCO_2 decreased, then metabolic rate must have decreased as well. Otherwise, PCO_2 would have had to increase. The validity of this assumption is best demonstrated by evidence in one client who "faked it." Figure 9 shows the breathing pattern and rate of a client at about 3 breaths per minute. $PETCO_2$ is about 6.5+. That is commonly observed in hyperventilators when their breathing rate is controlled by counting—another reason why a capnometer is indispensable.

Hypocapnia is also reduced by the RAR™. For instance, in a 20-year-

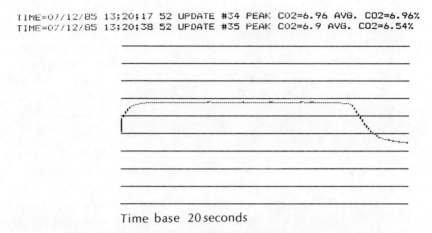

TIME=07/12/85 13;20;17 52 UPDATE #34 PEAK CO2=6.96 AVG. CO2=6.96%
TIME=07/12/85 13;20;38 52 UPDATE #35 PEAK CO2=6.9 AVG. CO2=6.54%

Time base 20 seconds

TIME=07/12/85 13;22;05 52 UPDATE #36 PEAK CO2=.24 AVG. CO2=4.2%

Figure 9. Capnograph of a 34-year-old woman showing breath holding rather than breath slowing.

old woman (Figure 10), the initial breathing rate was 24 breaths per minute. After 5 minutes of training, her inspiration rate was about 4 breaths per minute, and her PCO_2 was normal.

Respiratory Suspension

Numerous investigators have reported a breathing pattern in TM and Zen meditation not observed during relaxation, biofeedback, and hypnosis. They call it "respiratory suspension" (Badawi et al., 1984; Farrow & Hebert, 1982; Kesterson & Clinch, 1985), and it consists of episodes of breathing apparently suspended between 15 and 30 seconds. I have also observed it in clients during RAR℠. One such client began the session at about 21 breaths per minute, PETCO2 about 4.5. Twenty minutes later (see Figure 11), after 3 training sessions lasting about 3 minutes, PETCO2 was about 5.0, with suspended breathing periods lasting from 15 to 20 seconds.

Investigators who have reported such respiratory suspension periods equate it with the meditative state of "pure consciousness." Badawi et al. (1984) characterized it as having unique features differentiating it from other states of consciousness. It is important to note that these features occur during typical EEG configurations different from any found in biofeedback, relaxation, and hypnosis. The client whose breathing pattern is shown in Figure 11 reported this state, which she had never experienced

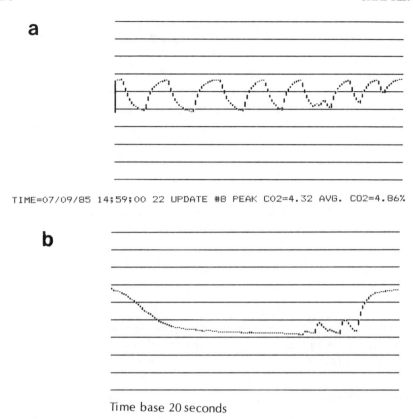

TIME=07/09/85 14;59;00 22 UPDATE #8 PEAK CO2=4.32 AVG. CO2=4.86%

Time base 20 seconds

TIME=07/09/85 15;02;09 22 UPDATE #14 PEAK CO2=6.42 AVG. CO2=6.42%

Figure 10. Capnographs of a 20-year-old woman before deep-diaphragmatic breathing training: (a) breathing rate is 21 breaths/minute; during training (b) it is around 2 breaths/minute, with some cardiac oscillation at end-tidal breath.

previously, during the respiratory suspension periods that coincided with the reported EEG configuration.

Electroencephalograph

TM and Zen meditation have produced a signature EEG, with predominant "coherent *alpha*"; decreased mean *theta*, with brief but relatively high-voltage *theta* transients; and decreased mean *beta* during *samadhi*, or "pure consciousness" (Anand, Chhina, & Singh, 1961; Banquet, 1972, 1973; Kasamatsu & Hirai, 1969). Kasamatsu and Hirai showed that this EEG

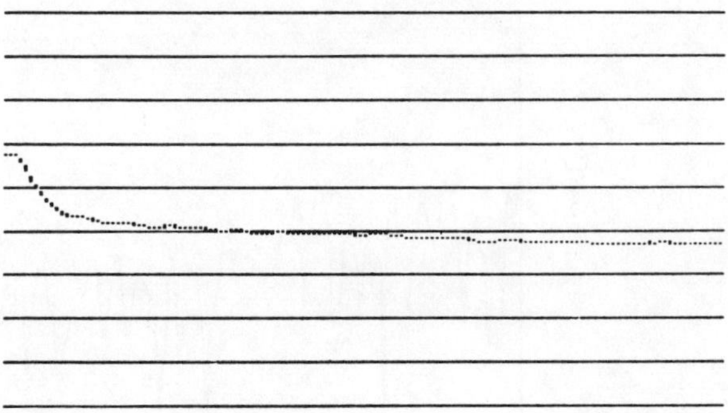

Time base 20 seconds

TIME=08/06/85 15;30;39 22 UPDATE #58 PEAK CO2=5.16 AVG. CO2=4.98%

Figure 11. Capnograph of a 30-year-old woman showing respiratory suspension during biofeedback-assisted breathing training with imagery.

pattern is absent in relaxation, biofeedback, and hypnosis. They stated that:

> Zen meditation is purely a subjective experience completed by a concentration which holds the inner mind calm, pure and serene. And yet, zen meditation produces a special psychological state based on the changes in the electroencephalogram. Therefore, zen meditation influences not only the psychic life but also the physiology of the brain. (p. 223)

The imagery method has also produced that state in several of my clients. In the client with respiratory suspension (Figure 11), mean *theta* is elevated at the beginning of the session (Figure 12a) and, as training progressed, it drops, as a distinct, coherent *alpha* emerged at 9.1 Hz (Figure 12b). As predicted (Badawi et al., 1984; Kasamatsu & Hirai, 1969; Wallace, Benson, & Wilson, 1971), there is a decrease in the frequency of *alpha* as she drifts into the "state." In another case (Figure 13) *Alpha* decreases to 8.9 Hz with the appearance of a transient *theta* at 6.4 Hz when breathing was about 3 breaths per minute.

The EEG of the client previously mentioned, who was holding her breath rather than breathing naturally and in synchrony to the beach image, was atypical. At the start of the session, it showed marked mean *theta*, elevated above *alpha* (Figure 14a), with a strong *beta* (at 17.3 Hz) as well as an elevated *theta* (at 5.0 Hz). This is a fairly typical pattern of hyperarousal. During "respiratory suspension" her EEG was unlike that of persons following instructions, or unlike those reported in TM, Zen, and so forth (see Figure 14b). *Theta* was elevated from 4 Hz to 7 Hz, and there was a peak at 12.7 Hz—which is a high *alpha* seldom seen in a meditative

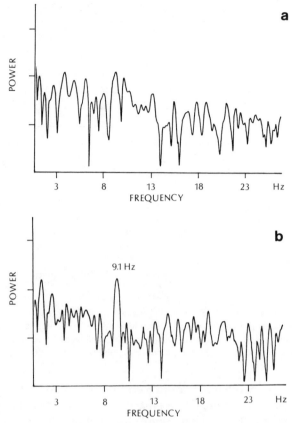

Figure 12. EEG power spectra in a 30-year-old woman before (a) and during (b) biofeedback-assisted deep-diaphragmatic breathing training with imagery. The spectrum in (a) shows diffuse general *theta* elevation; whereas in (b), *theta* decreases and there is a coherent *alpha* at 9.1 Hz.

state. *Beta* was elevated with peaks at 16.7 Hz and 18.4 Hz. The EEG confirmed the hypothesis that the slow breathing was not of the meditative type. Figures 15a and 5b show the pattern in an anxiety sufferer who reported extreme calmness during slow breathing with the surf imagery.

I recommend that breathing retraining be conducted by a professional with a good background in psychology and especially in the areas of biofeedback and clinical/counseling psychology. As clients begin to develop their new breathing patterns and a relationship with their trainer, emotional "clinical" material begins to emerge. In keeping with the general

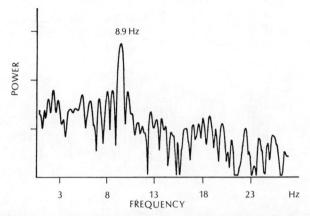

Figure 13. EEG power spectra in a 36-year-old woman during biofeedback-assisted deep-diaphragmatic breathing training with imagery, showing depressed *theta* with a coherent *alpha* at 8.9 Hz.

atmosphere of support and encouragement of clients as they learn this new task, a therapeutic relationship frequently develops. The management of this relationship requires the same clinical experience as any other therapeutic relationship. The importance of trained therapists, as clinical material comes to the client's awareness, is underscored by Stroebel and Glueck (1977), who reviewed some of the contraindications in clinical biofeedback and passive meditation techniques.

Breathing training involves clients who, in addition to HV, may have serious emotional problems. As is true of all biofeedback programs, the nonspecific effects of the client–trainer interaction and of the recognition that the symptoms have a physical basis, and can be self-controlled, are powerful variables in determining the outcome of the program. Nonspecific effects of therapeutic strategy are often considered to be placebo effects, but the concept of placebo control is not appropriate outside traditional blind and double-blind controlled studies of the effects of drugs (Fried, 1988; Surwit & Keefe, 1983). The self-regulation, biofeedback outcome studies cannot be faulted for contamination by the effects of the client–therapist interaction. That paradigm specifically calls for its use, wherever possible, in its most powerful form. That interaction may be the main effect. Clients should be encouraged to believe that correct breathing will make them feel better and that they can do it. This in no way alters the fact that, when they breathe correctly, they enhance peripheral and brain circulation, and help maintain the acid-base balance of the body, as well as

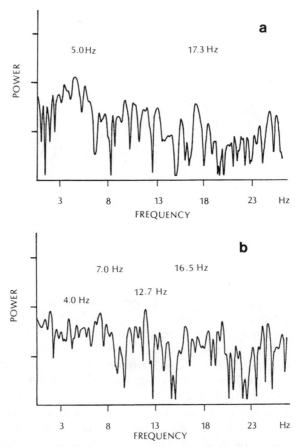

Figure 14. EEG power spectra showing elevated *theta* (a) in a 34-year-old woman before biofeedback-assisted deep-diaphragmatic breathing training with imagery; and (b) during training when she was holding her breath. Little *theta* reduction is evident during breath holding.

all other physiological mechanisms on which everything depends to function optimally.

The homeostatic mechanisms required by the body to correct the effects of chronic HV cause symptoms and discomfort. The nonspecific effects of believing that the program will help apply to the client's motivation to participate fully in the training program, an often difficult and frustrating task. The client should benefit from a regular regimen of

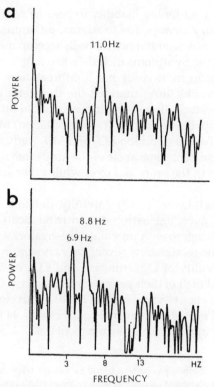

Figure 15. EEG power spectra of a 36-year-old female anxiety sufferer during (a) biofeedback-assisted deep-diaphragmatic breathing training with imagery. *Theta* is depressed and there is a coherent *alpha* at 11 Hz. After about 5 minutes (b) there was a highly coherent alpha, at 11.0 Hz, with increased *theta* and a high transient *theta* at 6.9 Hz, and *alpha* dropping to 8.8 Hz, as predicted (see Kasamatsu and Hiral, 1969).

breathing exercises even if she or he does not believe that there is any connection between the symptoms and breathing.

Asthma

Asthma, according to the *Merck Manual* (1982), is a "reversible airways obstruction not due to any other disease." It is one of the many somatic disorders that have been helped by clinical psychophysiologists employing behavioral methods including breathing training and biofeedback. An asthma attack is a frightening inability to breathe resulting from narrowing of the pulmonary airways due to edema, inflammation, and spasm of bronchial smooth muscle and mucosal wall, accompanied by an increased formation of mucous. Symptoms include wheezing, cough, and shortness of breath, and are in most cases not life-threatening. But in "intrinsic" asthma with irreversible lung changes, life-threatening crises may occur.

In an asthma attack, there is typically an initial phase of HV; airways restriction may impede ventilation (hypoventilation) to some areas of the lungs, reducing alveolar and blood O_2 and CO_2 perfusion and exchange. As the attack progresses, some areas of the lungs remain poorly ventilated due to obstruction in the bronchial tree, while other areas try to compensate by HV.

McFadden and Lyons (1968) carefully detailed arterial blood gas concentration in over 100 asthmatics during acute attacks of bronchospasm. They disagree with previous investigators who have stated that patients with only moderately severe bronchospasm only rarely show significant abnormality of O_2 saturation and CO_2 concentration. Hypoxemia was observed in 91 of their patients: mean arterial O_2 tension was 69.4 mm Hg (normal is about 98 mm Hg) (SD = 10.4 mm Hg). The lowest value observed was 49.1 mm Hg. Mean arterial pH was 7.44 (SD = 0.01), and 73 of them had respiratory alkalosis (mean pH = 7.46; SD = 0.03). They concluded that:

> . . . the characteristic blood gas pattern found in patients who are experiencing acute asthma attacks is hypoxemia associated with respiratory alkalosis. The most consistently observed abnormality was hypoxemia, which was encountered, to some degree, at all levels of airway obstruction. (p. 1030)

They further proposed that most asthmatic attacks are associated with alveolar HV, and that hypercapnia is not likely to occur until there are extreme degrees of airway obstruction. Their explanation for the discrepancy which they observed between levels of alveolar and minute ventilation is that inspired air is differentially directed to those areas in the lungs with the lowest flow resistance, which ordinarily amount to only about 25% to 40% of lung volume—which now receive between 80% and 90% of incoming air:

> Thus, a relatively small, but controlling number of alveolar units are hyperventilating in relation to their perfusion, giving rise to hypocarbia, a large physiologic dead space and a ventilation-perfusion ratio in excess of normal. The remaining 60 to 75 percent of the lung is poorly ventilated and hyperfused, with a ventilation-perfusion ratio that is markedly depressed. (p. 1031)

The following case from my patient files illustrates the relationship between PCO_2 and SaO_2 during an asthma attack. This young woman had a history of asthma, controlled most recently by a combination of medication and behavioral methods. She had lately come to rely less and less on medication but on one particular occasion, she was wheezy on entering the office, and she experienced an attack just prior to the breathing training session. Figure 16a shows her breathing pattern during the attack. Her breathing rate was about 26 breaths per minute and, as is typical, expirations were brief and incomplete. PETCO$_2$ was 3.6 and SaO$_2$ was 89.1%. Immediately following an application of albuterol inhalant (Figure 16b), breathing rate was 22 per minute, PETCO$_2$ rose somewhat (3.9), and SaO$_2$ rose sharply to the normal range (96.5%). Following six minutes of rest, she attempted abdominal breathing (Figure 16c). Three more breathing training trials, each lasting about three minutes, were distributed over a 25-minute period. On the last one (Figure 16d), her breathing rate was about 4 per minute, PETCO$_2$ normalized at 4.7, and SaO$_2$ was also in the normal range, at 97.5%.

It is reported by Gardner, Bass, and Moxham (1992) that even in some relatively mild cases of asthma, HV may result in sufficiently profound hypocapnia to trigger the symptoms characteristic of the HV syndrome. Their study was predicated on the contention that where HV is diagnosed,

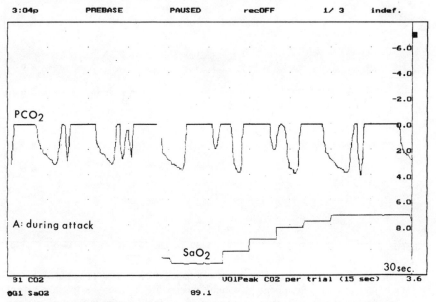

Figure 16a. Capnograph during asthma attack. Note rapid and uneven ventilation and low PETCO$_2$ and SaO$_2$.

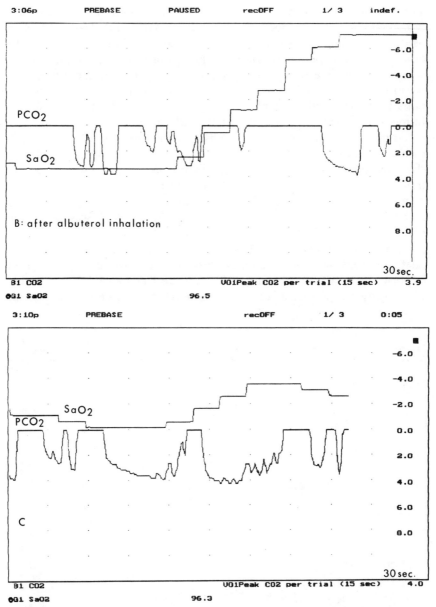

-6.0

-4.0

-2.0

PCO₂

0.0

SaO₂

2.0

4.0

6.0

B: after albuterol inhalation

8.0

30 sec.

B1 CO2   UO1Peak CO2 per trial (15 sec)   3.9

BG1 SaO2   96.5

-6.0

-4.0

SaO₂

-2.0

PCO₂

0.0

2.0

4.0

6.0

C

8.0

30 sec.

B1 CO2   UO1Peak CO2 per trial (15 sec)   4.0

BG1 SaO2   96.3

Figure 16b–c. (b) Capnograph immediately after inhalant. PETCO₂ is still low, but SaO₂ rises rapidly to normal level. (c) Capnograph 4 minutes later. PETCO₂ rises slowly as the patient attempts abdominal breathing. Breathing slows with some diaphragmatic spasms evident.

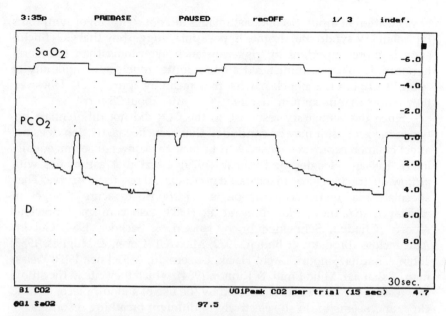

Figure 16d. Abdominal breathing normalizes PETCO$_2$, and SaO$_2$ remains at the high-normal level. Trace reversal in first expiration indicates diaphragmatic fatigue.

contrary to popular opinion, it is not invariably associated with anxiety and psychiatric disorders. Their case study illustrates an example of mild asthma presenting as HV in the absence of clinical features of airflow obstruction and anxiety. The authors conclude that:

> Hyperventilation implies excessive drive to breathe which can be due to a wide range of psychogenic, physiological and organic causes. Initiating and sustaining factors may be different. We believe that in every case of hyperventilation, an attempt should be made to document the cause or causes of excessive respiratory drive. A diagnosis of "hysterical hyperventilation" or "hyperventilation syndrome" discourages search for such causes, is unhelpful or even dangerous. (p. 351)

I couldn't agree more. Their article follows that of Hormbrey, Jacobi, Patil, and Saunders (1988), who compared the CO$_2$ response and breathing pattern in three subject groups: (a) symptomatic HV, (b) asthma, and (c) normal controls.

Their asthmatic group had a significantly higher baseline respiratory frequency and tidal volume and, predictably, lower PETCO$_2$ than either the control or the symptomatic HV groups. A number of their conclusions are especially germane. First, airway obstruction may cause increased ventilatory drive, in the absence of chemical stimuli, suggesting the action of vagal afferent input. Second, asthmatics did not complain of symptoms typical in HV syndrome, despite hypocapnia, suggesting that CO_2 fluctuation is more important in triggering such symptoms than long-term hypocapnia. They administered a one-minute undetectable quantity of "pure" CO_2; but it is not clear what they mean by "pure" CO_2. However, they report that maximum inspired PCO_2 was about 35 torr.

Since the ventilatory response to the CO_2 did not differentiate between the groups, it may be concluded that bronchoconstriction does not affect chemoreceptor response. And in fact, the converse seems equally likely. Kelsen, Fleegler, and Altose (1979) assert that asthmatics with airflow obstruction have an increased nonchemical respiratory drive. They speculate that bronchoconstriction is a response to acute changes in resistance to airflow. Hormbrey et al. (1988) also confirmed previous reports (Chadha, Schneider, Birch, Jenouri, & Sackner, 1984; Gilbert, Auchincloss, Brodsky, & Boden, 1972; Maxwell, Cover, & Hughes, 1985; Tobin, Chadha, Jenouri, Birch, Hacik, Gazeroglu, & Sackner, 1983; Weissman, Askanazi, Milic-Emili, & Kinney, 1984), which they cite in the study, that resting breathing rate is affected by the use of a mouthpiece, or nose clips, and seems to do so selectively in different breathing disorders.

If asthmatic bronchoconstriction is not a response to pulmonary chemoreceptor activity, what causes it? A number of physiological theories have been proposed to account for it. Foremost among these is an imbalance in beta-adrenergic and cholinergic activity, with increased cholinergic receptor and decreased beta-adrenergic receptor responsiveness. Support for this theory comes from the observation that inhaling a cholinergic agent, such as metacholine (Chadha, Schneider, Birch, Jenouri, & Sackner, 1984), or administering a beta-adrenergic blocking agent (propranolol), may provoke an attack (Berkow, 1982; Weiner, 1977).

Asthma may take the forms extrinsic, intrinsic, or mixed, which can be further subclassified as intrinsic exercise-induced, intrinsic aspirin-intolerant, extrinsic pharmacologic asthma, and so on.

Common Types of Asthma

Sodeman and Sodeman (1979) describe the following types of asthma: Extrinsic immediate atopic asthma is a Type I immunopathologic reaction to allergens. Histamine, platelet activating factor, prostaglandins, and other chemical mediators are released into the bloodstream rapidly following exposure to common allergens including grass pollens, dust, mold, animal hair, and so forth.

Extrinsic late nonatopic allergic asthma begins at least one hour after exposure to airborne allergens. This form appears to be secondary to the Type I reaction, or to an immunoglobulin other than IgE.

Extrinsic irritant and pharmacologic asthma is precipitated by chemical exposure, sometimes acting directly on the bronchial mucosa. The definition applies if removal from the chemical trigger causes resolution of the condition and if reexposure causes exacerbation. Soldering flux is cited as a known trigger.

Intrinsic asthma is thought to be based on a defect in autonomic regulation of the bronchial tree, because no known immunologic abnormalities have been demonstrated in this form. Sodeman and Sodeman (1979) cite viral respiratory tract infections, meteorologic changes, exercise, and so on. The connection to meteorologic changes should not be surprising since (a) low barometric pressure presents a further profusion problem in a hypoventilated lung, and (b) positive and negative ion density has also been related to pulmonary gas exchange (see Chapter 2).

Intrinsic aspirin-intolerant asthma is associated with ingestion of aspirin, indomethacin, ibuprofen, and tartrazine (FD & C yellow #5 dye), among others. It is associated with chronic sinusitis and nasal polyps.

Intrinsic exercise-induced asthma is most common in children. However, wheezing and bronchospasm are common after vigorous exercise in many forms of asthma. Intrinsic infectious asthma is common in children susceptible to recurrent viral upper respiratory tract infections; and intrinsic asthmatic bronchitis is characterized by asthma and chronic bronchitis, in which cigarette smoking may or may not be a factor. Cigarette smoking is a factor, however, in intrinsic asthma, with both irreversible and reversible obstructive airways disease.

These forms of asthma include bronchitic intrinsic asthma, with reversible airways disease, emphysematous-intrinsic asthma, and various combinations of bronchitis, asthma, and emphysema (Sodeman & Sodeman, 1979). Both intrinsic and extrinsic asthma are factors in mixed asthma.

Psychological Factors in Asthma

There have been many psychological interpretations of asthma, especially in childhood asthma. One psychodynamic theory centers on the concept of conflict (Alexander, 1950) and the "muted cry." But Weiner (1979) concludes that while actual or anticipated separation or loss may play an important role in initiating attacks in about 50% of cases, attacks may also be triggered by many other emotions, both unpleasant and pleasant, as well as by physical exertion. These theories are sufficiently nonspecific to be indistinguishable from theories of stress.

The stress theory of Selye is well known, but Gantt (1953) postulated an "innate susceptibility of the individual to breakdown" due to inherent conflict between general emotional responses and the more perfectly adaptive responses. He calls this process "schizokinesis." It seems most appropriate in asthma, considering Purcell, Bernstein, & Bukantz's 1961 findings that asthmatics with a "high allergic potential," as measured by skin test and by the Allergic Potential Scale of Block and colleagues (1964), seem "healthier psychologically and have more benign mothers" (cited in Weiner, 1979, p. 257).

Regarding allergy, Ottenberg and Stein (1958) and Shim and Williams (1986) found that odors trigger asthma in a remarkably large number of sufferers. Weiner (1979) ascribes psychological properties to this phenomenon, but I am more inclined to see it as a further connection between asthma and migraine. I have reported in 1990 that, to all extents and purposes, asthma responds to many of the same things that migraine responds to, including nutritional control, and shares many of the same blood mediators. More relevant here is that migraine and, parenthetically, idiopathic seizures are not uncommonly triggered by odors.

I encourage my clients to think of asthma as pulmonary migraine, and I make the same recommendations to them, in either case: reduce exposure to known airborne allergens and adopt an oligoantigenic diet (Egger, Carter, Soothill, & Wilson, 1989; Egger, Carter, Wilson, Turner, & Soothill, 1983; Fried, 1990a); reduce muscle tension and stress (Green & Shellenberger, 1991; Peper, 1988); lower blood levels of stress hormones; and learn deep-diaphragmatic breathing.

Allergic Mediators in Bronchial Asthma

Extrinsic bronchial asthma is an immunological reaction to allergens resulting in the production of IgE antibodies. Only about 40% of those exposed to allergens develop hypersensitivity to them; of those who do, less than half develop bronchial asthma. But the formation of IgE antibodies has also been observed to occur in persons who do not suffer asthma. Thus, it may be a necessary but not sufficient predisposing factor (Weiner, 1979).

Weiner (1979) summarized the immunological mechanism whereby specific allergens are first recognized by B-lymphocytes in the nasal, bronchial, and gastrointestinal lymph tissues: They mature into plasma cells that form the specific IgE molecules, which attach to mast cells and basophils in the connective and epithelial tissue of the bronchi and bronchioles.

Following IgE formation, exposure to the allergen causes mast cells, basophils, and epithelial cells, to which IgE and the allergen have attached, to release mediators: Histamine causes contraction of bronchial smooth muscle, constricting bronchial airways; small blood vessels increase in permeability; mucous secretion increases; and there is an increase in catecholamine release.

The "slow-reactive-substance-of-anaphylaxis" (SRS-A) causes profound long-lasting smooth muscle and bronchial muscle constriction. SRS-A is broken down by a basophil enzyme, ECF-A. Platelet-activating factor (PAP) may be released by sensitized lung tissue, causing platelet aggregation and the release of serotonin which promotes contraction of bronchial smooth muscle. Bradykinin is released as part of anaphylaxis and causes bronchoconstriction, hypotension, increased sweating and salivation, and increased blood vessel permeability.

Prostaglandins, especially PGF2, potentiated by parasympathetic ANS discharge, stimulate both bronchoconstrictors and vasoconstriction. Catecholamines, especially epinephrine, inhibit PGF2, but another class of prostaglandins, PGE1 and PGE2, inhibits catecholamine release. PGEs dilate bronchial airways and blood vessels, while PGFs have the opposite effect.

Other mechanisms involve cyclic nucleotides (i.e, increased or decreased GMP) and neuropeptides (neuropeptide tyrosine [NPY]) (Sheppard, Polak, Allen, & Bloom, 1984). All factors considered, it certainly seems that the lungs perform multiple endocrine and other complex secretory functions and that their role, ordinarily viewed as a more or less passive site except for gas exchange, is astonishingly oversimplified. Asthma may be one of the best windows into that complexity.

Behavioral Treatment Strategies to Reduce Asthma: Breathing Training and Biofeedback

The behavioral therapeutic approach to the reduction of asthma is a three-pronged attack. It (a) reduces triggers, including those that are airborne, and/or foodborne; (b) reduces stress, dysponetic bracing, and other muscle tension with relaxation techniques, and/or EMG biofeedback; and (c) improves breathing efficiency and restores diaphragmatic and thoracic muscle control and tonus.

On the psychological side, reducing the frequency and severity of asthma attacks has the additional benefit that comes from gaining control, seen in persons with a health or other impairment. According to Peper's client (1988):

> The most meaningful part in the training occurred when I inhaled 4000 ml. It gave me the sense of control and hope that I never had before. (p. 20)

Reduction of food triggers, as well as airborne antigens such as pollen or common roach exoskeleton, has been detailed in *The Breath Connection* (Fried, 1987a). I will therefore mention here only those items on the Egger et al. (1989) list which had a provocation probability greater than 10%: cow milk and cow cheese; citrus fruit; wheat; food additives (tartrazine and benzoic acid); hen eggs; tomato; chocolate; corn; and grapes.

These common foods also trigger migraine and epileptic seizures because of the body's reaction to their allergenic effect. I have found that these same foods, and others in specific cases, to which clients showed sensitivity, also triggered asthma, presumably for the same reason. The release of "mediators" has a deleterious effect on circulation and tissue oxygenation leading to hypoxia. Clinical psychophysiologists are urged to consider the food connection.

But the focus here is on biofeedback and breathing training techniques, especially those pioneered by Erik Peper (Konuk & Peper, 1984; Peper, 1988; Peper & Crane-Gochley, 1990; Peper, Klomp, & Levy, 1983; Peper, Smith, & Waddell, 1987; Peper & Tibbetts, in press; Peper, Waddell, & Smith, 1987; Roland & Peper, 1987; Tibbetts & Peper, 1988) of San Francisco State University.

Diaphragmatic Breathing Training with Incentive Inspirometer Biofeedback. Diaphragmatic breathing training is enhanced by the use of an "incentive spirometer." Peper uses the *Voldyne* (Sherwood), a simple and inexpensive unit that permits the client to observe inspiratory volume with each training effort. Although the primary problem in most cases of asthma is not inspiratory but expiratory volume, increasing inspiratory volume has a salutary effect on expiration.

Asthma sufferers seem to hold air in reserve. That is, they can readily inhale, but they tend not to exhale quite as fully as most nonasthma clients. By teaching them deep-diaphragmatic breathing, especially pulling back the abdomen with each exhale, they improve expiratory volume. Inspiratory volume improves when they exhale more fully. Thus, teaching full inhale also teaches fuller exhale.

The inspirometer is a graduated, transparent cylinder and piston, from which protrudes a short, flexible tubing with a mouthpiece at the distal end. The trainee can observe maximum inspiratory volume at the end of breath. She or he sits upright facing the inspirometer placed at mouth level, and is instructed to loosen clothing, including upper part of pants zipper, where applicable. She or he is then instructed in the use of the Voldyne and permitted, by practice trials, to demonstrate to the trainer that she or he knows how to use it (i.e., in through the mouth, and out through the nose). Baseline recordings are made with the subject's eyes closed and her or his taking 5 normal breaths, with time in between to permit the piston to return to zero. Maximum volume is recorded each time. She or he is then instructed to take five maximum breaths through the Voldyne. A special procedure was installed if the trainee exceeded 4000 ml (see Roland & Peper, 1987).

Following baseline recording, the trainee is given an explanation of the benefits of diaphragmatic breathing; instructions in "complete exhalation" by pulling the stomach in slightly at the end of exhalation; is told to inhale slowly, letting the tummy "bubble out" completely before filing the chest; and is told to relax the shoulders and chest until the end of exhalation. Instructions are demonstrated several times by the trainer; then 5 maximum volume breaths are recorded from the trainee.

Parenthetically, I have learned not to allow the trainee to use the chest at all until I am satisfied that she or he has abdominal breathing well under control. Although Peper's procedure varies from mine, there is no hard evidence one way or the other. According to Peper (personal communication, 1991):

> . . . we use the incentive inspirometer to demonstrate that if subjects breathe in a different pattern (thoracic shifted to diaphragmatic) the inhalation volume increases remarkably. The incentive inspirometer is very useful because of its high "face validity." Namely, most subjects experience breathing difficulty as the inability to get enough air. Hence the demonstration that changing breathing pattern actually increases the inhalation volume demonstrates to them experientially that the effortless diaphragmatic breathing is much more effective. In fact when they learn to exhale and then relax and allow the air to flow back in, most are surprised by the remarkable reduction of effort. They now know that if they focus on the exhalation phase and then let go and allow the abdomen to expand the air will flow in effortlessly.

They also use a similar breathing strategy with clients with panic and anxiety, because the mastery of effortless breathing adds a sense of control. Their training and coaching procedure is as follows:

(1) Trainer assists exhalation by applying pressure to abdomen and/ or sides with her or his hand.
(2) Trainer assists inhalation by placing hands on abdomen and/or sides and encouraging subject to "bubble out."
(3) Trainer assists shoulder relaxation by applying slight pressure with hands.
(4) Trainer assists shoulder relaxation by gently shaking or rocking shoulders.
(5) Trainer assists shoulder relaxation by instructing subject to tense and relax (Jacobsonian Progressive Relaxation Technique).
(6) Discussion of the emotional feelings associated with letting the stomach expand.

(7) Practice increasing volume as primary objective, as opposed to keeping shoulders relaxed.

(8) Practice keeping shoulders relaxed as primary objective, as opposed to increasing volume. Trainer provides feedback about shoulder relaxation.

(9) Ask subject to take a large thoracic breath, observe the volume, then take a slow diaphragmatic breath and observe the volume.

(10) Have subject observe normal breathing pattern with the Voldyne.

(11) Have subject demonstrate any problems she or he has with breathing. Then do diaphragmatic breathing.

(12) Use imagery of the air coming up through the feet and legs, filling up the abdominal area, then the chest, and being exhaled down the arms and out the fingertips. (Roland & Peper, 1987, p. 93)

Average coaching time lasts about 16 minutes. Five normal diaphragmatic breaths, followed by five maximum volume diaphragmatic breaths, are recorded posttraining.

Roland and Peper (1987) report a posttraining increase in inspiratory volume of over 70%. In subsequent studies, they explore the use of EMG biofeedback to (a) reduce upper thorax tension and (b) teach abdominal breathing with lessened thoracic muscle involvement.

EMG Biofeedback: Upper Thorax versus Abdomen.   EMG monitoring and biofeedback helps to control the muscle tension in the neck and upper thorax (Johnston & Lee, 1976) (see Chapter 5). Regional muscles are the anterior scalenes, which arise from the transverse processes of the 3rd to 6th cervical vertebrae, and insert into the first rib; the medial scalenes, which arise from the transverse process of all cervical vertebrae and insert into the first rib, lateral to the anterior scalene; and the posterior scalenes, which arise from the transverse process of the 5th and 6th cervical vertebrae and insert into the upper border of the second rib (Figure 17). Associated nerves descend from the cervical and brachial plexus and innervate the thoracic muscles.

Considering the scalenes' anatomical and spatial relationship to the right and left trapezius, and pectoral, among the many fairly massive muscles of the neck, shoulder and upper thoracic region, it is unlikely that EMG electrode placement anywhere in the region can be specific to the scalenes. But that does not really matter because the concern is with action biopotentials in that region during chest breathing relative to that in which

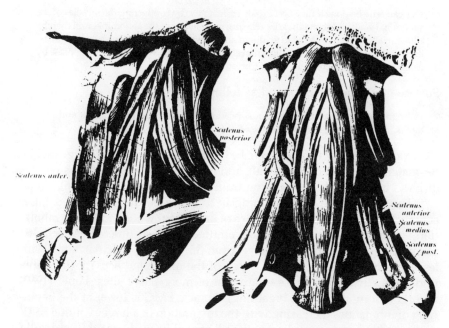

Scalenus posterior

Scalenus anter.

Scalenus anterior
Scalenus medius
Scalenus post.

Figure 17. Anatomy of the neck showing the location and attachment of the scalenes.

abdominal (diaphragmatic) breathing prevails. Peper makes this quite clear in a personal communication (1991), and in Tibbets and Peper (1988).

I have adopted his recommendation of the use of the scalene-trapezius EMG mainly as an *error signal* for thoracic breathing. According to Peper (personal communication, 1991):

> The task for our subjects was to breathe diaphragmatically and effortlessly. However they had to do this while reducing the upper thoracic EMG activity. Initially when we did this the subjects learned the feedback task very well. However, *they did this by breathing very shallowly.* This was the major reason for the addition of the incentive inspirometer feedback. The task was now to reduce thoracic EMG (Scalene-Trapezius) while at the same time increase inhalation volume. The only way the subjects could do this was to breathe diaphragmatically. This meant that they had to exhale more before allowing the inhalation to occur. This procedure automatically reduced (eliminated) the hyperinflation.

I have added the italics here to emphasize his warning. In the EMG biofeedback procedure, subjects are asked to inhale without increasing the EMG activity of the upper thorax. According to Peper (1988):

This can only be done if they first exhale sufficiently (by contracting the muscles of the abdominal wall) and then inhale by relaxing the muscles of the abdominal wall thereby allowing abdominal contents to go down and forward when the diaphragm contracts. If the abdominal wall does not allow movement, the person will tend to compensate by using the accessory chest muscles of breathing. (p. 114)

Surface electrodes were placed as follows:

. . . either over the bilateral trapezius, bilateral pectoralis, right trapezius and pectoralis, or left scalene and right trapezius. (p. 115)

Electrode placement is reported to be in accordance with that suggested by Basmajian and Blumenthal (1980), and is consistent with previous reports of EMG biofeedback in breathing training (Johnston & Lee, 1976).

The goal of the EMG training is to decrease the "integrated EMG activity" from the accessory muscles of breathing, while increasing inhalation volume. Muscle biopotentials emitted per unit time assess activity, ultimately in the form of voltage over time, at a particular site. With lessened muscle tension, the "slope" of the integrated activity (i.e., area under the curve) will be less than that of more active sites. Peper (1988) reports that in abdominal breathing, thoracic EMG is lower at the beginning of inhalation, increasing with the inspiration of a larger volume of air causing lifting and expanding of the rib cage. I have observed this also. In this 43-year-old woman (Figure 18), the EMG increases with inspiration as the chest rises, and falls as the chest drops with expiration. The EMG and $PETCO_2$ seem out of phase because it takes longer for CO_2 to register, since air must travel to the capnometer through the catheter. I have cautioned about this in Chapter 5.

Although Peper employs thoracic EMG biofeedback principally to provide an "error signal" for the tendency to inhale without abdominal excursion, in some cases EMG biofeedback from the lower abdomen was used to enhance relaxation of the lower rectus abdominis during inspiration, and contraction during the latter phase of expiration. The latter reportedly increased inspiration volume by about 24%, as EMG activity decreased. All subjects reported symptom relief, including reduction in shortness of breath, tightness of chest, wheezing, and reliance on medication.

In another study, Peper, Smith, and Waddell (1987) proposed symptom prescription (i.e., turning symptoms on and off). The subjects are first encouraged to produce or to simulate the symptoms, then to inhibit them with diaphragmatic breathing. This procedure is consistent with the practice of enhancing awareness of breathing patterns in retraining procedures, and provides a basis for desensitization to escalating asthma symptoms, and fear, as wheezing begins. Alternating self-induced asthma-like

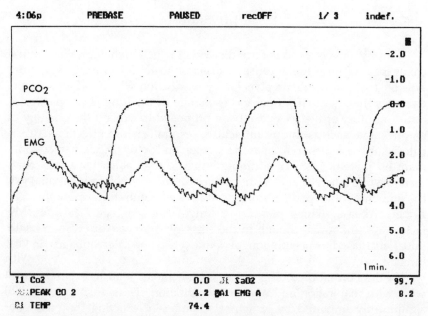

Figure 18. Capnograph (1-minute duration) of a 43-year-old woman asthma sufferer showing PETCO$_2$ and *trapezius* EMG at the beginning of biofeedback-assisted deep-diaphragmatic breathing training. An objective of training is to reduce the tendency to use ancillary breathing muscles (scaleni) to raise the chest with inspiration. This tendency is observed as EMG rises with inspiration.

symptoms and diaphragmatic breathing teaches the clients that they can abort an attack when wheezing begins, by shifting to abdominal (diaphragmatic) breathing.

U.S. government health agencies warn that the incidence of asthma is on the rise, and we have witnessed numerous media reports of the sudden and untimely death from asthma of notable public figures and celebrities. This can only be the tip of the iceberg. In all cases, reports suggested the sad inevitability of that death because no timely medical intervention was available. In no case was it suggested that the individual died despite his or her use of the breathing exercises which we routinely teach our asthma clients to use. My clients tell me that they were never told about them by their physician and, with notable exceptions, did not hear about them from any medical source. In every case that I have supervised, individuals with severe, even life-threatening asthma were able, after some training, to reduce medication (under their physician's supervision). I believe that it is tragic that this intervention was not available to others.

Emphysema

Emphysema is a pulmonary disease in which pathological structural changes in the bronchioles cause obstruction to air flow during expiration. This obstruction results in alveolar hyperinflation which, when chronic, damages them so that proper gas exchange in the lungs is jeopardized.

A number of theories have been proposed to explain the etiology of emphysema, such as chronic bronchitis, respiratory tract infections, tuberculosis, airborne irritants, cigarette smoke, and so on. (Sodeman & Sodeman, 1979; Stein, 1983). In addition, it is held that, at least in some cases, there may be a hereditary predisposition in the form of an inadequacy of the enzyme antitrypsin, leading to excess concentration of another enzyme, protease, which may cause lung tissue damage. The initiating factors are unknown, though in the early phases there appears to be an initial increased concentration of leukocytes and macrophages in the lungs.

In the normal breathing process, bronchioles tend to expand somewhat with inspiration and narrow at expiration. Thus, inspiration is not significantly impaired by structural changes obstructing the passages. However, on expiration, obstruction together with the narrowing bronchioles traps air in the alveoli. The combined efforts of the diaphragm and other respiratory muscles, exerted to evacuate the alveoli, together with bouts of paroxysmal coughing, result in a further pressure rise aggravating the obstruction. In the long run, this hyperinflation of the lungs causes them to enlarge, pushing the diaphragm downward into the configuration it usually assumes in normal maximal inspiration. Thus, diaphragmatic excursion is seriously limited and normal breathing is impaired.

Functionally, emphysema results in uneven ventilation of the lobes of the lungs, with variations in local gas mixture. Venous gas is, in many regions, exposed to low O_2 and high CO_2 concentrations. Consequently, arterial blood O_2 (SaO_2) may be depressed, and CO_2 ($PaCO_2$) may be elevated. Bearing in mind the suggestion by Sodeman and Sodeman (1979) that:

> An improvement in ventilation might be anticipated if the diaphragm could be returned to a more normal position on expiration—the rationale behind the use of emphysema belts, breathing exercises, and pneumoperitoneum. (p. 457)

I have undertaken the treatment of several persons with advanced emphysema. "Pneumoperitoneum," parenthetically, is the inflation of the peritoneal cavity.

The following case illustrates the procedure and outcome. A 72-year-old woman presented with extreme dyspnea, fatigue, paroxysmal coughing, and chronic heavy cigarette consumption, among other things. She reported that, despite the knowledge that it would "probably kill me soon," she was unable to stop smoking and had even tried hypnosis—unsuccessfully. The first session was taken up by routine intake protocol matters, and it was noted that her breathing was rapid (17 breaths per minute), of the high-chest, shallow type, interrupted frequently by violent coughing and mucous rales. Preliminary observation of SaO_2 ranging from 88% to 93% and $PETCO_2$ of 5.6 to 6.3 ($ETCO_2$ of 42.6 to 47.9 torr) were noted. The capnograms below illustrate the first training session.

The initial capnogram (Figure 19a) shows $PETCO_2$ at 5.1, SaO_2 at 93%, tachycardia (pulse rate is 116 per minute), and severe peripheral vaso-constriction (hand temperature is 73.1°F, in a room at 71.5°F). Her hands were so cold that the pulse plethysmograph sensor malfunctioned, as evidenced by the widely fluctuating excursions of the HR trace.

She was then taught deep-diaphragmatic breathing by the methods described earlier in this chapter. Her control of the mechanics of breathing was minimal at first—she found it difficult to restrain her chest. But gradually, she showed some improvement and, by successive, brief exer-cise segments consisting of 2 to 3 breaths (to avoid fatigue), she made

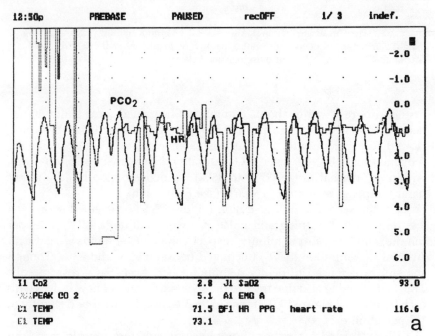

Figure 19a. First session pretraining PRP of a 72-year-old woman with emphysema: Breath-ing is rapid (17/minute), $ETCO_2$ is normal (5.1%), SaO_2 is well below normal (93%), pulse is rapid (116.6/minute), and hands are cold (73.1°F).

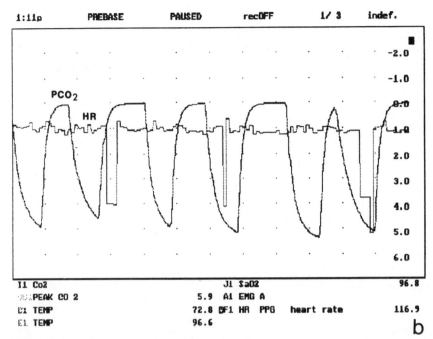

Figure 19b. First breathing training: After several breathing training trials spanning 20 minutes, breathing is deeper (6/minute), SaO_2 rose to high-normal (96.8%), and hand temperature soared (96.6%), but pulse remained elevated.

further progress within about 20 minutes. She gained some ability to use her abdominal muscles to push the diaphragm upward; her breathing slowed to 6 per minute; $PETCO_2$ rose somewhat to 5.9; her pulse rate remained high; but her arterial O_2 saturation (SaO_2) rose to 96.8%—well within the normal range (95% to 98%). Vasoconstriction lifted and her hand temperature soared to 96.6°F (see Figure 19b).

On the second training session (Figure 19c), she seemed somewhat less tense. Her breathing and pulse rate were still rapid (21 breaths per minute) and 114 beats per minute, respectively), but her hands were warm. Arterial O_2 saturation (SaO_2) fluctuated between 92% and 93%. Though she still experienced difficulty restraining her chest, SaO_2 rose rapidly. Thus, I decided to add that trace to the screen to show her how it rises with each breath (see Figure 19d). It rose to 98.3%, and HR dropped slightly to 112 per minute.

I have treated a number of emphysema sufferers, but do not claim extensive experience with this client population. They typically remain in training for only a few sessions and, though similar results were obtained

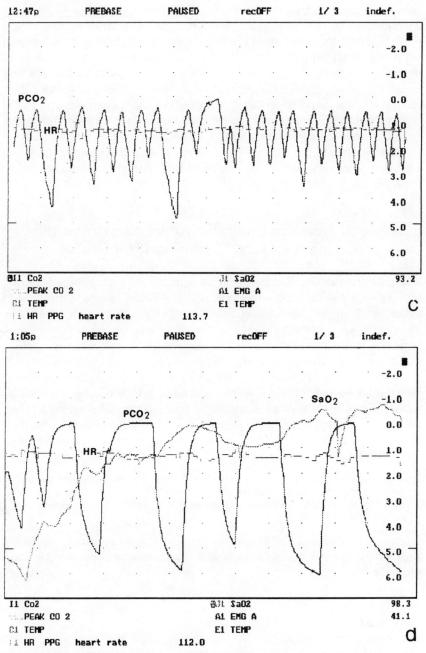

Figure 19c–d.   (c) Second session pretraining: Breathing is rapid (21/minute), SaO$_2$ is low (93.2%). (d) Second session posttraining: SaO$_2$ trace added to the biofeedback rises to 98.3%.

with other clients, I have no data on which to base a prediction of the long-term efficacy of this procedure. But I illustrate this case here because I think that it would be helpful to those who have such a client population to support their training procedure with the psychophysiological feedback of the within-session, and between-session, effectiveness of the training exercises. All my clients have reported that they were astonished that their blood O_2 levels could improve with simple breathing exercises and that it was helpful to see rising SaO_2 concentration. Its impairment is the major source of their concerns and anxiety. However, because of the structural fragility of alveoli, in emphysema, I have insisted that they do no home exercises. Exercises such as pursed lip breathing may increase alveolar air pressure.

A Recent Development in the Application of Breathing Training: Reducing Menopausal Hot Flushes

This chapter detailed methods integrating physiological monitoring with specific breathing training instructions, visual imagery, music, and biofeedback, applicable to functional as well as selected organic breathing disorders. Any new application of breathing training to reduce human suffering merits our attention. In this connection, I cite its recent application to reducing menopausal hot flushes.

Freedman (with Woodward, 1992a,b) reported that by using ambulatory monitoring of skin conductance changes, which reliably correspond to verbal reports of flushes experienced by menopausal women, a group taught paced-respiration had a significant decrease in hot flushes, as their breathing rate declined, while a muscle relaxation group showed neither breathing rate decline, nor reduced hot flushes. They concluded that:

> . . .training in a simple breathing procedure results in a significant reduction in menopausal hot flushes as measured over a 24-hour period. This technique may be useful for women with hot flushes who are unable to receive hormone replacement therapy. (1992a, p. 438)

Scientists are cautious and tend to make modest claims. I think that this is a very exciting finding and I hope that other innovative applications will follow it.

Chapter **10**

In Conclusion

I have contended that the sanative principle is in the man,
and is involved in the electro-nervous fluid, which is the posi-
tive force breathed in from the atmosphere. . . .
                                        —JOHN B. DODS

The metabolism of living beings gives rise, more or less continuously, to extremely small electrobiopotentials periodically varying in magnitude. Electrophysiological techniques amplify, filter, and record these biopotentials; and psychophysiologists employ them to assess physiological organ function and, in biofeedback, to treat somatic (i.e., psychophysiological) disorders by self-regulation methods.

Every bodily organ system has its own characteristic set of rhythmically varying electrobiopotentials, identifying it like a signature. Most biological biopotentials are amplitude modulated (AM), that is, the signal has a relatively low periodicity in which the process is represented by changes in its magnitude (usually microvoltage) over time. Frequency modulation (FM) is not characteristic of biopotentials but is common, for instance, in the physical world of sound and light. Biopotentials may have rhythmic variations beyond those of its characteristic amplitude changes. These rhythms, in the different body organs, are often attributable to *rhythm generators*, specialized cells or cell aggregates, which may integrate rhythms in positive or negative feedback loops. A feedback loop is a functional description of the modulating retroactive effect of events that have taken place on events about to occur. A positive loop enhances (excites) future activity in the system, while a negative loop inhibits it.

Breathing is, for the most part, controlled by involuntary feedback mechanisms regulated, in turn, by rhythm generators. This autonomous system can be overridden, up to a point, by voluntary activity. Air is periodically drawn into the body (inspiration), by the action of the diaphragm or of the rib muscles, through the nose or mouth, and conducted through airway passages which narrow significantly as they approach the functional respiratory units of the lungs—the alveoli. Gas exchange between the atmosphere and the blood takes place in the alveoli, which are relatively fragile and must be shielded against the intrusion of foreign matter. The upper segment of airway passages is lined with a mucous blanket which is antibacterial and which, by ciliary action of its epithelial cell wall, removes much foreign matter from air entering the lungs.

The O_2 content of blood in the vessels in the lungs is lower than that in the alveolar air, and the CO_2 content is higher. "Gas exchange" means that equilibration takes place across lung and blood vessel membranes between alveolar and blood O_2, and CO_2. After gas exchange has been effected, a process that takes only a fraction of a second, alveolar air is expelled (expiration). The rhythm of the breathing cycle is determined by the interactive effects of brain, and peripheral mechanisms, which appear to respond to chemoreceptors (predominantly to CO_2), and to stretch-reflexes in the lungs.

An increase in the periodicity of this breathing cycle inconsistent with metabolic demand may result in an increase in the amount of CO_2 expelled from the lungs (hypocapnia), reducing the blood CO_2 content below that required for proper function (hypocarbia). This process is called hyperventilation and results in a momentary shift of the acid-base equilibrium of blood toward alkalosis. If the process is extended, or even chronic, the blood alkalosis is compensated by renal (kidney) mechanisms to restore it to normal (pH = 7.38). Chronic compensation is often called "respiratory alkalosis," and has a rapid detrimental effect on metabolism.

Oxygenated blood is pumped through arteries to body organs and to the brain, and it returns to the lungs by the veins. The major portion of the resistance to blood flow occurs primarily in the arterioles and capillaries whose diameter depends, in the peripheral circulation, on autonomic nervous system function, and on the blood CO_2 content. In the brain, blood CO_2 content is the *only* determinant of vascular diameter (caliber) and blood flow. Decreased CO_2 content causes immediate vasoconstriction in both the peripheral and brain tissues. Breathing also regulates the lymphatic system of glands and ducts, which maintains intercellular (interstitial) fluid balance. Lymphatic fluid contributes to the immune system.

Circulating blood derives its red color from iron in the hemoglobin (Hb) within the red cell (erythrocyte), which transports the major share of O_2 and CO_2 in the blood. Though there are several forms of Hb, only one form combines with O_2, and its affinity for it depends on the pH of blood.

An upward shift from normal pH toward increased blood alkalinity causes Hb and O_2 to be bound more firmly to each other (OHb); a downward shift toward lessened alkalinity favors OHb dissociation and, therefore, greater O_2 delivery to tissues. Increased pH also increases blood levels of organic phosphates, which also compete with O_2 for binding on Hb, thus further jeopardizing delivery of O_2 in body tissues. Abnormal blood conditions may result in abnormal breathing patterns—for instance, a higher or lower red cell count may cause a disproportionate ratio of methemoglobin (which does not bind O_2) or variant forms of Hb. Some of these conditions may be side effects of medication, or may result from avitaminosis.

The assessment of breathing may be incorporated into a psychophysiological profile which permits functional evaluation of its role relative to that of other organs, including the heart and the brain. The profile simultaneously shows indices of common observable physiological parameters, such as rate, mode, rhythm, and end-tidal CO_2 concentration, over the course of time, in conjunction with the activity of the heart, brain, circulation, and muscles. Automated recording and analysis, as well as biofeedback protocols and procedures, may be implemented by computerized physiological interface units. Unfortunately, no present physiological interface module permits evaluation of breathing as a function of the effect of hormones, especially gonadal hormones in both men and women. For instance, increased progesterone leads to metabolic acidosis, which results in compensatory HV.

Hyperventilation is repeatedly causally implicated in stress syndromes, and in most mental disorders, including depression, anxiety, panic, and phobias. Its symptoms span those encountered in most such complaints, including anxiety, dizziness, faintness, apprehension, a feeling of unreality, vertigo, and often the fear of going crazy, or of dying. The numerous studies which link these disorders and symptoms, while by no means in unanimous agreement as to etiology, overwhelmingly point to respiratory patterns, and the physiological ventilatory response to CO_2.

The correction of a "functional" breathing disorder such as HV has been effected by various training methods, most of which derive from one or another form of yoga. *Functional* is in quotes here because that is not invariably the case. In common heart and kidney diseases, and in diabetes, potentially lethal metabolic acidosis prevails, and is compensated by breathing, which appears in the form of HV. To correct this compensation could have catastrophic results. In another instance, the assumption that HV is a benign process has led to its "therapeutic" use to provoke "latent" symptoms. Numerous sources caution against this procedure because the resultant hypocarbia may cause paroxysmal vasoconstriction in those who are subject to angina, stroke, or epileptic seizures. Many treatment methods emphasize deep-diaphragmatic breathing which can also be taught by biofeedback-assisted instructions, implemented with music and/or visual imagery.

This book describes an elaborate set of techniques, both traditional and original, which have been empirically verified and found to correct functional, as well as nonfunctional, disorders such as asthma and emphysema. These techniques describe capnometry (end-tidal CO_2 monitoring), and oximetry (arterial blood O_2 monitoring), in combination with computerized, multimodal, and traditional psychophysiological monitoring. The application of these methods has been shown to have a corrective effect on breathing and a salutary effect on the client, reducing tension, stress, anxiety, and the frequency and severity of symptoms, and in numerous cases, eliminating symptoms altogether.

In Chapter 6, *Clinical Psychoneuroimmunology,* in *Biofeedback: Principles and Practice for Clinicians,* 3d ed. (1983), edited by J.V. Basmajian, Norris writes:

> Good breathing is an essential part of good health, and many books have been written about the healing aspects of breathing exercises. . . . Proper *diaphragmatic* breathing promotes efficient gas exchange in the lungs and so rehabilitates oxygen deficiency disorders, balances the autonomic nervous system, reduces physiologic correlates of anxiety . . . and pumps the lymphatic system. I have come to believe that I would choose correct diaphragmatic breathing if we had to share only one tool or technique for maximally improving physical health. (p. 60) (author's italics)

Physical health! I couldn't be more in agreement, and it would be remiss not to quote the rest of that paragraph:

> The physiologic processes of respiration, and the critical role that breathing has in maintaining the body's metabolic processes, are covered comprehensively in *The Hyperventilation Syndrome: Research and Clinical Treatment* by Fried (13). (p. 60)

Thank you Dr. Norris! Very discerning. Behavioral medicine, or behavioral physiology, whichever you prefer in describing the reciprocal relationship between psychological and physical health, requires this integration and synchronization of physical and emotional factors. And many practitioners have come to realize that breathing may be the fulcrum for the balancing act that we call health. By analogy, in Chapter 6 of *The Federalist Papers,* by Alexander Hamilton, James Madison, and John Jay, Hamilton writes:

> A man must be far gone in Utopian speculations who can seriously doubt that if these States should either be wholly disunited, or only united in partial confederacies, the subdivisions into which they might be thrown would have frequent and violent contests with each other.

Had Hamilton been a physiologist instead of a federalist, might he not have said just about the same thing about how the body should work? Even though each has its own agenda, it's all about components working in harmony toward some common good, isn't it?

Getting the System to Hum. We are fascinated by energy, and we have certain very sensory ideas about it which transcend biology, physics, and mechanics. As Walt Whitman put it, in *Leaves of Grass*, "I sing the body electric. . . . " Considerably less poetically, we tune up the car. In 1852, John B. Dods, invited to address the U.S. Senate on *Electrical Psychology*, said that:

> Hence by Psychology we are to understand the Science of the Soul. And . . . all impressions are made upon the soul through the medium of electricity, as the only agent by which it holds communication with the external world. . . . (p. 19)

Chemistry teaches us that the physical world is made up of particles which are arranged spatially, in three dimensions, in accordance with the interplay of attracting and repelling forces which, in composite, we call "energy." Energy fluctuates periodically. One of its properties is "frequency." We often use the term "frequency" to describe breathing when we observe the periodicity of tidal volume. Yet it is nowhere more clear than in Cheyne-Stokes breathing, with its typical pattern of periodic, oscillatory, tidal volume changes, how that definition misses the point. A capnometer tracing of $ETCO_2$, by which we derive breathing frequency, is actually a tracing of the changing concentration of CO_2 in exhaled breath, as that concentration increases with the depth in the lungs, from which the air sample comes. Thus, $ETCO_2$ is ultimately a measure of the depth of pulmonary ventilation. This concept is entirely lost in its use as a measure of respiratory frequency.

The interplay of energy changes is dynamic and, in the aggregate, gives all things physical a continuous dynamic periodicity which we observe as rhythm. Most aspects of physical matter have their own rhythm, a signature, as it were, which interacts with other such rhythms to result in yet new rhythms for the aggregate. When physical matter is combined into a life form, we may observe it to have a complex interplay of these energy oscillations—something like the score of a symphony—where, at any moment in time, each component plays its characteristic "note" as part of its own melody and rhythm, and the aggregate creates a distinct new sound, superimposed on yet a new rhythm.

And so it is in psychophysiology that we begin with an assessment of the rhythm of the energy in an organ system, because we recognized dysrhythmia as dysfunction, and we believe that we can, like turning the pegs on a violin, restore the rhythm to the strings that will give the organ the proper pitch and harmonic composition. It is surely no coincidence that the word "organ," which can describe both an anatomical component and a musical instrument, is derived from the Greek word *organon*, from which we derive "*erg*," the unit of energy. In the dysrhythmic brain, we may alternatively try to locate the focus of disruption, extirpate it surgically, or medicate it into regulation, or self-regulate it by such methods as biofeedback or meditation. We do this with the heart, and we do it with muscles and other body organs. And most importantly, we do it with breathing.

Thus, on the one hand, the rather simplistic aphorism, "breathing is the rhythm of life," threadbare as it is, seems magically imbued with wisdom in direct proportion to how little we really know of the essential characteristics of frequency, periodicity, and synchrony at all levels in physiology. We know that there is something out there, and that it changes more or less predictably. We have faith in its importance because countless other aphorisms from admired, though inscrutable, sources also say so. For instance, a Tibetan saying is that "breath is the horse, and mind is the rider." It seems universal wisdom that the horse should be put before Descartes.

On the other hand, there is still an astonishing amount of controversy in some quarters over the role of breathing in clinical applications. In his book, *A Clinical Guide to the Treatment of the Human Stress Response* (1989), Everly writes:

> Unfortunately, there is no substantial body of research literature directed specifically towards one type of therapeutic breath pattern. . . . (p. 204)

Not only is he misinformed, as countless references in this and other books attest, but he contradicts his own previous assertion:

> Voluntary control of respiration patterns (breath control) is perhaps the oldest stress-reduction technique known. It has been used for thousands of years to reduce anxiety and to promote a generalized state of relaxation. (p. 201)

How would we know this if it were not documented? You can't have it both ways. But then again, breath control wasn't used for stress reduction for thousands of years. It was used in meditation, to transcend the conscious experience—not exactly the same thing. Its use in stress reduction is scientific, very recent, and thoroughly documented. Green and Shellenberger (1991) write that:

> Correct breathing is the foundation of relaxation, and some say that it is the foundation of good health. All relaxation exercises begin with a focus on breathing. (p. 197)

Would that it were so!

Appendix

Initial Intake Information

Date: _____   Referred by: _____

                              Address: _____

                                               _____

                                               _____

Name: _____

Sex: M ( ); F ( ).

Age: _____

Telephone: home–(   ) _____; work–(   ) _____.

Address: _____

                       _____

                       _____

Initial contact: Handshake: weak   ( ); strong ( ).

                                    cold   ( ); warm ( ).

                                    moist   ( );   dry ( ).

Grooming: _____; posture: _____

Demeanor/attitude: _____

Breathing mode: High chest shallow ( ); hyperpnea ( ).

Sighing: frequent (   ); occasional (   ); absent (   ).

Occupation: _____

Contact with: dust (   );   fibers (   );   paints (   );

                     solvents (   ); sprays (   ); detergents (   ).

   Other chemicals or airborne particles: _____

_____

Status: Married (   ); single (   ); divorced (   );

          other: _____

          children: No. Boys (   ); No. Girls (   ).

Physician(s) of record: _____

_____

Last medical examination: _____, 199____

Diagnos(e)s: _____

_____

_____

Treatment(s): _____

_____

_____

Medication(s): _____

_____

_____

Do you now have, have you ever had, or has any family member related to you by blood (mother, father, sister, brother, familial grandparents or uncles and aunts) had:

(   ) High blood pressure   (   ) Heart disease

( ) Low blood pressure   ( ) Angina

( ) Diabetes (insulin-dependent)   ( ) Anemia

( ) Diabetes (non-insulin-   ( ) Allergies

    dependent)   ( ) Dermatitis

( ) Colitis   ( ) Muscle spasms

( ) Gastritis   ( ) Tingling in hands and/or feet

( ) Ulcer   ( ) Fainting (syncope)

( ) Shortness of breath   ( ) Dizziness (vertigo)

( ) Asthma   ( ) Stroke

( ) Emphysema

( ) Headache   ( ) Hyperventilation

( ) TMJ/bruxism   ( ) Mitral valve prolapse

( ) Chronic low backache   ( ) Other heart murmur

( ) EB virus (mononucl.)   ( ) Heart arrhythmia

( ) PMS   ( ) Chronic vaginal yeast

( ) Chronic tiredness   ( ) Cystitis

( ) Menstrual irregul.   ( ) Raynaud's disease

( ) Tinnitus   ( ) Chronic pain

( ) Hyperthyroid   ( ) Eating disorder

( ) Hypothyroid   ( ) Cancer _____

( ) Herpes   _____

( ) Depression   ( ) Other _____

( ) Migraine   _____

Health status of:

Mother _____

Father _____

Brother(s) ————————————————————————

Sister(s) ————————————————————————

Exercise: *seldom* (   ); *moderately* (   ); *frequently* (   )

  Mode: ————————————————————————

————————————————————————

Injuries/fractures, etc.: ————————————————

————————————————————————

————————————————————————

————————————————————————

Do you consume:	*seldom*	*moderately*	*frequently*
Coffee	( )	( )	( )
Tea	( )	( )	( )
Herbal tea	( )	( )	( )
Cigarettes	( )	( )	( )
Alcohol	( )	( )	( )
Aspirin	( )	( )	( )
Cola	( )	( )	( )
Birth control pills	( )	( )	( )
Sedatives	( )	( )	( )
Tranquilizers	( )	( )	( )
Antidepressants	( )	( )	( )
Laxatives	( )	( )	( )
Steroids	( )	( )	( )
Hormones	( )	( )	( )
Vitamins/mineral suppl	( )	( )	( )
Cough/cold medicines	( )	( )	( )

Inhalants	( )	( )	( )
Antacids	( )	( )	( )
Diet pills	( )	( )	( )
Sleeping pills	( )	( )	( )
Muscle relaxants	( )	( )	( )
Other	( )	( )	( )

Do you have any food allergies or sensitivities? _____

Do you suffer from:

( ) Stress

( ) Tension

( ) Anxiety

( ) Panic attacks

( ) Phobias

( ) Depression

Are you suicidal?

Do you experience:	seldom	sometimes	frequent
	m m s*	m m s	m m s
Thirst	( )( )( )	( )( )( )	( )( )( )
Hunger	( )( )( )	( )( )( )	( )( )( )
Faintness	( )( )( )	( )( )( )	( )( )( )
Feeling unreal	( )( )( )	( )( )( )	( )( )( )
Urge to urinate	( )( )( )	( )( )( )	( )( )( )
Constipation	( )( )( )	( )( )( )	( )( )( )
Diarrhea	( )( )( )	( )( )( )	( )( )( )

*"m m s" = "mild," "moderate," "severe"

Blurred vision	( ) ( ) ( )	( ) ( ) ( )	( ) ( ) ( )
Insomnia	( ) ( ) ( )	( ) ( ) ( )	( ) ( ) ( )
Nightmares	( ) ( ) ( )	( ) ( ) ( )	( ) ( ) ( )
Sleep disturbance	( ) ( ) ( )	( ) ( ) ( )	( ) ( ) ( )
Sleep apnea	( ) ( ) ( )	( ) ( ) ( )	( ) ( ) ( )
Irritability	( ) ( ) ( )	( ) ( ) ( )	( ) ( ) ( )
Loss of memory	( ) ( ) ( )	( ) ( ) ( )	( ) ( ) ( )
Loss of work efficiency	( ) ( ) ( )	( ) ( ) ( )	( ) ( ) ( )
Irritability	( ) ( ) ( )	( ) ( ) ( )	( ) ( ) ( )
Sensation of smothering	( ) ( ) ( )	( ) ( ) ( )	( ) ( ) ( )
Tingling in hands and feet	( ) ( ) ( )	( ) ( ) ( )	( ) ( ) ( )

Other _____

Have you been told that any of the following clinical tests showed unusual (above or below average) results or problems:

Blood test _____

_____

ECG _____

_____

EEG _____

_____

Other _____

_____

_____

Psychophysiological Profile

Breathing:

    Mode _____

Rate _____ /min

$ETCO_2$ _____ %

Rhythm _____

Bronchitis _____

Asthma _____

COPD/emphysema _____

Other _____

SaO_2 _____ %

Cardiac:

Pulse rate _____ /min.

RSA _____

ECG _____

Cardiovascular:

Hand temperature [right ( ), left ( )] _____ deg. F

Head temperature [right ( ), left ( )] _____ deg. F

Room temperature _____ deg. F

Muscular:

Muscle group _____

_____

Electrode placement _____

_____

EEG:

Electrode placement _____

_____

_____ (International 10/20 system? ( )

Delta _____

Theta _____

Alpha _____

Beta ——————————————————————————————————

Comments: ————————————————————————————

——

Comments: ————————————————————————————

——

——

Training procedures: ————————————————————————

——

——

——

——

——

——

——

——

——

——

——

——

——

——

——

——

——

References

Ackerman, S. H. & Sachar, E. J. (1974). The lactate theory of anxiety: A review and reevaluation. *Psychosomatic Medicine*, 36:69–81.

Adrogue, H. J. & Madias, N. E. (1981). Changes in plasma potassium concentration during acute acid-base disturbances. *American Journal of Medicine*, 71:5 456–467.

Akselrod, S., Gordon, D., Ubel, F. A., Shannon, D. C., Barger, A. C., & Cohen, R. J. (1981). Power spectrum analysis of heart rate fluctuations: A quantitative probe of beat-to-beat cardiovascular control. *Science*, 213:220–222.

Albright, G. L., Andreassi, J. L., & Steiner, S. S. (1988). Interactive effects of type A personality and psychological and physical stressors on human cardiovascular function. *International Journal of Psychophysiology*, 6:315–326.

Alexander, F. (1950). *Psychosomatic Medicine*. New York: Norton.

Alford, B. A., Freeman, A., Beck, A. T., & Wright, F. D. (1990). Brief focused cognitive therapy of panic disorder. *Psychotherapy*, 27:230–234.

Allison, J. (1970). Respiratory changes during transcendental meditation. *Lancet*, 1:833–834.

Allison, R. D., Holmes, E. L., & Nyboer, J. (1964). Volumetric dynamics of respiration as measured by electrical impedance plethysmography. *Journal of Applied Physiology*, 19:166–173.

Allison, R. D. & Luft, U. C. (1964). Cardiopulmonary dynamics and electrical resistance changes in the thorax. *Federal Proceedings*, 23:116.

Altman, P. L. & Dittmer, D. S. (1971). *Respiration and Circulation*. Bethesda: Federation of American Societies for Experimental Biology.

Altura, B. M. (1982). Magnesium and regulation of contractility of vascular smooth muscle. In Altura, B. M., Davis, E., & Harders, H. (eds), *Advances in Microcirculation*. Basel: Karger, pp. 77–113.

Altura, M. B. & Altura, B. T. (1978). Magnesium and vascular tone and reactivity. *Blood Vessels*, 15:5–16.

Amery, W. K. (1982). Brain hypoxia: The turning point in the genesis of migraine? *Cephalalgia*, 2:83–89.

Amery, W. K. (1987). The oxygen theory of migraine. In Blau, N. J. (ed), *Migraine*. Baltimore: The Johns Hopkins University Press, pp. 403–431.

Ames, F. (1955). The hyperventilation syndrome. *Journal of Mental Science*, 101:466–525.

Anand, B. K., Chhina, G. S., & Singh, B. (1961). Some aspects of electroencephalographic studies of yogis. *EEG Clinical Neurophysiology*, 13:425–456.

315

Ancoli, S. & Kamiya, J. (1979). Respiratory patterns during emotional expression. *Biofeedback and Self-Regulation*, 4:242 (Abstract).

Andersen, P. & Andersson, S. A. (1968). *Physiological Basis of Alpha Rhythm*. New York: Appleton-Century-Crofts.

Angelone, A. & Coulter, N. A. (1964). Respiratory sinus arrhythmia: A frequency dependent phenomenon. *Journal of Applied Physiology*, 3:479–482.

Angst, J., Woggon, B., & Schoepf, J. (1977). The treatment of depression with L-5-hydroxytryptophan versus imipramine. *Archive für Psychiatrie und Nervenkrankheit*, 224:175–186.

Arbus, G. S., Herbert, L. A., Levesque, P. R., Etsten, B. E., & Schwartz, W. B. (1969). Characterization and clinical application of the "significance band" for acute respiratory alkalosis. *New England Journal of Medicine*, 280:117–123.

Aronson, P. R. (1966). Evaluation of psychotropic drug therapy in chronic hyperventilation syndrome. *Journal of New Drugs*, 6:305–307.

Askanazi, J., Silverberg, P. A., Foster, R. J., Hyman, A. J., Milic-Emili, J., & Kinney, J. M. (1980). Effects of respiratory apparatus on breathing pattern. *Journal of Applied Physiology*, 48:577–580.

Ask-Upmark, R. (1935). The carotid sinus and cerebral circulation. *Acta Psychiatrica Neurologica*, suppl. VI, pp. 1–374.

Astrup, J., Heuser, D., Lassen, N. A., Nilssen, B., Norberg, K., & Siesjo, B. K. (1978). Evidence against H⁺ and K⁺ as a main factor for the control of cerebral blood flow: A microelectrode study. In *Cerebral Smooth Muscle and Its Control*. Amsterdam: Elsevier–Excerpta Medica–North Holland, pp. 313–332.

Astrup, P. (1970). Red-cell pH and oxygen affinity of hemoglobin. *New England Journal of Medicine*, 283:202–204.

Bacon, J. & Poppen, R. (1985). A behavioral analysis of diaphragmatic breathing and its effects on peripheral temperature. *Journal of Behavior Therapy and Experimental Psychiatry*, 16:15–21.

Badawi, K., Wallace, R. K., Orme-Johnson, D., & Rouzere, A. M. (1984). Electrophysiologic characteristics of respiratory suspension periods occurring during the practice of the transcendental meditation program. *Psychosomatic Medicine*, 46:267–276.

Baldy-Moulinier, M. (1972). Cerebral blood flow and membrane ionic pump. *European Neurology*, 6:106–113.

Bali, L. R. (1979). Long-term effect of relaxation on blood pressure and anxiety levels of essential hypertensive males: A controlled study. *Psychosomatic Medicine*, 41:637–646.

Ballentine, R. M. (1979). Nasal functioning. In *Science of Breath: A Practical Guide*. See Rama, Ballantine, & Hymes (1979).

Banquet, J. P. (1972). EEG and meditation. *EEG Clinical Neurophysiology*, 33:454.

Banquet, J. P. (1973). Spectral analysis of EEG in meditation. *EEG Clinical Neurophysiology*, 35:143–151.

Barker, E. S., Singer, R. B., Elkinton, J. R., & Clark, J. K. (1957). The renal response in man to acute experimental respiratory alkalosis and acidosis. *Journal of Clinical Investigation*, 36:515–529.

Barolin, G. S. (1966). Migraines and epilepsies—A relationship? *Epilepsia*, 7:53–66.

Basmajian, J. V. (1978). *Therapeutic Exercises*, 3d ed. Baltimore: Williams & Wilkins.

Basmajian, J. V. (1989). *Biofeedback: Principles and practice for clinicians*. Baltimore: Williams & Wilkins.

Basmajian, J. V. & Blumenthal, R. (1980). *Electrode Placement in EMG Biofeedback*. Baltimore: Johns Hopkins University Press.

Bass, C. (1981). Diagnosis and treatment of breathlessness. *Lancet*, 1:220.

Bass, C. & Gardner, W. (1985a). Diagnostic issues in the hyperventilation syndrome. *British Journal of Psychiatry*, 146:101–102.

Bass, C. & Gardner, W. (1985b). Respiratory and psychiatric abnormalities in chronic somatic hyperventilation. *British Medical Journal*, 290:1387–1390.

Bass, C., Kartsounis, L., & Lelliott, P. (1987). Hyperventilation and its relationship to anxiety and panic. *Integrative Psychiatry*, 5:274–291.

Bass, C., Wade, C., Gardner, W. N., Causley, R., Ryan, D. C., & Hutchison, D. C. S. (1983). Unexplained breathlessness and psychiatric morbidity in patients with normal and abnormal coronary arteries. *Lancet*, 1:605–609.

Bates, J. H., Adamson, J. S., & Pierce, J. A. (1966). Death after voluntary hyperventilation. *New England Journal of Medicine*, 274:1371–1372.

Baxter, L. R., Phelps, M. E., Mazziotta, J. C., Schwartz, J. M., Gerner, R. H., Selin, C. E., & Sumida, R. M. (1985). Cerebral metabolic rates for glucose in mood disorder. *Archives of General Psychiatry*, 42:441–447.

Bazett, H. C., Love, L., Newton, M., Eisenberg, R., Day, R., & Forster, R. (1948). Temperature change in blood flowing in arteries and veins in man. *Journal of Applied Physiology*, 1: 3–19.

Beary, J. F., Benson, H., & Klemchuck, H. P. (1974). A simple psychophysiologic technique which elicits the hypometabolic changes of the relaxation response. *Psychosomatic Medicine*, 36:115–120.

Beauchemin, J. A. (1936). Allergic reactions in mental disease. *American Journal of Psychiatry*, 92:1191–1204.

Beh, H. C. & Nix-James, D. R. (1974). The relationship between respiratory phase and reaction time. *Psychophysiology*, 11:400–402.

Bell, G. J., Davidson, J. N., & Scarborough, H. (1968). *A Textbook of Physiology and Biochemistry*, 7th ed. Edinburgh: Livingstone.

Bendig, A. W. (1960). Extraversion, neuroticism, and student achievement in introductory psychology. *Journal of Educational Research*, 53:263–267.

Benesch, R. & Benesch, R. E. (1976). The effect of organic phosphates from the human erythrocyte on the allosteric properties of hemoglobin. *Biochemistry and Biophysics Research Committee*, 26:162–167.

Benesch, R. E. & Benesch, R. (1970). The reaction between diphosphoglycerate and hemoglobin. *Federal Proceedings*, 29:1101–1104.

Benson, H. (1974). Decreased blood pressure in pharmacologically treated hypertensive patients who regularly elicited the relaxation response. *Lancet*, 1:289–291.

Benson, H. (1975). *The Relaxation Response*. New York: Avon Books.

Benson, H., Beary, J. F., & Carol, M. P. (1974). The relaxation response. *Psychiatry*, 37:37–46.

Benson, H. & Friedman, R. (1985). A rebuttal to the conclusion of David Holmes's article: Meditation and somatic arousal reduction. *American Psychologist*, 40:725–728.

Benson, H., Rosner, B. A., Marzetta, B. R., & Klemchuck, H. P. (1974). Decreased blood pressure in borderline hypertensive subjects who practiced meditation. *Journal of Chronic Diseases*, 27:163–169.

Berger, H. (1929). Uber das elektrenkephalogramm des menschen. *Archives of Psychiatry*, 87:527–570.

Berkow, R. (1982). *The Merck Manual*, 14th ed. Rahway: Merck, Sharpe & Dohme.

Bernstein, D. A. & Borkovec, T. D. (1973). *Progressive Relaxation Training*. Champaign, Ill: Research Press.

Beubel, M. E. & Shannahoff-Khalsa, D. S. (1987). Hemispheric efficiency varies with the asymmetries of nasal air flow. *Biological Psychology*, 23:127–137.

Beumer, H. M. & Hardonk, H. J. (1971). Symptomatik und behandlung des hyperventila-tionssyndroms. *Munchner Medizinisher Wochenschrift*, 113:1225–1258.

Bevan, J. A., Halpern, W., & Mulvaney, M. J. (1991). *The Resistance Vasculature*. Totowa, N.J.: Humana Press.

Bin, H. (1970). *A Brief Introduction to the Science of Breathing Exercise*, rev. ed. Hong Kong: Hai Fen.

Birbaumer, N. (1988). Book review: The hyperventilation syndrome. *Biofeedback and Self-Regulation*, 13:271–273.

Bircher, M., Kohl, J., Nigg, B., & Koller, E. A. (1978). The microvibration of the body, and index for examination stress. *European Bulletin of Applied Physiology*, 39:99–109.

Birk, L. (1973). *Biofeedback: Behavioral Medicine*. New York: Grune & Stratton.

Birzis, L., & Tachibana, S. (1962). Measurement of local cerebral blood flow by impedance changes. *Life Sciences*, 11:587–598.

Blackwell, B., Bloomfield, S., Gartside, P., Robinson, A., Hanenson, I., Magenheim, H., Nidich, A., & Zigler, R. (1976). Transcendental meditation in hypertension. *Lancet*, 1:223–236.

Blair, D. A., Glover, W. E., & Rodie, I. C. (1961). Cutaneous vasomotor nerves to the head and trunk. *Journal of Applied Physiology*, 16:119–122.

Blanchard, E. B., Morrill, B., Wittrock, D. A., Scharff, L., & Jaccard, J. (1989). Hand temperature for headache, hypertension, and irritable bowel syndrome. *Biofeedback and Self-Regulation*, 14:319–331.

Blass, J. P., & Gibson, G. E. (1979). Consequences of mild, graded hypoxia. In Fahn, S. et al. (eds.), *Advances in Neurology*. New York: Raven Press.

Blau, J. N., Wiles, C. M., & Solomon, F. S. (1983). Unilateral somatic symptoms due to hyperventilation. *British Medical Journal*, 286:1108.

Blinn, K. A. & Noell, W. K. (1949). Continuous measurement of alveolar CO_2 tension during the hyperventilation test in routine electroencephalography. *EEG Clinical Neurophysiology*, 1:333–342.

Block, J., Jennings, P. H., Harvey, E., & Simpson, E. (1964). Interaction between allergic potential and psychopathology in childhood asthma. *Psychosomatic Medicine*, 26:307.

Bohr, C., Hasselbach, K., & Krogh, A. (1904). Uber einen biologischer Beziehung wichtigen Einfluss, den die Kohlensauerspannung des Blutes auf dessen Sauerstoff-bindung-ubt. *Scandinavian Archives of Physiology*, 16:402.

Bonjer, F. H., Van den Berg, J., & Dirken, M. N. J. (1964). The origin of variation of body impedance occurring during the cardiac cycle. *Circulation*, 6:414–420.

Bonn, J. A., Harrison, J., & Reese, W. L. (1971). Lactate induced anxiety: Therapeutic applications. *British Journal of Psychiatry*, 119:468–471.

Bonn, J. S., Readhead, C. P. A., & Timmons, B. H. (1984). Enhanced adaptive behavioral response in agoraphobic patients pretreated with breathing training. *Lancet*, 1:665–669.

Bowersox, S. S. & Sterman, M. B. (1981). Changes in sensorimotor sleep spindle activity and seizure susceptibility after somatosensory deafferentation. *Experimental Neurology*, 74:814–828.

Bradley, P. W. & Younes, M. (1980). Relaxation between respiratory value dead space and tidal volume. *Journal of Applied Physiology: Respiration, Environment and Exercise Physiology*, 49:528–532.

Brain, L. (1962). *Diseases of the Nervous System*. London: Oxford University Press.

Brain, L. (1964). *Clinical Neurology*. London: Oxford University Press.

Braithwaite, V. A. (1987). The scale of emotional arousability: Bridging the gap between the neuroticism construct and its measurement. *Psychological Medicine*, 17:217–225.

Brashear, R. E. (1983). Hyperventilation syndrome. *Lung*, 161:257–273.

Brautbar, N., Leibovici, H., Finader, P., Campese, V., Penia, C., & Massry, S. G. (1980). Mechanisms of hypophosphatemia during acute hyperventilation. *Clinical Research,* 28:387A.

Brazeau, P., Gilman, A., Denger, F. F., & Swords, M. T. (1953). Effect of plasma CO_2 tension on renal tubular reabsorption of bicarbonate. *American Journal of Physiology,* 175:33–38.

Breckenridge, C. G. & Hoff, H. E. (1950). Pontile and medullary regulation of respiration in the cat. *American Journal of Physiology,* 160:385–394.

Breggin, P. R. (1964). The psychophysiology of anxiety. *Journal of Nervous and Mental Disease,* 139:558–568.

Bremer, F. (1938). L'activité électrique de l'écorce cérebrale. *Actualités Scientifiques et Industrielles,* 658:46.

Breslav, I. S., Shmeleva, A. M., & Normatov, A. T. (1986). Biofeedback control of alveolar carbon dioxide tension to eliminate hypocapnia in man in the presence of hypoxia. *Kosmicheskaya Biologiya I Aviakosmicheskaya Meditsina,* 21:74–77.

Brewer, G. J. (1972). *Proceedings of the International Conference on Red Cell Metabolism and Function,* 2nd ed. New York: Plenum.

Brewer, G. J. (1974). Red cell metabolism and function. In *The Red Cell.* Ed. G. M. Surgeon. New York: Academic Press.

Brewer, G. J. & Eaton, J. W. (1971). Erythrocyte metabolism: Interaction with oxygen transport. *Science,* 171:1205–1211.

Brewis, R. A. L. (1969). Clinical measurement relevant to the assessment of hypoxia. *British Journal of Anaesthesia,* 41:742–750.

Brick, H. (1958). Carbon dioxide therapy in prison with some comparisons in private practice. See Meduna (1950).

Brigo, B., Campacci, R., Avesani, R., Fambito, A., & Schinina, V. (1968). Voluntary regularization method of respiration applied to chronic obstructive pulmonary disease. *International Journal of Rehabilitation Research,* 6:283–288.

Brill, N. G. & Seidmann, H. (1942). Electroencephalographic changes during hyperventilation in epileptic and non-epileptic disorders. *Annals of Internal Medicine,* 16:451.

Brobeck, J. R. (1979). *Best and Taylor's Physiological Basis of Medical Practice,* 10th ed. Baltimore: Williams & Wilkins.

Brodtkorb, E., Gimse, R., Antonaci, F., Ellersten, B., Sand, T., Sulg, I., & Sjaastad, O. (1990). Hyperventilation syndrome: Clinical, ventilatory, and personality characteristics as observed in neurological practice. *Acta Neurologica Scandinavica,* 81:307–313.

Brody, B. S. & Dusser de Barenne, J. G. D. (1932). Effect of hyperventilation on the excitability of the motor cortex in cats. *Archives of Neurology and Psychiatry,* 28:571–585.

Bronk, D. W. (1966). Influence of circulation on the activity of nerve cells. See Cobb, S., Frantz, A. M., Penfield, W., & Riley, H. A. (eds.) (1966).

Brown, E. B. (1953). Physiological effects of hyperventilation. *Physiology Review,* 33:445.

Browse, N. L. & Hardwick, P. J. (1969). The deep breath-venoconstrictive reflex. *Clinical Science,* 37:125–135.

Buchsbaum, M. S., De Lisi, L. E., Holcomb, H. H., Cappelletti, J., King, A. C., Johnson, J., Hazlett, E., Dowling-Zimmermann, S., Post, R. M., Morihisa, J., Carpenter, W., Cohen, R., Pickar, D., Weinberger, D. R., Margolin, R., & Kessler, R. M. (1984). Anteroposterior gradients in cerebral glucose use in schizophrenia and affective disorders. *Archives of General Psychiatry,* 4:1159–1166.

Budzynski, T. H. (1983). Biofeedback strategies in headache treatment. In Basmajian, J. V. (ed.), *Biofeedback Principles and Practice for Clinicians.* Baltimore: Williams & Wilkins.

Bulkley, G. H., Klacsmann, P. G., & Hutchins, G. M. (1978). Angina pactoris, myocardial infarction and sudden cardiac death with normal coronary arteries: A clinicopathological study of 9 patients with progressive systemic sclerosis. *American Heart Journal,* 95:563–569.

Bunn, H. F. & Jandi, J. H. (1970). Control of hemoglobin function within the red cell. *New England Journal of Medicine,* 282:1414–1421.

Burch, G. E. & Winsor, T. (1955). *A Primer of Electrocardiography.* Philadelphia: Lea & Febiger.

Burnell, J. M., Villamil, M.F., Uyeno, B. T., & Scribner, B. H. (1956). The effect in humans of extracellular pH change on the relationship between serum potassium concentration and intracellular potassium. *Journal of Clinical Investigation,* 35:935–939.

Burns, B. H. (1971). Breathlessness in depression. *British Journal of Psychiatry,* 119:45–49.

Burns, B. H. & Howell, J. B. L. (1969). Disproportionately severe breathlessness in chronic bronchitis. *Quarterly Journal of Medicine,* 38:277–294.

Burnum, J. F., Hickam, J. B., & McIntosh, H. D. (1954). The effect of hypocapnia on arterial blood pressure. *Circulation,* 9:89.

Cacioppo, J. T., & Petty, R. E. (1982). *Perspectives in Cardiovascular Psychophysiology.* New York: Guilford Press.

Campbell, E. J. M. & Howell, J. B. L. (1963a). The sensation of breathlessness. *Journal of Applied Physiology Bulletin,* 18:36–40.

Campbell, E. J. M. & Howell, J. B. L. (1963b). The sensation of dyspnea. *British Medical Journal,* 2:868.

Cannon, W. B. (1927). The James-Lange theory of emotion: A critical examination and an alternative theory. *American Journal of Psychology,* 39:106–124.

Cannon, W. B. (1932). *The Wisdom of the Body.* New York: W. W. Norton.

Carlson, N. R. (1981). *Physiology of Behavior.* Boston: Allyn and Bacon.

Carlton, R. M., Fried, R., & Rubin, S. R. (1983). Intracellular magnesium deficiencies in epilepsy. *Journal of the American College of Nutrition,* abstract 48.

Carmichael, E. A., Doupe, J., & Williams, D. J. (1937). The cerebro-spinal fluid pressure of man in the erect posture. *Journal of Physiology,* 91:186–201.

Carr, D. G. & Sheehan, D. V. (1984). Panic anxiety: A new model. *Journal of Clinical Psychiatry,* 45:323–330.

Carrington, P. (1984). Modern methods of meditation. In Woolfolk, R. L. & Lehrer, P. M. (eds.), *Principles and Practice of Stress Management,* New York: Guilford Press.

Carryer, H. M. (1943). Syndrome of hyperventilation with tetany: Report of a case. *Proceedings of the Staff Meetings of the Mayo Clinic,* 18:522.

Caspers, H. & Speckmann, E. J. (1972). Cerebral PO_2, pCO_2 and pH: Changes during convulsive activity and their significance for spontaneous arrest of seizures. *Epilepsia,* 13:699–725.

Catlin, G. (1869). *Shut Your Mouth.* London: Tubner.

Chadha, T. S., Schneider, A. W., Birch, S., Jenouri, G., & Sackner, M. A. (1984). Breathing pattern during induced bronchoconstriction. *Journal of Applied Physiology: Respiration, Environment and Exercise Physiology,* 56:1053–1059.

Chadha, T. S., Watson, H., Birch, S., Jenouri, G. A., Schneider, A. W., Cohen, M. A., & Sackner, M. A. (1982). Validation of the respiratory inductive plethysmography using different calibration procedures. *American Review of Respiratory Diseases,* 125:644–649.

Chanutin, A. & Curnish, R. R. (1967). Effect of organic phosphates on the oxygen equilibrium of human erythrocytes. *Archives of Biochemistry and Biophysics,* 121:96–102.

Charry, J. M. & Kavet, R. (1989). *Air Ions: Physical and Biological Effects.* Boca Raton: CRC Press.

Chase, M. H. & Harper, R. M. (1971). Somatomotor and visceromotor correlates of operantly conditioned 12–14 c/sec sensorimotor cortical activity. *EEG and Clinical Neurophysiology,* 31:85–92.

Chernick, R. M. & Raber, M. B. (1972). Normal standards for ventilatory function using an automated wedge spirometer. *American Review of Respiratory Disease*, 106:38–46.

Chernick, V. (1981). Endorphin and ventilatory control. *New England Journal of Medicine*, 304:1227–1228.

Chernick, V., Madansky, D. L., & Lawson, E. E. (1980). Nalaxone decreases the duration of primary apnea with neonatal asphyxia. *Pediatric Respiration*, 13:357–359.

Chobot, R., Dundy, H. D., & Pacella, B. L. (1950). The incidence of abnormal electroencephalographic patterns in allergic children. *Journal of Allergy*, 21:334–338.

Christensen, B. D. (1946). Studies on hyperventilation: II. Electrocardiographic changes in normal man during voluntary hyperventilation. *Journal of Clinical Investigation*, 25: 880–889.

Christie, R. V. (1935). Some types of respiration in the neuroses. *Quarterly Journal of Medicine*, 16:427–432.

Christophers, B. (1961). The hyperventilation syndrome. *Medical Journal of Australia*, 2:490–516.

Clark, D. M. & Hemsley, D. R. (1982). The effects of hyperventilation: Individual variability and its relation to personality. *Journal of Behavior Therapy and Experimental Psychiatry*, 13:41–47.

Clark, D. M., Salkovskis, P. M., & Shalkley, A. J. (1983). Respiratory control as a treatment for panic attacks. *Biological Psychology*, 16:285–297.

Clark, D. M., Salkovskis, P. M., & Chalkley, A. J. (1985). Respiratory control as a treatment for panic attacks. *Journal of Behavior Therapy and Experimental Psychiatry*, 16:23–30.

Clark, F. J. & von Euler, C. (1972). On the regulation of depth and rate of breathing. *Journal of Physiology*, 222:267–295.

Clark, M. E. & Hirschman, R. (1990). Effect of paced respiration on anxiety reduction in clinical populations. *Biofeedback and Self-Regulation*, 15:273–284.

Clark, T. J. H. & Cochrane, G. M. (1970). Effect of personality on alveolar ventilation in patients with chronic airways obstruction. *British Medical Journal*, 1:273–275.

Clausen, O. (1951). Respiratory movements in normal, neurotic, and psychotic subjects. *Acta Psychiatrica Scandinavica*, suppl. 168.

Cobb, S., Frantz, A. M., Penfield, W., & Riley, H. A. (eds.). (1966). *The Circulation of the Brain and Spinal Cord*. New York: Hafner Publishing Co.

Cobb, S., Sargant, W. W., & Schwab, R. S. (1938). Simultaneous respiratory and electroencephalographic recording in petit mal. *Archives of Neurology and Psychiatry*, 42:1189–1191.

Coca, A. F. (1956). *The Pulse Test*. New York: Lyle Stuart.

Cogen, P. H. & Zimmermann, E. A. (1979). Ovarian hormones and cerebral function. In Fahn S. et al. (eds.), *Advances in Neurology*. New York: Raven Press, pp. 123–133.

Cohen, J. J., Madias, N. E., Wolf, C. L., & Schwartz, W. B. (1976). Regulation of acid-base equilibrium in chronic hypocapnia. Evidence that the response of the kidney is not geared to the defense of extracellular [H$^+$]. *Journal of Clinical Investigation*, 57:1483–1489.

Cohen, M. E., & White, P. D. (1950). Life situations, emotions and neurocirculatory asthenia (anxiety neurosis, neurasthenia, effort syndrome). *Archives of Research in Nervous and Mental Diseases*, Proccedings 29:832–869.

Cohen, M. E., White, P. D., & Johnson, R. E. (1948). Neurocirculatory asthenia, anxiety neurosis or the effort syndrome. *Archives of Internal Medicine*, 81:260.

Cohen, M. I. (1968). Discharge patterns of brain-stem respiratory neurons in relation to carbon dioxide tension. *Journal of Neurophysiology*, 31:142–165.

Cohen, M. I. (1979). Neurogenesis of respiratory rhythm in mammals. *Physiological Review*, 59:1105–1173.

Cohen, M. I. & Wang, S. C. (1969). Respiratory neuronal activity in the pons of the cat. *Journal of Neurophysiology*, 22:33–50.

Cohen, R. D. & Woods, H. F. (1976). *Clinical and Biochemical Aspects of Lactic Acidosis*. Oxford: Blackwell.

Cohn, M. A., Rao, A. S. V., Broudy, M., Birch, S., Watson, H., Atkins, N., Davis, B., Stott, F. D., & Sackner, M. A. (1982). The respiratory inductive plethysmograph: A new non-invasive monitor of respiration. *Bulletin of European Physiopathology and Respiration*, 18:643–658.

Cohn, M. A., Rao, B. V. A., Davis, B., Watson, H., Broudy, M. J., Sackner, J. D., & Sackner, M. A. (1979). *Measurement of Tidal Ventilation and Forced Vital Capacity in Normals and Patients with Obstructive Lung Disease with a Respiratory Inductive Plethysmograph*. Presented at the 3rd International Symposium on Ambulatory Monitoring, Harrow, Middlesex, U. K.

Colantuoni, A., Bertuglia, S., & Inaglietta, M. (1985). Variations of rhythmic diameter changes at the arterial microvascular bifurcations. *European Journal of Physiology*, 403:289–295.

Collier, C. R., Affeldt, J. E., & Farr, A. F. (1955). Continuous rapid infrared CO_2 analysis. *Journal of Laboratory and Clinical Medicine*, 45:526–539.

Collier, R. J., Densham, H. B. A. R., & Wells, H. M. (1927). The influence of respiratory movement on the cutaneous circulation. *Quarterly Journal of Experimental Physiology*, 18:192–196.

Compernolle, T., Hoogduin, K., & Joelle, L. (1979). Diagnosis and treatment of the hyperventilation syndrome. *Psychosomatic Medicine*, 20:612–625.

Comroe, J. H. (1939). The location and function of the chemoreceptors of the aorta. *American Journal of Physiology*, 127:176.

Comroe, J. H. (1964). The peripheral chemoreceptors. In *Handbook of Physiology*. Sec. 3, Respiration. See Fenn & Rahn (1964).

Comroe, J. H. (1974). *Physiology of Respiration*, 2nd ed. Chicago: Year Book Medical Publishers.

Comroe, J. H., et al. (1962). *The Lung*, 2nd ed. Chicago: Year Book Medical Publishers.

Comstock, G. W., Stone, R. W., Tonascia, J. A., & Johnson, D. H. (1981). Respiratory survey findings as predictors of disability from respiratory disease. *American Review of Respiratory Disease*, 124:367–371.

Conway, J., Greenwood, D. T., & Middlemiss, D. N. (1978). Central nervous action of β-adrenoreceptor antagonists. *Journal of Clinical Science and Molecular Medicine*, 54: 119–124.

Cooper, R., Moskalenko, Y. E., & Walter, W. G. (1964). The pulsation of the human brain. *Journal of Physiology*, 172:540–560.

Corwin, W. & Barry, H. (1940). Respiratory plateaus in "daydreaming" and in schizophrenia. *American Journal of Psychiatry*, 97:308–318.

Cowen, M. A. (1967). Elementary functional correlates of the transcephalic dc circuit. *Psychophysiology*, 3:262–272.

Cowen, M. A. (1974). The brain as a generator of transcephalic measured direct current potentials. *Psychophysiology*, 11:321–335.

Cowen, M. A. (1975). CO_2: A possible missing link between regional cortical metabolism and transcephalic direct current potentials. *Psychophysiology*, 12:693–701.

Cowen, M. A. (1976). CO_2 and the cephalic direct current systems: Studies on humans and a biophysical analysis. *Psychophysiology*, 13:572–580.

Cowen, M. A., Ross, J., & McDonald, R. (1967). Some aspects of the transcephalic dc circuit. *Psychophysiology*, 4:207–215.

Cowley, D. S. & Roy-Byrne, P. P. (1987). Hyperventilation and panic disorder. *American Journal of Medicine*, 83:929–937.

Damas-Mora, J., Davies, L., Taylor, W., & Jenner, F. A. (1980). Menstrual respiratory changes and symptoms. *British Journal of Psychiatry*, 136:492–497.

Damas-Mora, J., Grant, L., Kenyon, P., Patel, M. K., & Yenner, F. A. (1976). Respiratory ventilation and carbon dioxide levels in syndromes of depression. *British Journal of Psychiatry*, 129:457–464.

Damas-Mora, J., Jenner, F. A., Sneddon, J., & Addis, W. A. (1978). Ventilatory response to carbon dioxide in syndromes of depression. *Journal of Psychosomatic Research*, 22: 473–476.

Danskin, D. G. & Crow, M. A. (1981). *Biofeedback—An Introduction and Guide*. Palo Alto, California: Mayfield.

Darrow, C. W. & Graf, C. C. (1945). Relation of electroencephalogram to photometrically observed vasomotor changes in the brain. *Journal of Neurophysiology*, 8:449–461.

Darrow, C. W. & Pathman, J. H. (1944). Relation of heart rate to slow waves in the electroencephalogram during overventilation. *American Journal of Physiology*, 140:583–588.

Das, N. N. & Gastaut, H. (1957). Variations de l'activité électrique du cerveau, du coeur, et des muscles squélétiques au cours de la méditation et de l'extase yogique. *EEG and Clinical Neurophysiology*, suppl. 6:211–219.

Datey, K. K., Deshmukh, S. N., Dalvi, C. P., & Vinekar, S. L. (1969). "Shavasan": A yogic exercise in the management of hypertension. *Angiology*, 20:325–333.

Davidson, H. M. (1952). Allergy of the nervous system. *Quarterly Review of Allergy and Applied Immunology*, 6:157–188.

Davidson, R. J. & Schwartz, G. E. (1976). The psychobiology of relaxation and related states: A multi-process theory. In Mostofsky, D. I. (ed.), *Behavior Control and Modification of Physiological Activity*. Englewood Cliffs, NJ: Prentice-Hall.

Davies, C. T. M. & Neilson, J. M. M. (1967). Sinus arrythmia in man at rest. *Journal of Applied Physiology*, 22:947–955.

Davis, C. A. (1987). A psychophysiological and psychometric study of temperament and arousal from an Eysenckian and "strength and nervous system" perspective. *Dissertation Abstracts International*, February, 47 (8-b):3560.

Davis, H. & Wallace, W. (1942). Factors affecting changes produced by standard hyperventilation. *Archives of Neurology and Psychiatry*, 47:606–625.

Davis, J. A. (1981). Endorphin and ventilatory control. *New England Journal of Medicine*, 305:958–959.

Davis, J. N. & Carlsson, A. (1973). Effect of hypoxia on monoamine synthesis, level, and metabolism in rat brain. *Journal of Neurochemistry*, 21:783–790.

Davison, G. D. & Neale, J. M. (1982). *Abnormal Psychology*. New York: Wiley.

de Boer, R. W., Karemaker, J. M., & Strackee, J. (1985). Description of heart-rate variability data in accordance with a physiological model of the genesis of heart-beats. *Psychophysiology*, 22:147–155.

DeJours, P. (1964). *Control of respiration in muscular exercise*. See Fehn & Rahn.

Demany, M. A. & Zimmermann, H. A. (1966). Hyperventilation vs. chest pain of coronary origin: Frequently a diagnostic dilemma [sic]. *Medical Times*, 94:1222–1226.

Dempsey, J. A., Forster, H. V., & doPico, G. A. (1974). Ventilatory acclimatization to moderate hypoxemia in man. The role of spinal fluid [H^+]. *Journal of Clinical Investigation*, 53:1091–1100.

Denavit-Saubie, M., Champagnat, J., & Zieglgansberger, W. (1978). Effect of opiates and methionine-enkephalin on pontine and bulbar respiratory neurones in the cat brain. *Brain Research*, 155:55–67.

Dent, R., Yates, D., & Higenbottam, T. (1983). Does the hyperventilation syndrome exist? *Thorax*, 38:223.

de Rutter, C., Rijken, H., Garssen, B., & Kraaimaat, F. (1989). Breathing retraining, exposure and a combination of both, in the treatment of panic disorder with agoraphobia. *Behavior Therapy and Research*, 27:647–655.

Deutsch, F., Ehrentheil, O., & Pierson, O. (1941). Capillary studies in Raynaud's disease. *Journal of Laboratory and Clinical Medicine*, 26:1729–1750.

Discher, D. P. & Steinborn, J. (1970). LS/MFT: Lung screening by meaningful function testing—Part II. *American Journal of Public Health*, 12:2361–2385.

Dods, J. B. (1852). *The Philosophy of Electrical Psychology*. New York: Fowler and Wells.

Donhoffer, Sz., Szegvari, Gy., Jarai, I., & Farkas, M. (1959). Thermoregulatory heat production in the brain. *Nature*, 4691:993–994.

Douglas, W. W. (1975). Histamine and antihistamine: 5-hydroxytriptamine and antagonists. In Goodman, L. S. & Gilman, A. G. (eds.) *The Pharmacological Basis of Therapeutics*, 5th ed. New York: Macmillan.

Douglas, W. W. (1980). Histamine and 5-hydroxytriptamine (serotonin) and their antagonists. In Goodman, L. S. & Gilman, A. G. (eds.), *The Pharmacological Basis of Therapeutics*, 6th ed. New York: Macmillan.

Drevets, W. C., Videen, T., O., Price, J. L., Preskorn, S. H., Carmichael, S. T., & Raichle, M. E. (1992). A functional anatomical study of unipolar depression. *Journal of Neuroscience*, 12:3628–3641.

Dripps, R. D. (1947). The effect of inhalation of high and low oxygen concentrations on respiration, pulse rate, ballistocardiogram, and arterial oxygen saturation (oximeter) of normal individuals. *American Journal of Physiology*, 149:227.

Dripps, R. D. & Comroe, J. H. (1944). The clinical significance of the carotid and aortic bodies. *American Journal of Physiology*, 208:681–694.

Dudley, D. L., Holmes, T. H., Martin, C. J., & Ripley, H. S. (1964). Changes in respiration associated with hypnotically induced emotions, pain, and exercise. *Psychosomatic Medicine*, 26:46–57.

Dudley, D. L., Martin, C. J., Masuda, M., Ripley, H. S., & Holmes, T. H. (1969). *Psychophysiology of Respiration in Health and Disease*. New York: Appleton-Century-Crofts.

Dudley, D. L. & Pitts-Poarch, A. R. (1980). Psychophysiologic aspects of respiratory control. *Clinical Chest Medicine*, 1:131–143.

Duffy, F. H., Denckla, M. B., Bartels, P. H., & Sandini, G. (1980). Dyslexia: Regional differences in brain electrical activity by topographic mapping. *Annals of Neurology*, 7:412–420.

Durlach, J. (1969). *Spasmophilia and Magnesium Deficit*. Paris: Masson.

Eckberg, D. L., Drabinsky, M., & Braunwald, E. (1971). Defective parasympathetic control in patients with heart disease. *New England Journal of Medicine*, 285:877–883.

Edlund, M. J., Swann, M. O. H., & Clothier, J. (1987). Patients with panic attacks and abnormal EEG results. *American Journal of Psychiatry*, 144:508–509.

Edvinsson, L., Hardebo, J. E., & Owman, C. (1978). *Influence of the cerebrovascular sympathetic innervation on regional flow, autoregulation, and blood-brain barrier function*. See Heistad, Marcus, & Abboud (1978).

Edwards, R. H. T. & Clode, M. (1970). The effect of hyperventilation on lactic acidemia of muscular exercise. *Clinical Science*, 8:269–276.

Egan, D. F. (1973). *Respiratory Therapy*. St. Louis: Mosby.

Egger, J., Carter, C. M., Soothill, J. F., & Wilson, J. (1989). Oligoantigenic diet treatment of children with epilepsy and migraine. *The Journal of Pediatrics*, 114:51–58.

Egger, J., Carter, C. M., Wilson, J., Turner, M. W., & Soothill, J. F. (1983). Is migraine a food allergy? A double-blind controlled trial of oligoantigenic diet treatment. *Lancet*, 2: 865–869.

Elam, M., Yoa, J., Thoren, P., & Svensson, T. H. (1981). Hypercapnia and hypoxia: chemoreceptor-mediated control of the locus ceruleus neurons and splanchnic, sympathetic nerves. *Brain Research*, 222:373–381.

Ellis, A. (1962). *Reason and Emotion in Psychotherapy*. Secaucus: Lyle Stuart.

Elson, B. D., Hauri, P., & Cunis, D. (1977). Physiological changes in yoga meditation. *Psychophysiology*, 14:52–57.

Elul, R. (1962). Dipoles of spontaneous activity in the cerebral cortex. *Experimental Neurology*, 6:285.

Engel, B. T. & Chism, R. A. (1967). Effect of increase and decrease in breathing rate on heart rate and finger pulse volume. *Psychophysiology*, 4:83–89.

Engel, G. L., Ferris, E. B., & Logan, M. (1947). Hyperventilation: Analysis of clinical symptomatology. *Annals of Internal Medicine*, 27:683–704.

Engel, G. L., Romano, J., Ferris, E. B., Webb, J. P., & Stevens, C. D. (1944). A simple method of determining frequency spectrums in the electroencephalogram. Observations on effects of physiologic variations in dextrose, oxygen, posture, and acid-base balance on normal encephalogram. *Archives of Neurology and Psychiatry*, 51:134–146.

Engel, G. L., Romano, J., & McLin, T. R. (1944). Vasodepressor and carotid sinus syncope. *Archives of Internal Medicine*, 74:100–119.

Engel, J. (1984). The use of positron emission tomographic scanning in epilepsy. *Annals of Neurology*, suppl. S:180–191.

England, S. J. & Farki, L. E. (1976). Fluctuations in alveolar CO_2 and base excess during the menstrual cycle. *Respiratory Physiology*, 26:157–161.

Ernesting, J. (1966). The effect of hypoxia upon human performance and the electroencephalogram. In Payne, J. P. & Hill, D. W. (eds.), *Oxygen Measurement in Blood and Tissue and Their Significance*. London: Churchill.

Erslev, A. J. & Gabuzda, T. G. (1975). *Pathophysiology of Blood*. Philadelphia, Pa: W.B. Saunders.

Evans, D. W. & Lum, L. C. (1977). Hyperventilation: An important cause of pseudoangina. *Lancet*, 1:155–157.

Evans, D. W. & Lum, L. C. (1981). Hyperventilation as a cause of chest pain mimicking angina. *Practical Cardiology*, 7:131–136.

Evans, F. J. (1977). The control of altered states of awareness. In Edmonston, W. E. (ed.), *Conceptual and Investigative Approaches to Hypnosis and Hypnotic Phenomena. Annals of the New York Academy of Sciences*, 296:162–174.

Everly, G. S. (1989). *A Clinical Guide to the Treatment of the Human Stress Response*. New York: Plenum Press.

Eysenck, H. J. (1970). *The Structure of Human Personality*. London: Methuen.

Eysenck, H. J. & Eysenck, S. B. G. (1968). *Manual: Eysenck Personality Inventory*. San Diego: Educational and Industrial Testing Service.

Fair, P. L. (1983). Biofeedback-assisted relaxation strategies in psychotherapy. In Basmajian, J. V. (ed.), *Biofeedback—Principles and Practices for Clinicians*. Baltimore: Williams & Wilkins.

Farrow, J. T. & Hebert, J. R. (1982). Breath suspension during transcendental meditation. *Psychosomatic Medicine*, 44:133–135.

Fazekas, J., McHenry, L., Alman, R., & Sullivan, J. (1961). Cerebral hemodynamics during brief hyperventilation. *Archives of Neurology*, 4:132–138.

Fenn, W. O. & Rahn, H. (eds.). (1964). *Handbook of Physiology*, Sec. 3, Respiration, Vol. 1. Washington DC: American Physiology Society.

Fensterheim, H. (1983). Clinical treatment of the hyperventilation syndrome. Paper presented at the annual meeting of the American Psychological Association, Anaheim, Ca.

Fensterheim, H. (1989). Ninth International Symposium on Respiratory Psychophysiology. Keynote address: Symposium on Hyperventilation and Asthma. Charing Cross Hospital, London, U.K.

Fenwick, P. B. C., Donaldson, S., Gillis, L., Bushman, J., Fenton, G. W., Tilsley, I. P., & Serafinowicz, H. (1977). Metabolic and EEG changes during transcendental meditation: An explanation. *Biological Psychology*, 5:101–118.

Ferguson, A., Addington, W. W., & Gaensler, E. A. (1969). Dyspnea and bronchospasm from inappropriate postexercise hyperventilation. *Annals of Internal Medicine*, 71:1063–1072.

Fernstrom, J. D. & Wurtman, R. J. (1972). Brain serotonin content: Physiological regulation by plasma neural amino acids. *Science*, 178:414–416.

Ferris, E. B. (1941). Objective measurement of relative intracranial blood flow in man—with observations concerning the hydrodynamics of the craniovertebral system. *Archives of Neurology and Psychiatry*, 46:377–401.

Finesinger, J. E. (1943). The spirogram in certain psychiatric disorders. *American Journal of Psychiatry*, 100:159–169.

Finesinger, J. E. (1944). The effect of pleasant and unpleasant ideas on the respiratory pattern (spirogram) in psychoneurotic patients. *American Journal of Psychiatry*, 100:659–667.

Finesinger, J. E. & Mazick, S. G. (1940). The effect of a painful stimulus and its recall upon respiration in psychoneurotic patients. *Psychosomatic Medicine*, 2:333–368.

Fink, B. R., Katz, R., Reinhold, H., & Schoolman, A. (1962). Suprapontine mechanisms in regulation of respiration. *American Journal of Physiology*, 202:217–220.

Finley, W. W. (1976). Operant conditioning of the EEG in two patients with epilepsy: Methodological considerations. *Pavlovian Journal of Biological Science*, 12:93–111.

Fischer, V. H. (1965). *Detecting Physiological Conditions by Measuring Bioelectric Output Frequency*. U.S. Patent No. 3,195,533.

Folgering, H. P. & Braakhekke, J. (1980). Ventilatory response to hypocapnia in normal subjects after propranolol, metoprolol, and oxprenolol. *Respiration*, 39:139–143.

Folgering, H. P. & Colla, P. (1978). Some anomalies in the control of $PaCO_2$ in patients with hyperventilation syndrome. *Bulletin of European Physiopathology Research*, 14:503–512.

Folkow, B. (1955). Nervous control of blood vessels. *Physiological Review*, 35:629–663.

Forbes, H. S. & Cobbs, S. (1966). *Vasomotor Control of Cerebral Vessels*. See Cobb, Frantz, Penfield, & Riley (eds.).

Forster, H. V., Dempsey, J. A., Thomson, J., Vidruk, E., & doPico, G. A. (1972). Estimation of arterial PO_2, PCO_2, pH, and lactate from arterialized venous blood. *Journal of Applied Physiology*, 32:134–137.

Fox, M. C. (1991). *Interaction among five psychophysiological variables and a psychosoma inventory: The EPI, SEA, JAS, and MMPI-HO under a cognitive and perceptual-motor stressor*. New York: City University of New York, Ph.D. Dissertation.

Fox, R. H., Goldsmith, R., & Kidd, D. J. (1959). Cutaneous vasomotor nerves in the human ear and forehead. *Proceedings of the Physiological Society*, pp. 12–13.

Fox, R. H., Goldsmith, R., & Kidd, D. J. (1960). The cutaneous vasomotor control in the human nose, lip and chin. *Proceedings of the Physiological Society*, 150:22P–23P.

Fox, R. H., Goldsmith, R., & Kidd, D. J. (1962). Cutaneous vasomotor control in the human head, neck and chest. *Journal of Physiology*, 161:298–312.

Fox, S. S. & Simpson, D. L. (1973). Biofeedback and analog coding in brain behavior. In Mostofsky, D. I. (ed.), *Behavior Control and Modification of Physiological Activity*. Englewood Cliffs: Prentice-Hall.

Franks, C. M. (1957). Personality factors and the rate of conditioning. *British Journal of Psychology,* 48:119–126.

Franks, C. M. (1961). Conditioning and abnormal behavior. In Eysenck, H. J. (ed.), *Handbook of Abnormal Behavior.* New York: Basic Books.

Freedman, R. R. & Woodward, S. (1992a). Behavioral treatment of menopausal hot flushes: Evaluation by ambulatory monitoring. *American Journal of Obstetrics and Gynecology,* 167:436–439.

Freedman, R. R. & Woodward, S. (1992b). Behavioral treatment of menopausal hot flushes: Evaluation by ambulatory monitoring. *American Journal of Obstetrics and Gynecology,* 17:305–306.

Freeman, L. J., Conway, A., & Nixon, P. G. F. (1986). Physiological responses to psychological challenge under hypnosis in patients considered to have the hyperventilation syndrome: Implications for diagnosis and therapy. *Journal of the Royal Society of Medicine,* 79: 76–83.

Freeman, L. & Nixon, P. G. F. (1985). Chest pain and the hyperventilation syndrome—Aetiological considerations. *Postgraduate Medical Journal,* 61:957–961.

Fried, R. (1969). *Introduction to Statistics.* New York: Oxford University Press.

Fried, R. (1972). *Cardiac Arrythmia Computer.* U.S. Patent No. 3,698,386.

Fried, R. (1973). Psychophysiological correlates of desensitization of phobias. *Psychotherapy and Psychosomatics,* 21:12–24.

Fried, R. (1985). Behavioral control of idiopathic epileptic seizures. In Entmacher, P. S. (ed.), *President's Committee on Employment of the Handicapped: Management of Chronic Disabilities.* Washington DC: U.S. Government Printing Office.

Fried, R. (1987a). *The Hyperventilation Syndrome—Research and Clinical Treatment.* Baltimore: Johns Hopkins University Press.

Fried, R. (1987b). Relaxation with biofeedback-assisted guided imagery: The importance of breathing rate as an index of hypoarousal. *Biofeedback and Self-Regulation,* 12:273–279.

Fried, R. (1988). Letter to the Editor. *Biofeedback and Self-Regulation,* 13:181–183.

Fried, R. (1989). Letter to the Editor. *Biofeedback and Self-Regulation,* 14:259–261.

Fried, R. (1990a). *The Breath Connection.* New York: Insight/Plenum.

Fried, R. (1990b). Integrating music in breathing training and relaxation: I. Background, rationale, and relevant elements. *Biofeedback and Self-Regulation,* 15:161–169.

Fried, R. (1990c). Integrating music in breathing training and relaxation: II. Applications. *Biofeedback and Self-Regulation,* 15:171–177.

Fried, R. (1992). PCO_2 biofeedback to control idiopathic epileptic seizures. Paper presented at the Eleventh International Symposium on Respiratory Psychophysiology. Bordeaux, France.

Fried, R. (1993a). Breathing training for the self-regulation of alveolar CO_2 in the behavioral control of idiopathic epileptic seizures. In Mostofsky, D. I. & Loyning, Y. (eds.), *Neurobehavioral Treatment in Epilepsy.* Hillsdale, New Jersey: Lawrence Erlbaum & Assoc., Inc.

Fried, R. (1993b). The role of respiration in stress control: Towards a theory of stress as a hypoxic phenomenon. In Lehrer, P. M. & Woolfolk, R. L. (eds.), *Principles and Practice of Stress Management.* New York: Guilford Press, pp. 301–331.

Fried, R., Fox, M. C., Carlton, R. M., & Rubin, S. R. (1984). Method and protocols for assessing hyperventilation and its treatment. *Journal for Drug Research and Therapy,* 9:280–288.

Fried, R., Fox, M. G., & Carlton, R. M. (1990). Effect of diaphragmatic respiration with end-tidal CO_2 biofeedback on respiration, EEG, and seizure frequency in idiopathic epilepsy. *Annals of the New York Academy Sciences,* 602:67–96.

Fried, R. & Fried, B. (1981). Cardiac activity in a simple reaction time task. *Pavlovian Journal of Biological Science,* 16:457–487.

Fried, R. & Gluck, S. (1966). Conditioned galvanic skin response in the chick embryo: Preliminary report. *Psychonomic Science*, 6:319–320.

Fried, R. & Golden, W. L. (1989). The role of psychophysiological hyperventilation assessment in cognitive behavior therapy. *Journal of Cognitive Psychotherapy*, 3:5–14.

Fried, R., Korn, S., & Welch, L. (1966). The effect of change in sequential visual stimuli on GSR adaptation. *Journal of Experimental Psychology*, 72:325–327.

Fried, R. & Rubin, S. R. (1984). Efecto de la biorretroalimentacion del dioxido de carbono del volumen respiratorio final sobre la hiperventilacion cronica y la epilepsia idiopatica. *Revista Latinoamericana de Psicologia*, 16: 421–433.

Fried, R., Rubin, S. R., Carlton, R. M., & Fox, M. C. (1984a). Behavioral control of intractable idiopathic seizures: I. Self-regulation of end-tidal carbon dioxide. *Psychosomatic Medicine*, 46:315–332.

Fried, R., Rubin, S. R., Carlton, R. M., & Fox, M. C. (1984b). Diaphragmatic respiration with end-tidal percent carbon dioxide biofeedback treatment in chronic hyperventilation in idiopathic seizure sufferers: I. Effect on the EEG. *American Journal of Clinical Biofeedback*, 7:13–21.

Fried, R., Welch, L., & Friedman, M. (1967). High and low anxiety and GSR habituation. *Psychonomic Science*, 9:635–636.

Fried, R., Welch, L., Friedman, M., & Gluck, S. (1967). The effect of change in sequential visual stimuli on GSR habituation: II. The novel stimulus as a disinhibiting stimulus. *Perception and Psychophysics*, 2:419–420.

Friedman, A. P. & Merritt, H. H. (1959). Migraine. In Friedman, A. P. & Merritt, H. H. (eds.), *Headache: Diagnosis and Treatment*. Philadelphia, Pennsylvania: Davis, pp. 201–249.

Friedman, M. (1945). Studies concerning the etiology and pathogenesis of neurocirculatory asthenia: The respiratory manifestations of neurocirculatory asthenia. *American Heart Journal*, 3:557.

Friedman, M. & Rosenman, R. H. (1969). The possible general causes of coronary artery disease. In Friedman, M. (ed.), *Pathogenesis of Coronary Artery Disease*. New York: McGraw-Hill.

Froese, G. & Burton, A. C. (1957). Heat losses from the human head. *Journal of Applied Physiology*, 10:235–241.

Gallego, J. & Perruchet, P. (1991). Effect of practice on the voluntary control of a learned breathing pattern. *Psychophysiology and Behavior*, 49:315–319.

Gallego, J., Perruchet, P., & Camus, J-F. (1991). Assessing attentional control of breathing by reaction time. *Psychophysiology*, 28:219–227.

Gamble, J. L. (1982). *Acid-Base Physiology*. Baltimore: Johns Hopkins University Press.

Gantt, W. H. (1953). Principles of nervous breakdown—schizokinesis and autokinesis. *Annals of the New York Academy of Sciences*, 56:143–163.

Gardin, J. M., Isner, J. M. Ronan, J. A., & Fox, S. M. (1980). Pseudoischemic "false positive" S'T segment changes induced by hyperventilation in patients with mitral valve prolapse. *American Journal of Cardiology*, 45:952–958.

Gardner, W. N., Bass, C., & Moxham, J. (1992). Recurrent hyperventilation tetany due to mild asthma. *Respiratory Medicine*, 86:349–351.

Gardner, W. N., Meah, M. S., & Bass, C. (1986). Controlled study of respiratory responses during prolonged measurement in patients with chronic hyperventilation. *Lancet*, 2:826–830.

Garssen, B., de Ruiter, C., & van Dyck, R. (1992). Breathing retraining: A rational placebo? *Clinical Psychology Review*, 12:141–153.

Garssen, B., van Veenendaal, W., & Bloemink, R. (1983). Agoraphobia and the hyperventilation syndrome. *Behavior Research and Therapy*, 21:643–649.

Gaskell, P. (1956). Are there sympathetic vasodilator nerves to the vessels of the hands? *Journal of Physiology*, 131:647–656.

Gastaut, H. (1975). Comments on "Biofeedback in epileptics: Equivocal relationship of reinforced EEG frequency to seizure reduction," by Bonnie Kaplan. *Epilepsia*, 16:477–485.

Gault, J. E. (1969). Dyspnea and angina: A clinical study. *Medical Journal of Australia*, 1:1066–1068.

Gautier, H. & Bertrand, F. (1975). Respiratory effects of pneumotaxic center lesions and subsequent vagotomy in chronic cats. *Respiratory Physiology*, 23:71–85.

Geddes, L. A., Hoff, H. E., Hickman, D. M., & Moore, A. G. (1962). The impedance pneumograph. *Aerospace Medicine*, 33:28–33.

Gellhorn, E. & Loofbourow, G. (1963). *Emotions and Emotional Disorders*. New York: Harper & Row.

Genazzani, A. R., Nappi, G., Facchinetti, F., Mazzella, G. L., Parrini, D., Sinforiani, E., Petraglia, F., & Savoldi, F. (1982). Central deficiency of β-endorphin in alcohol addicts. *Journal of Clinical Endocrinology and Metabolism*, 55:583–586.

Gennari, F. J., Goldstein, M. B., & Schwartz, W. B. (1972). The nature of the renal adaptation to chronic hypocapnia. *Journal of Clinical Investigation*, 51:1722–1730.

Gentry, W. D., (ed.). (1984). *Handbook of Behavioral Medicine*. New York: Guilford Press.

George, W. K., George, W. D., Smith, J. P., Gordon, F. T., Baird, E., & Mills, G. C. (1964). Change in serum calcium, serum phosphate and red cell phosphate during hyperventilation. *New England Journal of Medicine*, 270:726–728.

Gerard, R. W. (1938). *Brain Metabolism and Circulation*. (See Cobb, Frantz, Penfield, & Riley). pp. 317–345.

Gesell, R., Bricker, J., & Magee, C. (1936). Structural and functional organization of the central mechanisms controlling breathing. *American Journal of Physiology*, 117:423–452.

Giannini, A. J., Castellani, S., & Dvoredshy, A. E. (1983). Anxiety states: Relationship to atmospheric cations and serotonin. *Journal of Clinical Psychiatry*. 44:262–264.

Giannini, A. J., Malone, D. A., & Piotrowski, T. A. (1986). Serotonin irritation syndrome—A new clinical entity? *Journal of Clinical Psychiatry*, 47:25.

Gibbs, D. M. (1992). Hyperventilation-induced cerebral ischemia in panic disorder and effects of nimodipine. *American Journal of Psychiatry*, 149:1589–1591.

Gibbs, E. L., Lennox, W. G., & Gibbs, F. A. (1940). Variations in the carbon dioxide content of the blood in epilepsy. *Archives of Neurology and Psychiatry*, 43:223–239.

Gibbs, F. A., Maxwell, H., & Gibbs, E. L. (1947). Volume flow of blood through the human brain. *Archives of Neurology and Psychiatry*, 57:137–144.

Gibbs, F. A., Williams, D., & Gibbs, E. L. (1949). Modification of the cortical frequency spectrum by changes in CO_2, blood sugar, and O_2. *Journal of Neurophysiology*, 3:49–58.

Giebisch, G., Berger, L., Pitts, R. F., Parks, M. E., & MacLeod, M. B. (1955). The extrarenal response to acute acid-base disturbance of respiratory origin. *Journal of Clinical Investigation*, 34:231–245.

Gilbert, R., Auchincloss, J. H., Brodsky, J., & Boden, W. (1972). Changes in tidal volume, frequency, and ventilation induced by their measurement. *Journal of Applied Physiology*, 33:252–254.

Gilman, A. & Brazeau, P. (1953). The role of kidney in the regulation of acid-base metabolism. *American Journal of Medicine*, 15:765.

Glass, L. & Mackey, M. C. (1988). *From Clocks to Chaos—The Rhythms of Life*. Princeton University Press.

Gledhill, N., Beirne, G. J., & Dempsey, J. A. (1975). Renal response to short-term hypocapnia in man. *Kidney International*, 8:376–386.

Gliebe, P. A. & Auerbach, A. (1944). Sighing and other forms of hyperventilation simulating organic disease. *Journal of Nervous and Mental Diseases*, 99:600–615.

Glueck, B. S. & Stroebel, C. F. (1975). Biofeedback and meditation in the treatment of psychiatric illness. *Comparative Psychiatry*, 16:303–321.

Goldberg, G. J. (1958). Psychiatric aspects of hyperventilation. *South African Medical Journal*, 32:447–449.

Goldensohn, E. S. (1976). Paroxysmal and other features of the electroencephalogram in migraine. *Research and Clinical Studies in Headache*, 4:118–128.

Goldensohn, E. S., Schoenfeld, R. L., & Hoefer, P. F. A. (1951). The slowly changing voltage of the brain and the electrocorticogram. *EEG and Clinical Neurophysiology*, 3:231–336.

Goldensohn, E. S. & Zablow, L. (1959). An electrical impedance spirometer. *Journal of Applied Physiology*, 14:463–464.

Goldman, M. J. (1967). *Principles of Electrocardiography*. Los Altos: Lange Medical Publications.

Goodland, R. L. & Pommerenke, W. T. (1952). Cyclic fluctuations of the alveolar carbon dioxide tension during the normal menstrual cycle. *Fertility and Sterility*, 3:394–401.

Goodland, R. L., Reynolds, J. G., McCord, A. G., & Pommerenke, W. T. (1953). Respiratory and electrolyte effects induced by estrogen and progesterone. *Fertility and Sterility*, 4:300–317.

Gorman, J. M., Askanazi, J., Leibowitz, M. R., Fyer, A. J., Stein, J., Kinney, J. M., & Klein, D. F. (1984). Response to hyperventilation in a group of patients with panic disorder. *American Journal of Psychiatry*, 141:857–861.

Gorman, J. M., Cohen, B. S., Liebowitz, M. R., Fyer, A. J., Ross, D., Davies, S. O., & Klein, D. F. (1986). Blood gas changes in hypophosphatemia in lactate-induced panic. *Archives of General Psychiatry*, 43:1067–1071.

Gorman, J. M., Fyer, A. F., Glicklich, J., King, D. L., & Klein, D. F. (1981). Mitral valve prolapse and panic disorders: Effects of imipramine. In Klein, D. F. & Rabkin, J. (eds.), *Anxiety: New Research and Changing Concepts*. New York: Raven Press, pp. 317–326.

Gorman, J., Fyer, M. R., Goetz, R., Askanazi, J., Liebowitz, M. R., Fyer, A. J., Kinney, J., & Klein, D. F. (1988). Ventilatory physiology of patients with panic disorder. *Archives of General Psychiatry*, 45:31–39.

Gorman, J. M., Levy, G. F., Leibowitz, M. R., McGrath, P., Appleby, I. L., Dillon, D. J., Davies, S. O., & Klein, D. F. (1983). Effect of acute β-adrenergic blockade on lactate-induced panic. *Archives of General Psychiatry*, 40:1079–1082.

Gotoh, F., Meyer, J. S., & Takagi, Y. (1965). Cerebral effects of hyperventilation in man. *Archives of Neurology*, 12:410–423.

Gotoh, F., Tazaki, Y., & Meyer, J. S. (1961). Transport of gases through brain and their extravascular vasomotion action. *Experimental Neurology*, 4:48–58.

Gottstein, U., Berghoff, W., Held, K., Gabriel, H., Textor, T., & Zahn, U. (1970). Cerebral metabolism during hyperventilation and inhalation of CO_2. In Russel, R. W. R. (ed.), *Proceedings of the Fourth International Symposium on Regulation of Cerebral Blood Flow*. London: Pitman.

Gowers, W. G. (1907). *The Borderland of Epilepsy*. London: Churchill.

Granholm, L., Lukjanova, L., & Siesjo, B. K. (1968). Evidence of cerebral hypoxia in pronounced hyperventilation. *Scandinavian Journal of Laboratory Investigation*, suppl. 2.

Green, J. & Shellenberger, R. (1991). *The Dynamics of Health and Wellness—A Biopsychosocial Approach*. Philadelphia: Holt, Rinehart & Winston.

Griesheimer, E. M. (1963). *Physiology and Anatomy*, 8th ed. Philadelphia: Lippincott.

Griez, E., Zandbergen, J., Lousberg, H., & van den Hout, M. (1988). Effects of low pulmonary CO_2 on panic anxiety. *Comprehensive Psychiatry*, 29:490–497.

Grollman, A. (1931). Physiological variations in the cardiac output of man: IX. The effect of breathing carbon dioxide, and of voluntary forced ventilation on the cardiac output of man. *American Journal of Physiology*, 94:287–299.

Grossman, P. (1983). Stress and cardiovascular function. *Psychophysiology*, 20:284–300.

Grossman, P. (1991). Respiratory mediation of cardiac function within a psychophysiological perspective. In Carlson, J. G. & Seifert, A. R. (eds.), *International Perspectives on Self-Regulation and Health*. New York: Plenum Press.

Grossman, P. & DeSwart, J. C. G. (1984). Diagnosis of hyperventilation syndrome on the basis of reported complaints. *Journal of Psychosomatic Research*, 28:97–104.

Grossman, P., DeSwart, J. C. G., & Defares, P. B. (1985). A controlled study of a breathing therapy treatment of hyperventilation syndrome. *Journal of Psychosomatic Research Abstract*, 29:97.

Grossman, P., Karemaker, J., & Wieling, W. (1991). Prediction of tonic parasympathetic cardiac control using respiratory sinus arrhythmia: The need for respiratory control. *Psychophysiology*, 28:201–216.

Grote, J., Zimmer, K., & Schubert, R. (1981). Effects of severe arterial hypocapnia on regional blood flow regulation, tissue PO_2 and metabolism in the brain of cats. *Pflugers Archives*, 391:195–199.

Grunhaus, L., Rabin, D., & Greden, J. F. (1986). Simultaneous panic and depressive disorder: Response to antidepressant treatment. *Journal of Clinical Psychiatry*, 47:4–7.

Guthrie, D., Moeller, T., & Guthrie, R. (1983). Biofeedback and its application to the stabilization and control of diabetes mellitus. *American Journal of Clinical Biofeedback*, 6:82–87.

Guttman, E. & Jones, M. (1940). Hyperventilation and the effort syndrome. *British Medical Journal*, 2:736.

Guyton, A. C. (1981). *Textbook of Medical Physiology*, 6th ed. Philadelphia: W. B. Saunders.

Guyton, A. C., Cromwell, J. W., & Moore, J. W. (1956). Basic oscillating mechanism of Cheyne-Stokes breathing. *American Journal of Physiology*, 187:395–398.

Guz, A., Mier, A., & Murphy, K. (1988). Does the cortex play a role in the ventilatory response to inhaled CO_2 in man? *Journal of Physiology*, 403:105P.

Haas, A., Pineda, H., Haas, F., & Axen, K. (1979). *Pulmonary Therapy and Rehabilitation: Principles and Practice*. Baltimore: Williams & Wilkins.

Hadjiev, D. (1968). A new method of quantitative evaluation of cerebral blood flow by rheoencephalography. *Brain Research*, 8:213–215.

Haldane, J. S. & Poulton, E. P. (1908). The effects of want of oxygen on respiration. *Proceedings of the Physiology Society*, 37:390.

Hamilton, J. A. & Shock, N. W. (1936). Experimental study of personality, physique, and acid-base equilibrium of blood. *American Journal of Psychology*, 48:467.

Hamilton, L. H., Beard, J. D., & Kory, R. C. (1965). Impedance measurement of tidal volume and ventilation. *Journal of Applied Physiology*, 20:565–568.

Hanington, E. (1982). Migraine as a blood disorder: Preliminary studies. In Critchley, M. (ed.), *Advances in Neurology*, vol. 33. New York: Raven, pp. 253–256.

Hanington, H. (1987). The Platelet Theory. In Blau, J. N. (ed.), *Migraine*. Baltimore: The Johns Hopkins University Press, pp. 331–353.

Hardonk, H. J. & Beumer, H. M. (1979). Hyperventilation syndrome. In Vinken, P. J. & Bruyn, G. W. (eds.), *Handbook of Clinical Neurology*. Vol. 38, Neurological Manifestations of Systemic Disease, pt. 1. Amsterdam: North Holland.

Harper, M. A. & Bell, R. A. (1963). The effect of metabolic acidosis and alkalosis on blood flow through the cerebral cortex. *Journal of Neurology, Neurosurgery and Psychiatry*, 26:341–344.

Harper, R. M. & Sterman, M. B. (1972). Subcortical unit activity during conditioned 12–14 Hz sensorimotor rhythm in cats. *Federation Proceedings*, 31:404.

Harris, J. B., Hoff, H. E., & Wise, R. A. (1954). Diaphragmatic flutter as a manifestation of hysteria. *Psychosomatic Medicine*, 16:56–66.

Harris, P. & Heath, D. (1962). *The Human Pulmonary Circulation*. Baltimore: Williams & Wilkins.

Hattingberg, H. (1931). Das Atemkorsett. *Berichte uber d: VI. Allgemeine arztlichen Kongress f. Psychotherapie.* Leipzig: Kretchmer und Cimbal, pp. 129–135.

Hauge, A., Thorensen, M., & Walloe, L. (1980). Changes in cerebral blood flow during hyperventilation and CO_2-breathing measured transcutaneously in humans by a bidirectional, pulsed, ultrasound doppler blood velocimeter. *Acta Physiologica Scandinavica*, 110:167–173.

Hauptmann, A. & Myerson, A. (1948). Studies of finger capillaries in schizophrenia and manic-depressive psychoses. *Journal of Nervous and Mental Diseases.* 108:81–108.

Heim, E., Blaser, A., & Waidlich, A. (1972). Dyspnea: Psychophysiologic relationships. *Psychosomatic Medicine*, 34:405.

Heistad, D. D., Marcus, M. L., & Abboud, F. M. (1978). Experimental attempts to unmask the effects of neural stimuli on cerebral blood flow. In Purves, M. J. et al. (eds.), *Cerebral Vascular Smooth Muscle and Its Control*. Amsterdam: Elsevier Excerpta Medica.

Helsing, K. J., Comstock, G. W., Speizer, F. E., Ferris, B. G., Lebowitz, M. D., Tockman, M. S., & Burrows, B. (1979). Comparison of three standardized questionnaires on respiratory symptoms. *American Review of Respiratory Disease*, 120:1221–1231.

Hering, E. & Breuer, J. (1968). Die Selbststeuerung der atmung durch den Nervus vagus. *Sitzbericht der Akademie Wissenschaft Wien*, 57:672–677.

Hersen, M., Eisler, R. M., & Miller, P. M. (1977). *Progress in Behavior Modification*. New York: Academic Press.

Hertzman, A. B. (1959). Vasomotor regulation of cutaneous circulation. *Physiological Review*, 39:280–306.

Hertzman, A. B. & Dillon, J. G. (1939). Selective vascular reaction patterns in the nasal septum and the skin of the extremities and head. *American Journal of Physiology*, 127:617–684.

Hertzman, A. B. & Roth, L. W. (1942). The absence of vasoconstrictor reflexes in the forehead circulation: Effects of cold. *American Journal of Physiology*, 136:692–697.

Hess, D. (1989). *A Guide to Understanding Capnography*. Louisville, Colorado: Ohmeda—The BOC Group, Inc.

Hess, W. R. (1957). *Functional Anatomy of the Brain*. New York: Grune & Stratton.

Heyck, H. (1969). Pathogenesis of migraine. *Research and Clinical Studies in Headache*, 2:1–28.

Heymans, C. & Neill, E. (1958). *Reflexogenic Areas of the Vascular System*. Boston: Little, Brown.

Hibbert, G. A. (1984). Hyperventilation as a cause of panic attacks. *British Medical Journal*, 288:263–264.

Hibbert, G. & Chan, M. (1989). Respiratory control: Its contribution to the treatment of panic attacks—A controlled study. *British Journal of Psychiatry*, 154:232–236.

Hibbert, G. & Pilsbury, D. (1988). Hyperventilation and panic attacks—Ambulant monitoring and transcutaneous carbon dioxide. *British Journal of Psychiatry*, 153:76–80.

Hill, O. (1979). The hyperventilation syndrome. *British Journal of Psychiatry*, 135:367–368.

Himwich, H. E. (1951). *Brain Metabolism and Cerebral Disorders*. Baltimore: Williams & Wilkins.

Hinkle, L. E., Carver, S. T., & Plakun, A. (1972). Slow heart rates and increased risk of cardiac death in middle-aged men. *Archives of Internal Medicine*, 129:732–748.

Hirsh, J. S. & Bishop, B. (1981). Respiratory sinus arrhythmia in humans: How breathing pattern modulates heart rate. *American Journal of Physiology*, 241:H620–629.

Hirsh, J. S. & Bishop, B. (1982). Human breathing patterns on mouthpiece or face mask during air, CO_2, or low O_2. *Journal of Applied Physiology: Respiration, Environment and Exercise Physiology*, 53:1281–1290.

Hockaday, J. M. (1978). Late outcome of childhood onset migraine and factors affecting outcome with partial reference to early and late EEG findings. In Greene, R. (ed.), *Current Concepts in Migraine*. New York: Raven Press.

Hoefer, P. F. A. (1967). The electroencephalogram in cases of headache of various etiology. *Research and Clinical Studies in Headache*, 1:165–183.

Hoes, J. J. (1983). Pharmacotherapy of the hyperventilation syndrome. *Journal of Drug Research and Therapy*, 8:1881–1887.

Hoes, M., Colla, P., & Folgering, H. (1980). Clomipramine treatment of hyperventilation syndrome. *Pharmacopsychology and Neuro-Psychopharmacology*, 13:25–28.

Hoes, M. (1981). Hyperventilation syndrome: Treatment with L-tryptophan and pyridoxine: Predictive value of xanturenic acid excretion. *Journal of Orthomolecular Psychiatry*, 10:7–15.

Hofbauer, L. (1921). *Atmungs-Pathologie und Therapie*. Berlin: Julius Springer.

Holmberg, G. (1953). Electroencephalogram during hypoxia and hyperventilation. *EEG and Clinical Neurophysiology*, 5:371.

Holmes, D. S. (1984). Meditation and somatic arousal reduction. *American Psychologist*, 39: 1–10.

Holmes, T. H., Goodell, H., Wolf, S., & Wolff, H. (1950). *The Nose*. Springfield, IL: Charles C Thomas.

Holt, P. E. & Andrews, G. (1989). Hyperventilation and anxiety in panic disorder, social phobia, GAD and normal controls. *Behavior Research and Therapy*, 27:453–460.

Hormbrey, J., Jacobi, M. S., Patil, C. P., & Saunders, K. B. (1988). Co_2 response and pattern of breathing in patients with symptomatic hyperventilation, compared to asthmatic and normal subjects. *European Respiratory Journal*, 1:846–852.

Hosaka, T., Shirakura, K., Iga, T., Ohsuga, H., Noji, K., & Nezu, S. (1987). Clinical application of biofeedback treatment with a microvibration transducer. *Tokai Journal of Medical Science*, 12:319–324.

Howell, J. B. (1990). Behavioural breathlessness. *Thorax*, 45:287–292.

Hrushesky, W. J. M., Fader, D., Schmitt, O., & Gilbertsen, V. (1984). The respiratory sinus arrhythmia: A measure of cardiac age. *Science*, 224:1001–1004.

Huckabee, W. E. (1961). Abnormal resting blood lactate. *American Journal of Medicine*, 30: 833–840.

Huey, S. R. (1983). Hyperventilation: Its relation to symptom experience and anxiety. *Journal of Abnormal Psychology*, 92:422–432.

Huey, S. R. & Sechrest, L. (1981). *Hyperventilation Syndrome and Psychopathology*. Center for Research on the Utilization of Scientific Knowledge, Institute for Social Research, University of Michigan. Unpublished manuscript.

Huey, S. R. & West, S. G. (1983). Hyperventilation: Its relation to symptom experience and to anxiety. *Journal of Abnormal Psychology*, 92:422–432.

Hughes, J. (1975). *Opiate receptor mechanisms*. In Snyder, S. H. & Matisse, S. (eds.), *Neurosciences Research Program Bulletin*, 1:55–58.

Hughes, R. L. (1979). Does abdominal breathing affect regional gas exchange? *Chest*, 76: 288–293.

Hunt, H. F. & Brady, J. V. (1955). Some effects of punishment and intercurrent "anxiety" on a simple operant. *Journal of Comparative and Physiological Psychology*, 48:305–310.

Hymes, A. & Nuernberger, P. (1980). Breathing patterns found in heart attack patients. *Research Bulletin of the Himalaya International Society*, 2:10–12.

Jacobson, E. (1934). *You Must Relax*. New York: McGraw-Hill.

Jacobson, E. (1935). *Progressive Relaxation*. Chicago: University of Chicago Press.

Jacquy, J., Dekoninck, W. J., Piraux, A., Calay, R., Bacq, J., Levy, D., & Noel, G. (1974). Cerebral blood flow and quantitative rheoencephalography. *EEG and Clinical Neurophysiology*, 37:507–511.

Jacquy, J., Piraux, A., Noel, G., & Henriet, M. (1973). A tentative study of regional vasomotor capacitance variations by rheoencephalography. *European Journal of Neurology*, 10:12–24.

Jammes, Y., Auran, Y., Gouvernet, J., Delpierre, S., & Grimaud, C. (1979). The ventilatory pattern of conscious man according to age and morphology. *Bulletin of European Physiopathology and Respiration*, 15:527–540.

Javaheris, S., Shore, N. J., Rose, B., & Kazemi, H. (1982). Compensatory hypoventilation in metabolic acidosis. *Chest*, 81:296–301.

Jay, G. W., (1982). Epilepsy, migraine, and EEG abnormalities in children: A review and hypothesis. *Headache*, 22:110–114.

Jellinek, M. S., Goldenheim, P. D., & Jenike, M. A. (1985). The impact of grief on ventilatory control. *American Journal of Psychiatry*, 142:121–122.

Jenkins, C. D. (1971). Psychological and social precursors of coronary disease. *New England Journal of Medicine*, 284:307–317.

Jenkins, C. D. (1978). Behavioral risk factors in coronary artery disease. *Annual Review of Medicine*, 29:543–562.

Jenkins, C. D. (1979). *Manual: Jenkins Activity Survey*. New York: Psychological Corp.

Jensen, D. (1971). *Intrinsic Cardiac Regulation*. New York: Appleton-Century-Crofts.

Jevning, R., Fernando, G., & Wilson, A. F. (1989). Evaluation of consistency among different electrical impedance indices of relative cerebral blood flow in normal resting individuals. *Journal of Biomedical Engineering*, 11:53–56.

Jevning, R., Wilson, A. F., Smith, W. R., & Morton, M. E. (1978). Redistribution of blood flow in acute hypo-metabolic behavior. *American Journal of Physiology*, 235:R89–92.

Jitsuiki, S., & Bauer, H. (1973). Preliminary study on microvibration (MV). *Hiroshima Journal of Medical Science*, 22:365–375.

Johnson, G. B. (1982). The environment and HVDC transmission lines. In Charry, J. M. (ed.), *Conference on Environment: Ions and Related Biological Effects*. Philadelphia: American Institute of Medical Climatology.

Johnston, R. & Lee, K. (1976). Myofeedback—A new method of teaching breathing exercises in emphysematous patients. *Physical Therapy*, 56:826–829.

Juan, G., Calverley, P., Talamo, C., Schnader, J., & Fousso, C. (1984). Effects of carbon dioxide on diaphragmatic function in human beings. *New England Journal of Medicine*, 10:874–879.

Juszczak, N. M. & Andreassi, J. L. (1987). Performance and physiological response of type A and type B individuals during a cognitive and perceptual-motor task. *International Journal of Psychophysiology*, 5:81–89.

Kamyia, J. (1979). Autoregulation of the EEG rhythm: A program for the study of consciousness. In Peper, E., Ancoli, S., & Quinn, M. (eds.), *Mind–Body Integration: Essential Readings in Biofeedback*. New York: Plenum.

Kane, J. M., Woerner, M., Zeldis, S., Kramer, R., & Saravay, S. (1981). Panic and phobic disorders in patients with mitral valve prolapse. In Klein, D. F. & Rabkin, J. (eds.), *Anxiety: New Research and Changing Concepts*. New York: Raven Press.

Kanellakos, D. P. & Lukas, J. S. (1974). *The Psychobiology of Transcendental Meditation: A Literature Review*. Menlo Park: Benjamin.

Kaplan, B. J. (1975). Biofeedback in epileptics: Equivocal relationship of reinforced EEG frequency to seizure reduction. *Epilepsia*, 16:477–485.

Kasamatsu, A. & Hirai, T. (1966). An electroencephalographic study of Zen meditation. *Folia Psychiatrica et Neurologia Japonica*, 20:315–336.

Kasamatsu, A. & Hirai, T. (1969). An electroencephalographic study of Zen meditation (Zazen). *Psychologia*, 12:205–225.

Kassabian, J., Miller, K. D., & Lavietes, M. H. (1982). Respiratory center output and ventilatory timing in patients with acute airway (asthma) and alveolar (pneumonia) disease. *Chest*, 81:536–543.

Katz, I. R. (1982). Is there a hypoxic affective syndrome? *Psychosomatics*, 23:846–853.

Kavet, R. (1989). Hypothetical neural substrates for biological response to air ions. In Charry, J. M. & Kavet, R. (eds.), *Air Ions: Physical and Biological Aspects*. Boca Raton: CRC Press.

Keatinge, W. R. (1978). How vascular smooth muscle works. In Purves, M. J. (ed), *Cerebral Vascular Smooth Muscle and Its Control*. Amsterdam: Elsevier Exerpta Medica.

Kelson, S. G., Fleegler, B., & Altose, M. B. (1979). The respiratory neuromuscular response to hypoxia, hypercapnia, and obstruction to airflow in asthma. *American Review of Respiratory Diseases*, 120:517–527.

Keltz, H., Samortin, T., & Stone, D. J. (1972). Hyperventilation: A manifestation of exogenous beta—adrenergic stimulation. *American Review of Respiratory Diseases*, 105:637–640.

Kempf, E. (1930). Affective-respiratory factors in catatonia. *Medical Journal Record*, 131:181–185.

Kenardy, J., Oei, T. P. S., & Evans, L. (1990). Hyperventilation and panic attacks. *Australian and New Zealand Journal of Psychiatry*, 24:261–267.

Kenin, R. & Wintle, J. (1978). *The Dictionary of Biographical Quotation*. New York: Dorset Press.

Kennealy, J. A., McLennan, J. E., London, R. G., & McLaurin, R. L. (1980). Hyperventilation-induced cerebral hypoxia. *American Review of Respiratory Disease*, 122:407–411.

Kerr, W. J., Dalton, J. W., & Gliebe, P. A. (1937). Some physical phenomena associated with anxiety states and their relationship to hyperventilation. *Annals of Internal Medicine*, 11:961–992.

Kesterson, J. & Clinch, N. (1985). Peripheral and central control mechanisms during respiratory suspension in transcendental meditation as evidenced by latency, hypoxia, and RQ change. *Society for Neurosciences Abstract*, 11:1144.

Kety, S. S. & Schmidt, C. F. (1946). The effect of active and passive hyperventilation on cerebral blood flow, cerebral oxygen consumption, cardiac output, and blood pressure of normal young men. *Journal of Clinical Investigation*, 24:107–109.

Kety, S. S. & Schmidt, C. F. (1948). The effects of altered arterial tensions of carbon dioxide and oxygen on cerebral blood flow and cerebral oxygen consumption of normal young men. *Journal of Clinical Investigation*, 27:484–492.

Keuning, J. (1968). On the nasal cycle. *Journal of International Rhinology*, 6:99–136.

Khan, A. U. (1977). Effectiveness of biofeedback and counter conditioning in the treatment of bronchial asthma. *Journal of Psychosomatic Research*, 21:97–104.

Kilburn, K. H. (1965). Tachypnea and hyperpnea. *Annals of Internal Medicine*, 62:486–498.

King, D. S. (1981). Can allergic exposure provoke psychological symptoms? A double-blind test. *Biological Psychology*, 16:19.

King, N. J. & Montgomery, R. B. (1980). Biofeedback-induced control of human peripheral temperature: A critical review of the literature. *Psychological Bulletin*, 88:738–751.

King, N. J. & Montgomery, R. B. (1981). The self-control of human peripheral (finger) temperature: An exploration of somatic maneuvers as aids to biofeedback training. *Behavior Therapy*, 12:263–273.

King, R. J., Bayon, E. P., Clark, D. B., & Taylor, C. B. (1988). Tonic arousal and activity: Relationship to personality disorder traits in panic patients. *Psychiatry Research* (Ireland), 25:65–72.

Klee, W., Ziouchou, A., & Streaty R. A. (1977). Exorphins: Peptides with opioid activity isolated from wheat gluten, and their possible role in the etiology of schizophrenia. In Usdin, E., Bunney, W. E., & Kline, N. S. (eds.), *Endorphins in Mental Health Research*. New York: Oxford University Press, pp. 209–218.

Klein, D. F. (1992). *Suffocation false alarm theory of panic*. Paper presented at the Eleventh International Symposium on Respiratory Psychophysiology, Bordeaux, France.

Klein, D. F. & Gorman, J. M. (1984). Panic disorder and mitral valve prolapse. *Journal of Clinical Psychiatry Monograph*, 2:14–20.

Klein, D. F., Zitrin, C. M., & Woerner, M. (1978). Anti-depressants, anxiety, panic, and phobia. In Lipton, M. A., DiMascio, A., & Williams, K. F. (eds.), *Psychopharmacology: A Generation of Progress*. New York: Raven Press.

Klein, R., Pilton, D., Possner, S., & Shannahoff-Khalsa, D. S. (1986). Hemispheric performance efficiency varies with nasal airflow. *Biological Psychology*, 23:127–137.

Kleinfelter, H. F. (1973). Letter to the Editor: Hyperventilation and sphygmomanometry. *Journal of American Medical Association*, 226:81–82.

Kling, V. & Szekely, G. (1968). Stimulation of rhythmic nervous activities: I. Function of networks with cyclic inhibitions. *Kybernetik*, 5:89–103.

Kluver, H. & Bucy, P. C. (1939). Preliminary analysis of functions of the temporal lobes in monkeys. *Archives of Neurology and Psychiatry*, 4:261–267.

Kohlrausch, W. (1940). Wesen und Bedeutung der Krankengymnastik bei psychischen und organischen Nervenkrankheiten. *Fortschrift dehr Neurologie und Psychiatrie*, 12: 235–262.

Koizumi, K., Terui, N., & Kollai, M. (1984). Relationship between vagal and sympathetic activities in rhythmic fluctuations. In Miyaka, K., Koepchen, H. P., & Polosa, C. (eds.), *Mechanisms of Blood Pressure Waves*. Berlin: Springer-Verlag, pp. 43–55.

Kolb, L. C. (1968). *Noyes' Modern Clinical Psychiatry*, 7th ed. Philadelphia: W. B. Saunders.

Konuk, E. & Peper, E. (1984). Developing multimodal procedures in asthma management through diaphragmatic breathing and EMG feedback. In *Proceedings of the 15th Annual Meeting of the Biofeedback Society of America*, Wheat Ridge, Colorado, pp. 122–125.

Kooi, K. A. (1971). *Fundamentals of Electroencephalography*. New York: Harper & Row.

Kopp, M. S. & Koranyi, L. (1982). Autonomic and psychological correlates in hypertension and duodenal ulcer. *Pavlovian Journal of Biological Research*, 17:178–187.

Koshtoyants, Kh. S. (1950). *I. P. Pavlov—Selected works*. Moscow: Foreign Language Publishing House.

Kossowsky, W. A. (1984). Cocaine and acute myocardial infarction. *Chest*, 86:729–731.

Kotzes, H., Rawson, J. C., & Wigal, J. K. (1987). Respiratory airway changes in response to suggestion in normal individuals. *Psychosomatic Medicine*, 49:536–541.

Kraft, A. R. & Hoogduin, C. A. L. (1984). The hyperventilation syndrome—A pilot study of the effectiveness of treatment. *British Journal of Psychiatry*, 145:538–542.

Krantz, D. S. & Glass, D. C. (1984). Personality, behavior patterns, and physical illness: Conceptual and methodological issues. In Gentry, W. D. (ed.), *Handbook of Behavioral Medicine*. New York: Guilford Press.

Krapf, R., Beeler, I., Hertner, D., & Hulter, H. N. (1991). The effect of sustained hyperventilation on renal regulation of acid-base equilibrium. *New England Journal of Medicine*, 324:1394–1401.

Kreisberg, R. A. (1980). Lactate homeostasis and lactic acidosis. *Annals of Internal Medicine*, 92:227.

Kristof, M., Servit, Z., & Manas, K. (1981). Activating effect of nasal airflow on epileptic electrographic abnormalities in the human EEG. Evidence for the reflex origin of the phenomenon. *Physiolog Bohemoslov*, 30:73–77.

Krueger, A. P. & Reed, E. J. (1976). Biological impact of small air ions. *Science*, 193:1209.

Krueger, A. P. & Smith, R. F. (1960). The biological mechanism of air-ion action. I. 5-Hydroxytryptamine as the endogenous mediator of positive air ion effects on the mammal trachea. *Journal of General Physiology*, 43:533–540.

Krueger, T. P., Rockoff, S. D., Thomas, L. J., & Ommaya, A. K. (1963). The effect of change of end-expiratory carbon dioxide tension on the normal cerebral angiogram. *American Journal of Roentgenography*, 90:506–511.

Kubicek, W. G., Kinnen, E., & Edin, A. (1964). Calibration of an impedance pneumograph. *Journal of Applied Physiology*, 19:560–577.

Kuhlman, W. N. (1979–80). EEG feedback training of epileptic patients: Clinical and electroencephalographic analysis. In Shapiro, D., Stoyva, J., Kamiya, J., Barber, T. S., Miller, N. R., & Schwartz, G. E. (eds.), *Biofeedback and Behavioral Medicine*. New York: Aldine Press.

Kuhlman, W. N. & Allison, T. (1977). EEG feedback training in the treatment of epilepsy: Some questions and some answers. *Pavlovian Journal of Biological Science*, 12:112–122.

Lacey, J. I. (1956). The evaluation of autonomic responses: Toward a general solution. *Annals of the New York Academy of Sciences*, 67:123–164.

Lacey, J. I., Kagan, J., Lacey, B. C., & Moss, H. A. (1963). The visceral level: Situational determinants and behavioral correlates of autonomic response patterns. In Knapp, P. H. (ed.), *Expression of Emotions in Man*. New York: International Universities Press.

Laitinen, G., Johnasson, G., & Sipponen, P. (1966). Recording of regional cerebral circulation by an impedance method. Preliminary report. *Brain Research*, 2:184–187.

Lambertsen, C. J. (1960). Carbon dioxide and respiration in acid-base homeostasis. *Anesthesiology*, 21:642–651.

Lambertsen, C. J., Semple, S. J. G., Smyth, M. G., & Gelfand, R. (1961). H^+ and pCO_2 as chemical factors in respiratory and cerebral circulatory control. *Journal of Applied Physiology*, 16:473–484.

Lassen, N. A. (1959). Cerebral blood flow and oxygen consumption in man. *Physiological Reviews*, 39:183–238.

Lassen, N. A. (1963). Regional cerebral blood flow measurement in man. *Archives of Neurology*, 9:615–623.

Lathrop, R. G. (1966). First order response dependencies at a differential brightness threshold. *Journal of Experimental Psychology*, 72:120–124.

Lauritzen, M., Olsen, T. S., Lassen, N. A., & Paulson, O. B. (1983). Regulation of regional cerebral blood flow during and between migraine attacks. *Annals of Neurology*, 14:569–572.

Lawson, E. E., Waldrop, T. G., & Eldridge, F. L. (1979). Nalaxone enhances respiratory output in cats. *Journal of Applied Physiology*, 47:527–531.

Lawson, N. W., Butler, G. H., & Ray, C. T. (1973). Alkalosis and cardiac arrhythmias. *Anaesthesia and Analgesia*, 52:951–962.

Lazarus, H. R. & Kostan, J. J. (1969). Psychogenic hyperventilation and death anxiety. *Psychosomatics*, 10:14–22.

Lechner, H., Geyer, N., Lugaresi, E., Martin, F., Lifshitz, L., & Markowich, S. (1969). *Rheoencephalography and Plethysmographical Methods*. Amsterdam: Excerpta Medica Foundation.

Lechner, H., Geyer, N., & Rodler, H. (1967). Rheography of function. *EEG and Clinical Neurophysiology*, 23:185.

Lechtenberg, R. (1982). *The Psychiatrist's Guide to Diseases of the Nervous System*. New York: Wiley.

Lee, C. T. & Wei, L. Y. (1983). Spectrum analysis of human pulse. *IEEE Transactions of Biomedical Engineering*, 30:348–352.

Lehrer, P. M., Woolfolk, R. L., Rooney, A. J., McCann, G., & Carrington, P. (1983). Progressive relaxation and meditation: A study of psychophysiological and therapeutic differences between two techniques. *Behavior Therapy and Research*, 21:651–721.

Leitenberg, H. (1976). *Handbook of Behavior Modification and Behavior Therapy*. Englewood Cliffs, Prentice-Hall.

Lennox, W. G. (1928). The effects on epileptic seizures of varying the composition of respired air. *Journal of Clinical Investigation*, 6:23.

Lennox, W. G., Gibbs, F. A., & Gibbs, E. L. (1938). The relationship in man of cerebral activity to blood flow and blood constituents. *Journal of Neurology and Psychiatry*, 1: 221–225.

Lennox, W. G. & Lennox, M. A. (1960). *Epilepsy and Related Disorders*, vols. 1 and 2. Boston: Little, Brown, and Co.

Lennox, W. G. & Leonardt, E. (1931). The effect of mental work. *Archives of Neurology and Psychiatry*, 26:725–730.

Leon-Sotomayor, L. A. (1974). Cardiac migraine—report of twelve cases. *Angiology*, 25: 161–171.

Levander, V. L., Benson, H., Wheeler, R. C., & Wallace, R. K. (1972). Increased forearm blood flow during a wakeful hypometabolic state. *Federation Proceedings*, 31:405.

Levine, B. S. & Coburn, J. W. (1984). Magnesium, the mimic/antagonist of calcium. *New England Journal of Medicine*, 310:1253–1255.

Levine, H. J. (1978). Mimics of coronary disease. *Postgraduate Medicine*, 64:58–67.

Lewis, B. I. (1957). Hyperventilation syndrome: Clinical and physiological observations. *Postgraduate Medicine*, 53:259–271.

Lewis, B. I. (1964). Mechanisms and management of hyperventilation syndrome. *Clinical Biochemistry*, 4:68–96.

Lewis, R. A. & Howell, J. B. (1986). Definition of hyperventilation syndrome. *Bulletin of European Physiopathology and Respiration*, 22:201–205.

Ley, R. (1985a). Agoraphobia, the panic attack, and the hyperventilation syndrome. *Behavior Therapy and Research*, 23:79–81.

Ley, R. (1985b). Blood, breath, and fears: A hyperventilation theory of panic attacks and agoraphobia. *Clinical Psychological Review*, 5:271–285.

Ley, R. & Walker, H. (1973). Effects of carbon dioxide-oxygen inhalation on heart rate, blood pressure, and subjective anxiety. *Journal of Behavior Therapy and Experimental Psychiatry*, 4:223–228.

Liberson, W. T. & Strauss, H. (1941). EEG studies: Slow activity during hyperventilation in relation to age. *Proceedings of the Society for Experimental Biological Medicine*, 48:674.

Liebowitz, M. R. & Klein, D. F. (1981). Differential diagnosis and treatment of panic attacks and phobic states. *Annual Review of Medicine*, 32:583–599.

Little, R. C. (1964). Cardiovascular response to acute hypocapnia due to overventilation. *American Journal of Physiology*, 206:1025.

Lobel, T. E. (1988). Personality correlates of type A coronary-prone behavior. *Journal of Personality Assessment*, 52:434–440.

Loevenhart, A. S., Lorenz, W. F., Martin, H. G., & Malone, J. Y. (1918). Stimulation of the respiration by sodium cyanid and its clinical application. *Archives of Internal Medicine*, 92:109–129.

Loevenhart, A. S., Lorenz, W. F., & Waters, R. M. (1929). Cerebral stimulation. *Journal of the American Medical Association*, 16:880–883.

Lombard, J. S. (1879). *The Regional Temperature of the Head*. London: H. K. Lewis.

Lorente de No, R. (1934): Studies on the structure of the cerebral cortex. II. Continuation of the study of the ammonic system. *Journal of Psychology and Neurology*, 46:113–177.

Lou, H. C., Henriksen, L., & Bruhn, P. (1984). Focal cerebral hypoperfusion in children with dysphasia and/or attention deficit disorder. *Archives of Neurology*, 41:825–829.

Lowenstein, H. A. (1968). A clinical investigation of phobias. *British Journal of Psychiatry*, 114:1196–1197.

Lowry, T. P. (1967). *Hyperventilation and Hysteria*. Springfield, Illinois: Charles C Thomas.

Lubar, J. F. (1991). Discourse on the development of EEG diagnostics and biofeedback for attention-deficit/hyperactivity disorders. *Biofeedback and Self-Regulation*, 16:201–225.

Lubar, J. F. & Bahler, W. W. (1976). Behavioral management of epileptic seizures following EEG biofeedback training of the sensorimotor rhythm. *Biofeedback and Self-Regulation*, 1: 77–104.

Lubar, J. F., Shasbin, H. S., Natelson, S. E., Holder, G. S., Whitsett, S. F., Pamplin, W. E., & Krulikowksi, D. I. (1981). EEG operant conditioning in intractable epileptics. *Archives of Neurology*, 38:700–704.

Lubbers, D. W. & Leniger-Follert, E. (1978). *Capillary flow in the brain cortex during change in oxygen supply and state of activation*. See Purves.

Lugaresi, E. & Coccagna, G. (1971). The usefulness of REG in clinical practice. *Annals of the New York Academy of Sciences*, 170:645–651.

Lum, L. C. (1975). Hyperventilation—The tip and the iceberg. *Journal of Psychosomatic Research*, 19:375–383.

Lum, L. C. (1976). The syndrome of habitual hyperventilation. In Hill, O. W. (ed.), *Modern Trends in Psychosomatic Medicine*. London: Butterworth.

Lum, L. C. (1978–1979). Respiratory alkalosis and hypocarbia. *Chest, Heart, Stroke Journal*, 3:31–34.

Lum, L. C. (1981). Hyperventilation and anxiety state. *Journal of the Royal Society of Medicine*, 74:4.

Lum, L. C. (1983). Physiological considerations in the treatment of hyperventilation syndromes. *Journal of Drug Research*, 8:1867–1872.

Lundberg, D., Mueller, R., & Breese, G. (1980). An evaluation of the mechanism by which serotonergic activation depresses respiration. *Journal of Pharmacology and Experimental Therapeutics*, 212:397–404.

Lykken, D. T. (1965). The role of individual differences in psychophysiological research. In Venables, P. E. & Christie, M. J. (eds.), *Research in Psychophysiology*. New York: John Wiley & Sons.

Lynch, J. J. (1985). *The Language of the Heart*. New York: Basic Books.

Lyons, H. A. (1969). Respiratory effect of gonadal hormones. In Salhanick, H. A., Kipnis, D. M., & Vande Wiele, R. L. (eds.), *Metabolic Effect of Gonadal Hormones and Contraceptive Steroids*. New York: Plenum.

Lysebeth, A. V. (1979). *Pranayama: The Yoga of Breathing*. London: Mandala Books (Unwin Paperbacks).

Mackenzie, A. I. (1979). Naloxone in alcohol intoxication. *Lancet*, 1:733–734.

Macklem, P. T. & Mead, J. (1967). The physiologic basis of common pulmonary function tests. *Archives of Environmental Health*, 14:5.

Magarian, G. (1982). Hyperventilation syndromes: Infrequently recognized common expressions of anxiety and stress. *Medicine*, 61:210–236.

Magnaes, B. & Nornes, H. (1974). Circulatory and respiratory changes in spontaneous epileptic seizures in man. *European Neurology*, 12:104–115.

Mahesh, M. (1963). *Transcendental Meditation*. New York: New American Library (Signet).

Mairbaurl, H. & Humpeler, E. (1981). In vitro influences of adrenaline on erythrocyte metabolism and on oxygen affinity of hemoglobin. In Brewer, G. J. (ed.), *The Red Cell: Fifth Annual Ann Arbor Conference*. New York: Liss, pp. 311–319.

Mangold, R., Sokoloff, L., Conner, E., Kleinerman, J., Therman & Kety, S. S. (1955). *Journal of Clinical Investigation*, 34:1092–1100.

Manzotti, M. (1958). The effect of some respiratory maneuvers on heart rate. *Journal of Physiology*, 144:541–557.

Margraf, J., Ehlers, A., & Roth, W. T. (1986). Sodium lactate infusion and panic attacks. A review and critique. *Psychosomatic Medicine*, 48:23–51.

Masserman, J. H. & Yum, K. S. (1946). An analysis of the influence of alcohol on the experimental neuroses in cats. *Psychosomatic Medicine*, 8:36.

Masucci, E. F., Seipel, J. H., & Kurtzke, J. K. (1970). Clinical evaluation of "quantitative" rheoencephalography. *Neurology*, 20:642–648.

Mathew, R. & Wilson, W. H. (1990). Anxiety and cerebral blood flow. *American Journal of Psychiatry*, 147:838–849.

Mattson, R. H., Henniger, G. R., Gallagher, B. B., & Glaser, G. H. (1970). Psychophysiologic precipitants of seizures in epileptics. *Neurology*, 20:407.

Maxwell, D. L., Cover, D., & Hughes, J. M. B. (1985). Effect of respiratory apparatus on timing and depth of breathing in man. *Respiratory Physiology*, 61:255–264.

McCabe, P. M., Yongue, B. G., Ackles, P. K., & Porges, S. W. (1985). Changes in heart period, heart-period variability, and a spectral analysis estimate of respiratory sinus arrhythmia in response to pharmacological manipulation of the baroreceptor reflex in cats. *Psychophysiology*, 22:195–203.

McFadden, E. R. & Lyons, H. A. (1968). Arterial blood gas tension in asthma. *New England Journal of Medicine*, 278:1027–1032.

McHenry, L. C. (1965). Rheoencephalography. *Neurology*, 15:507–517.

McKell, T. E. & Sullivan, A. J. (1947). The hyperventilation syndrome in gastroenterology. *Gastroenterology*, 9:6–16.

Mead, J. (1960). Control of respiration frequency. *Journal of Applied Physiology*, 15:325–336.

Meduna, L. J. (1958). *Carbon Dioxide Therapy*, 2d ed. Springfield: Charles C Thomas.

Melcher, A. (1976). Respiratory sinus arrhythmia in man. *Acta Physiologica Scandinavica*, suppl. 435:7–31.

Mellman, T. A. & Uhde, T. W. (1989). Sleep panic attacks: New clinical findings and theoretical implications. *American Journal of Psychiatry*, 146:1204–1207.

Merritt, H. H. & Putnam, T. J. (1938). Sodium diphenyl hydantoin in the treatment of convulsive disorders. *Journal of the American Medical Association*, 111:1068–1073.

Meyer, J. S. & Gotoh, F. (1960). Metabolic and electroencephalographic effects of hyperventilation. *AMA Archives of Neurology*, 3:539–552.

Meyer, J. S., Hata, T., & Imai, A. (1987). Evidence supporting a vascular pathogenesis of migraine and cluster headache. In Blau, J. N. (ed.), *Migraine*. Baltimore: Johns Hopkins University Press.

Meyer, J. S. & Waltz, A. G. (1961). Relationship of cerebral anoxia to functional electroencephalographic abnormality. In Gasteau, H. & Meyer, J. S. (eds.), *Cerebral Anoxia and the Electroencephalograph*. Springfield: Charles C Thomas.

Meyer, J. U., Lindbom, L., & Intaglietta, M. (1987). Coordinated diameter oscillations at the arteriolar bifurcations in skeletal muscle. *American Journal of Physiology*, 253:H568–573.

Meyers, F. H., Jawetz, E., & Goldfien, A. (1978). *Review of Medical Pharmacology*, 6th ed. Los Altos, California: Lange Medical Publications.

Meyers, R. E. (1979). A unitary theory of causation of anoxic and hypoxic brain pathology. In Fahn et al. (eds.), *Advances in Neurology*, vol. 26. New York: Raven Press.

Michael, M. I. & Williams, J. M. (1962). Migraine in children. *Journal of Pediatrics*, 41: 18–24.

Milic-Emili, J. (1982). Recent advances in clinical assessment of control of breathing. *Lung*, 160:1–17.

Miller, D., Waters, D. D., Warnica, W., Szlachcic, J., Kreeft, J., & Theroux, P. (1981). Is variant angina the coronary manifestation of a generalized vasospastic disorder? *New England Journal of Medicine*, 13:763–766.

Miller, N. E. (1989). Biomedical foundations of biofeedback as a part of behavioral medicine. In Basmajian, J. V. (ed.), *Biofeedback: Principles and Practice for Clinicians*, 3d ed. Baltimore: Williams & Wilkins.

Millon, T. (1987). *MCMI—II*, 2nd ed. Minneapolis, National Computer Systems.

Missri, J. C. & Alexander, S. (1978). Hyperventilation syndrome: A brief review. *Journal of the American Medical Association*, 240:2093–2096.

Morgan, J., Baidevan, B., Petty, T. L., & Zwillich, C. W. (1979). The effect of unanesthetized arterial puncture on PCO_2 and pH. *American Review of Respiratory Diseases*, 120:795–796.

Morrice, J. K. W. (1956). Slow wave production in the EEG with reference to hyperpnea, carbon dioxide, and autonomic balance. *EEG and Clinical Neurophysiology*, 8:49–72.

Morris, J. F. (1976). Spirometry in the evaluation of pulmonary function. *Western Journal of Medicine*, 125:110–118.

Morris, W. (ed.). (1980). *The American Heritage Dictionary of the English Language*. New York: Houghton Mifflin.

Morse, D. R., Martin, J. S., Furst, M. L., & Dubin, L. L. (1977). A physiological and subjective evaluation of meditation, hypnosis, and relaxation. *Psychosomatic Medicine*, 39:304–324.

Moss, I. R. & Friedman, E. (1978). β-endorphin: Effects on respiratory regulation. *Life Sciences*, 23:1272–1276.

Moss, I. R. & Scarpelli, E. M. (1981). To the editor. *New England Journal of Medicine*, 305:959.

Mostofsky, D. I. (1981). Recurrent paroxysmal disorders of the central nervous system. In Turner, S. M., Calhoun, K. S., & Adams, H. E. (eds.), *Handbook of Clinical Behavior Therapy*. New York: Wiley.

Mostofsky, D. I. & Balaschak, B. A. (1977). Psychobiological control of seizures. *Psychological Bulletin*, 84:723–750.

Mustchin, C. P., Gribbin, H. R., Tattersfield, A. E., & George, C. F. (1976). Reduced respiratory response to carbon dioxide after propranolol: A central action? *British Medical Journal*, 2:1229–1231.

Naifeh, K .H., Kamyia, J., & Sweet, M. (1982). Biofeedback of alveolar carbon dioxide tension and level of arousal. *Biofeedback and Self-Regulation*, 7:283–300.

Nakamura, T. (1981). *Oriental Breathing Therapy*. Tokyo: Japan Publications.

Neill, W. A. & Hattenhauer, M. (1975). Impairment of myocardial O_2 supply due to hyperventilation. *Circulation*, 52:854–858.

Ngai, S. H. & Wang, S. C. (1957). Organization of respiratory mechanisms in the brain stem of the cat: Localization by stimulation. *American Journal of Physiology*, 190:343–349.

Nicoli, P. A. & Webb, R. L. (1955). Vascular patterns and active vasomotion as determinants of flow through minute vessels. *Angiology*, 6:291–308.

Nilsson, B., Rehncrona, S. & Siesjo, B. K. (1978). Coupling of cerebral metabolism and blood flow in epileptic seizures, hypoxia and hypoglycemia. See Purves.

Nishizawa, Y., Olsen, T. S., Larsen, B., & Lassen, N. A. (1982). Left-right cortical asymmetries of regional cerebral blood flow during listening of word. *Journal of Neurophysiology*, 48:458–466.

Nixon, P. G. F. (1989). Hyperventilation and cardiac symptoms. *Internal Medicine for the Specialist*, 10:67–84.

Nixon, P. G. F. (1986). Exhaustion: Cardiac rehabilitation's starting point. In Maes, S., Speilberger, C. D., Defares, P. B., & Sarason, I. G. (eds), *Topics in Health Psychology*. New York: John Wiley & Sons, pp. 129–139.

Nixon, P. G. F. & Freeman, L. J. (1988). The "Think" test: A further technique to elicit hyperventilation. *Journal of the Royal Society of Medicine*, 81:277–279.

Noyes, R., Kathol, R., Clancy, J., & Crowe, R. W. (1981). Antianxiety effects of propranolol: A review of clinical studies. In Klein, D. F. & Rabkin, J. (eds.), *Anxiety: New Research and Changing Concepts*. New York: Raven Press.

Okel, B. B. & Hurst, J. W. (1961). Prolonged hyperventilation in man. *Archives of Internal Medicine*, 108:757–762.

Olsten, A. B. (1902). *Mind Powers and Privileges*. New York: Crowell.

Orme-Johnson, D. & Farrows, J. (eds.). (1977). *Scientific Research on the Transcendental Meditation Program*, vol. 1. Los Altos, California: Maharishi European Research Press.

Ornstein, R. E. (1972). *The Psychology of Consciousness*. San Francisco: Freeman.

Oski, F. A., Gottlieb, A. J., Miller, W. W., & Delivoria-Papadopoulos, M. (1970). The effects of deoxygenation of adult and fetal red cell 2,3-diphosphoglycerate and its in vivo consequences. *Journal of Clinical Investigation*, 49:400–407.

Otis, A. B. (1964). Quantitative relationships in steady-state gas exchange. See Fenn & Rahn.

Ottenberg, P. & Stein, M. (1958). Role of odors in asthma. *Psychosomatic Medicine*, 20:60.

Owman, C. & Edvinsson, L. (1978). Cited in Purves, J. J. (ed.), *Cerebral Vascular Smooth Muscle and Its Control*. Amsterdam: Elsevier.

Ozaki, T. & Konda, Y. (1968). On the application of the interval histogram for the analysis of the microvibration (MV). *Journal of the Physiological Society of Japan*, 30:353–354.

Pain, M. C. F., Biddle, N., & Tiller, J. W. G. (1988). Panic disorder, the ventilatory response to carbon dioxide and respiratory variables. *Psychosomatic Medicine*, 50:541–548.

Papp, L. A., Goetz, R., Cole, R., Klein, D. F., Jordan, F., Liebowitz, M. R., Fyer, A. J., Hollander, E., & Gorman, J. (1989). Hypersensitivity to carbon dioxide in panic disorder. *American Journal of Psychiatry*, 146:779–781.

Parade, G. W. (1966). Herzkranke, Die es nicht sind. *Munchner Medizinischer Wochenschrift*, 108:1385–1392.

Park, R. & Arief, A.I. (1980). Lactic acidosis. *Advances in Internal Medicine*, 25:33.

Patel, C. (1973). Yoga and biofeedback in the management of hypertension. *Lancet*, 2:1035–1055.

Patel, C. (1975a). 12-month follow-up of yoga and biofeedback in the management of hypertension. *Lancet*, 1:62–64.

Patel, C. (1975b). Randomized controlled trial of yoga and biofeedback in management of hypertension. *Lancet*, 2:93–95.

Patterson, A. S. (1933). The depth and rate of respiration in normal and psychotic subjects. *Journal of Neurology and Psychopathology*, 14:323–331.

Pavlov I. P. (1927). *Conditioned Reflexes*. New York: Oxford University Press.

Pavlov, I. P. (1928). *Lectures on Conditioned Reflexes*, vol. 1. New York: International Publishers.

Pelletier, K. R. (1977). *Mind as Healer, Mind as Slayer*. New York: Dell (Delta Books).

Pelletier, K. R. (1978). *Toward a Science of Consciousness*. New York: Dell (Delta Books).

Penfield, W. (1933). The evidence for a cerebral vascular mechanism in epilepsy. *Annals of Internal Medicine*, 7:303–310.

Penfield, W. (1939). The epilepsies: With a note on radical therapy. *New England Journal of Medicine*, 221:209–218.

Penfield, W. & Jasper, H. (1954). *Epilepsy and the Functional Anatomy of the Brain*. Boston: Little, Brown.

Peniston, E. G. & Kulkosky, P. J. (1989). Brain wave training and endorphin levels in alcoholics. *Alcoholism: Clinical and Experimental Research*, 13:271–279.

Peper, E. (1985). Hope for asthmatics. Biofeedback systems teaching: The combination of self-regulation strategies and family therapy in the self-healing of asthma. *Somatics*. 2: 56–62.

Peper, E. (1988). Strategies to reduce the effort of breathing: Electromyographic and in-spirometry biofeedback. In von Euler, C. & Katz-Salamon, M. (eds.), *Respiratory Psychophysiology*. London: The Macmillan Press, pp. 113–122.

Peper, E. & Crane-Gochley, V. (1990). Toward effortless breathing. *Medical Psychotherapy*, 3:135–140.

Peper E., Klomp, K., & Levy, J. (1983). Breath and symptoms: Gasping, diaphragmatic breathing and EMG feedback. *Proceedings of the 14th Annual Meeting of the Biofeedback Society of America*. Wheat Ridge, Colorado, pp. 172–175.

Peper, E., Smith, K., & Waddell, D. (1987). Voluntary wheezing versus diaphragmatic breathing with inhalation (Voldyne) feedback: A clinical intervention in the treatment of asthma. *Clinical Biofeedback and Health*, 10:83–88.

Peper, E. & Tibbets, V. (in press). 15 month follow up with asthmatics utilizing EMG/incentive inspirometer feedback. *Biofeedback and Self-Regulation*.

Peper, E., Waddell, D., & Smith, K. (1987). EMG and incentive inspirometer (Voldyne) feedback to reduce symptoms in asthma. *Proceedings of the 18th Annual Meeting of the Biofeedback Society of America*. Wheat Ridge, Colorado, pp. 75–78.

Perez-Borja, C. & Meyer, J. S. (1964). A critical evaluation of rheoencephalography in control subjects and in proven cases of cerebrovascular disease. *Journal of Neurology, Neurosurgery and Psychiatry*, 26:66–72.

Phillipson, E. A. & Sullivan, C. E. (1978). Editorial, Arousal: The forgotten response to stimuli. *American Review of Respiratory Diseases*, 118:807–809.

Piggott, L. R., Ax, A. F., Bamford, J. L., & Fetzner, J. M. (1973). Respiratory sinus arrhythmia in psychotic children. *Psychophysiology*, 10:401–414.

Pilsbury, D. & Hibbert, G. (1987). An ambulatory system for long-term continuous monitoring of transcutaneous PCO_2. *European Journal of Physiopathology of Respiration*, 23: 9–13.

Pinciroli, F., Rossi, R., Vergani, L., Carnevali, P., Mantero, S., & Parigi, O. (1986). Remark and experiments on the construction of respiratory waveforms from electrocardiographic tracings. *Computers and Biomedical Research*, 19:391–409.

Pincus, J. H. (1978). Disorders of conscious awareness: Hyperventilation syndrome. *British Journal of Hospital Medicine*, 19:312.

Pincus, J. H. & Tucker, G. J. (1974). *Behavioral Neurology*. New York: Oxford University Press.

Pitts, F. N. (1984). Lactate, beta-antagonists, beta-blockers, and anxiety. *Journal of Clinical Psychiatry Monograph*, 2:25–39.

Pitts, F. N. & McClure, J. N. (1967). Lactate metabolism in anxiety neurosis. *New England Journal of Medicine*, 277:1329–1336.

Pitts, R. F. (1939). The origin of respiratory rhythmicity. *American Journal of Physiology*, 127:654–660.

Pitts, R. F. (1946). Organization of the respiratory center. *Physiological Review*, 26:609–630.

Pitts, R. F. (1949). Organization of the neural mechanisms responsible for rhythmic respiration. In Fulton, J. F. (ed.) *Textbook of Physiology*. Philadelphia: W. B. Saunders.

Pitts, R. F., Magoun, H. W., & Ranson, S. W. (1939). Inter-relations of the respiratory centers in the cat. *American Journal of Physiology*, 126:689–707.

Poincare, H. (1954). *Oeuvres I.* Paris: Gautier-Villar.

Pollock, G. H. (1949). Central inhibitory effects of carbon dioxide. *Journal of Neurophysiology*, 12:315–324.

Pollock, L., McDonald, K. E., Kjartansson, K. B., Delin, N. A., & Schenck, W. G. (1964). Influence of hyperventilation, cardiac output, and renal blood flow. *Surgery*, i55:299.

Pollock, V. E., Volavka, J., Goodwin, D. W., Mednick, S. A., Gabrielli, W. F., Knop, J., & Schulsinger, F. (1983). The EEG after alcohol administration in men at risk for alcoholism. *Archives of General Psychiatry*, 40:857–861.

Porges, S. W., McCabe, P. M., & Yongue, B. G. (1982). Respiratory-heart rate interactions: Psychophysiology—Implications for pathophysiology and behavior. See Cacioppo & Petty.

Prohovnik, I. & Risberg, J. (1979). Inter- and intra-hemispheric functional relationships in resting normal subjects. *Acta Neurologica Scandinavica*, Suppl. 60:26–27.

Purcell, K., Bernstein, L., & Bukantz, S. C. (1961). A preliminary comparison of rapidly remitting and persistently "steroid dependent" asthmatic children. *Psychosomatic Medicine*, 23:305.

Purves, M. J. (ed.). (1978). *Cerebral Vascular Smooth Muscle and Its Control.* Amsterdam: Elsevier—Excerpta Medica—North Holland.

Qui, R. J., Hutt, S. J., & Forrest, S. (1979). Sensorimotor rhythm feedback training and epilepsy: Some methodological and conceptual issues. *Biological Psychology*, 9:129–149.

Radford, E. P. Jr. (1955). Ventilation standards for use in artificial respiration. *Journal of Applied Physiology*, 7:451–460.

Rafferty, G. F., Saisch, S. G. N., & Gardner, W. N. (1992). Relation of hypocapnic symptoms to rate of fall of end-tidal PCO_2 in normal subjects. *Respiratory Medicine*, 86:355–340.

Raichle, M. E. & Plum, F. (1972). Hyperventilation and cerebral blood flow. *Stroke*, 3:566–575.

Raichle, M. E., Posner, J. B., & Plum, F. (1970) Cerebral blood flow during and after hyperventilation. *Archives of Neurology*, 23:394–403.

Rama, S., Ballentine, R., & Hymes, A. (1979). *Science of Breath: A Practical Guide.* Honesdale, PA: Himalayan Institute.

Ramacharaka, Y. (1905). *Science of Breath.* Chicago: Yogi Publications.

Rampil, I. J. (1984). Fast Fourier transformation of EEG data. *Journal of the American Medical Association*, 251:601.

Rapee, R. (1986). Differential response to hyperventilation in panic disorder and generalized anxiety disorder. *Journal of Abnormal Psychology*, 95:24–28.

Rapoport, S. I. (1978). *Osmotic Opening of the Blood-Brain Barrier.* See M. Y. Purves.

Rapoport, S., Stevens, C.D., Engel, G. L., Ferris, E. B., & Logan, M. (1946). The effect of voluntary overbreathing on the electrolyte equilibrium of arterial blood in man. *Journal of Biological Chemistry*, 163:411–427.

Rasmussen, K., Jull, S., Bagger, J. P., & Henningsen, P. (1987). Usefulness of ST deviation induced by hyperventilation as a predictor of cardiac death in angina pectoris. *American Journal of Cardiology*, 59:763–768.

Read, D. J. C. (1967). A clinical method of assessing the ventilatory response to carbon dioxide. *Australian Annals of Medicine*, 16:20–32.

Rebuck, A. S., Kangalee, M., Pengelly, L. D., & Campbell, E. J. M. (1973). Correlation of ventilatory response to hypoxia and hypercapnia. *Journal of Applied Physiology*, 35:173–177.

Reiman, E. M., Raichle, M. E., Butler, F. K., Herscovitch, P., & Robbins, E. (1984). A focal brain abnormality in panic disorder, a severe form of epilepsy. *Nature*, 310:683–685.

Relman, A. S., Etsten, B., & Schwartz, W.B. (1953). The regulation of renal reabsorption by plasma carbon dioxide tension. *Journal of Clinical Investigation*, 32:972–978.

Rice, R. L. (1950). Symptom patterns of hyperventilation syndrome. *American Journal of Medicine*, 8:691–700.

Richardson, D. W., Wasserman, A. J., & Patterson, J. L., Jr. (1961). General and regional circulatory response to change in blood pH and carbon dioxide. *Journal of Clinical Investigation*, 40:31.

Richter-Heinrich, E., Homuth, V., Heirichk, B., Schmidt, K. H., Wiedemann, R., & Gohlke, H. R. (1981). Long-term application of behavioral treatments in essential hyperventilation. *Physiology of Behavior*, 26:915–920.

Riley, T. L. (1982). Epilepsy—or merely hyperventilation? *Emergency Medicine*, 14:162–167.

Robinson, L. J. (1944). Electroencephalographic study during epileptic seizure related to hyperventilation. *Diseases of the Nervous System*, 5:87.

Rockoff, S. D., Doppman, J., Kreuger, T. P., Thomas, L. J., & Ommaya, A. K. (1966). Altered opacification of the external carotid circulation by changes of end-tidal expiratory carbon dioxide tension: An angiographic study in man. *Investigative Radiology*, 1: 123–129.

Roddie, I. C., Sheperd, J. T., & Whelan, R. F. (1957). Humoral vasodilation in the forearm during voluntary hyperventilation. *Journal of Physiology*, 137:80–85.

Rohracher, H. & Inanaga, K. (1969). *Die Mikrovibration*. Bern: Hans Huber.

Roland, M. & Peper, E. (1987): Inhalation volume changes with inspirometer feedback and diaphragmatic breathing coaching. *Clinical Biofeedback and Health*, 10:89–97.

Romer, G. A. (1931). *Atmung als ausdruckssymptom und als aetiologischer Faktor by psychischen zustandsbildern*. Berichte uber d: VI. Allgem arztlichen Kongress f Psychother Leipzig: Kretschmer und Cimbal, pp. 18–28.

Rosen, S. D., King, J. C., Wilkinson, J. B., & Nixon, P. G. F. (1990). Is chronic fatigue syndrome synonymous with effort syndrome. *Journal of the Royal Society of Medicine*, 83: 761–764.

Rosenbaum, J. F. (1982). The drug treatment of anxiety. *New England Journal of Medicine*, 306:401–404.

Rosenthal, J. S., Strauss, A., Minkoff, L. A., & Winston, A. (1985). Variations in red blood cell proton T1 relaxation times that correspond to menstrual cycle changes. *American Journal of Obstetrics and Gynecology*, 153:812–813.

Rosenthal, T. B. (1948). The effect of temperature on the pH of blood and plasma in vitro. *Journal of Biological Chemistry*, 173:25–30.

Rosett, J. (1924). The experimental production of rigidity, of abnormal involuntary movements and of abnormal states of consciousness in man. *Brain*, 47:293–336.

Rosser, R. & Guz, A. (1981). Psychological approaches to breathlessness and its treatment. *Journal of Psychosomatic Research*, 25:439–447.

Roughton, F. J. W. (1964). *Transport of Oxygen and Carbon Dioxide*. See Fenn & Rahn.

Royer, F. L. (1965). Cutaneous vasomotor component of the orienting reflex. *Behavior Research and Therapy*, 3:161–170.

Rubin, M. A. & Turner, E. (1942). Blood sugar level and influence of hyperventilation on slow activity in electroencephalogram. *Proceedings for the Society for Experimental Medicine and Biology*, 50:270–272.

Rubin, R. T. (1984). Neuroendocrine aspects. *Psychosomatic Medicine*, suppl. 225:21–26.

Ruch, T. C. & Fulton, J. F. (1961). *Medical Physiology and Biophysics*. Philadelphia: W. B. Saunders.

Rushmer, R. F. (1961). *Cardiovascular Dynamics*. Philadelphia: W. B. Saunders.

Sackner, J. D., Broudy, M. J., Davis, B., Cohn, M. A., & Sackner, M. A. (1979). *Ventilation at Rest and during Exercise Measured without Physical Connection to the Airway.* Presented at the 3rd International Symposium on Ambulatory Monitoring, Harrow, Middlesex, U. K.

Sackner, J. D., Nixon, A. S., Davis, B., Atkins, N., & Sackner, M. A. (1980). Effects of breathing through dead space on ventilation at rest and during exercise. *American Review of Respiratory Disease,* 122:933–940.

Sackner, M. A. (1980). Monitoring ventilation without a physical connection to the airway. In Sackner, M. A. (ed.) *Diagnostic techniques in pulmonary disease,* part I. New York: Marcel Dekker.

Salkovskis, P. M., Clark, D. M., & Chalkley, J. (1983). The use of respiratory control in the behavioral treatment of panic attacks. *Biological Psychology,* 16:285–297.

Salkovskis, P. M., Jones, D. R. O., & Clark, D. M. (1985). Respiratory control in the treatment of panic attacks: Replication and extension with concurrent measurement of behavior and pCO_2. *British Journal of Psychiatry,* 148:526–532.

Salkovskis, P. N., Warwick, M. C., Clark, D. M., & Wessel, D. J. (1986). A demonstration of acute hyperventilation during naturally occurring panic attack. *Behavior Research and Therapy,* 24:91–94.

Salter, A. (1961). *Conditioned Reflex Therapy.* New York: Capricorn Books.

Saltzman, H. A., Heyman, A., & Sieker, H. O. (1963). Correlation of clinical and physiologic manifestations of sustained hyperventilation. *New England Journal of Medicine,* 268:1431–1436.

Samet, J. M. (1978). Review and commentary—A historical and epidemiological perspective on respiratory symptoms questionnaires. *American Journal of Epidemiology,* 108:435–446.

Samuel, J. R., Grange, R. A., & Hawkins, T. D. (1968). Anaesthetic technique for carotid angiography, *Anaesthesia,* 23:543–551.

Sanderson, W. C. & Wetzler, S. (1990). Five percent carbon dioxide challenge: Valid analogue and marker of panic disorder? *Biological Psychiatry,* 27:689–701.

Sandman, C. A., O'Halloran, J. P., & Isenhart, R. (1984). Is there an evoked vascular response? *Science,* 224:1355–1357.

Saunders, N. A., Heilpern, S., & Rebuck, A. S. (1972). Relation between personality and ventilatory response to carbon dioxide in normal subjects: A role in asthma. *British Medical Journal,* 1:719–721.

Sayers, B. M. (1973). Analysis of heart rate variability. *Ergonomics,* 16:17–32.

Schachter, S. & Singer, J. E. (1962). Cognitive, social and physiological determinants of emotional state. *Psychology Review,* 69:379–399.

Schafmeister, A., Richter, R., Andersen, B., & Thom, E. (1983). Methodological study to predict the spirometric volume curve and parameters of the breathing cycle from thoracic and abdominal girth changes. Paper presented at the 2nd International Symposium on Respiratory Psychophysiology. Abstract in *Biological Psychology,* 16:285–297.

Schalling, D., Asberg, M., Edman, G., & Orland, L. (1987). Markers for vulnerability to psychopathology: Temperament traits associated with platelet MAO activity. *Acta Psychiatrica Scandinavica,* 767:172–182.

Schlossberg, L., & Zuidema, G. D. (1986). *The Johns Hopkins Atlas of Human Functional Anatomy,* 3rd ed. Baltimore: The Johns Hopkins University Press.

Schmidt, C. F. (1966). The influence of cerebral blood flow on respiration: I. The respiratory response to changes in cerebral blood flow. *American Journal of Physiology,* 84:202–222.

Schmidt, C. F. (1934). The intrinsic regulation of the circulation in the hypothalamus of the cat. *American Journal of Physiology,* 10:572–585.

Schmidt, C. F. & Hendrix, J. P. (1938). *The Action of Chemical Substances on the Cerebral Blood Vessels.* See Cobb, Frantz, Penfield, & Riley.

Schneider, J. (1961). Urinary excretion of electrolytes in centrencephalic epileptics. *Epilepsia*, 2:358–366.

Schwab, R. S., Grunwald, A., & Sargant, W. W. (1941). Regulation of the treatment of epilepsy by synchronized recording of respiration and brain waves. *Archives of Neurology and Psychiatry*, 46:1017–1034.

Schwartz, G. E. & Beatty, J. (1977). *Biofeedback Theory and Research*. New York: Academic Press.

Schwartz, M. (1987). *Biofeedback*. New York: Guilford Press.

Seelig, M. S. (1980). *Magnesium Deficiency in the Pathogenesis of Disease*. New York: Plenum.

Selby, G. & Lance, J. W. (1960). Observations on 500 cases of migraine and allied vascular headache. *Journal of Neurosurgery and Psychiatry*, 23:23–32.

Servit, Z., Kristof, M., & Strejckova, A. (1981). Activating effect of nasal and oral hyperventilation on epileptic electrographic phenomena: Reflex mechanisms of nasal origin. *Epilepsia*, 22:321–329.

Severinghaus, J. W. & Lassen, N. (1967). Step hypocapnia to separate arterial from tissue PCO_2 in the regulation of cerebral blood flow. *Circulation Research*, 20:272–279.

Shader, R. I., Goodman, M., & Gever, J. (1982). Panic disorders: Current perspectives. *Journal of Clinical Psychopharmacology*, 25:105.

Shapiro, B. A., Harrison, R. A., & Walton, J. R. (1982). *Clinical Application of Blood Gases* 3d ed. Chicago: Year Book Medical Publishers.

Shapiro, D. H. (1982). Overview: Clinical and physiological comparison of meditation with other self-regulation control strategies. *American Journal of Psychiatry*, 139:267–274.

Shapiro, D. H. (1985): Clinical use of meditation as a self-regulation strategy: Comments on Holmes' conclusions and implications. *American Psychologist*, 40:719–720.

Sheehan, D. V. (1982). Panic attacks and phobias. *New England Journal of Medicine*, 307:156–158.

Shehi, M. & Patterson, W. M. (1984). Treatment of panic attacks with aprazolam and propranolol. *American Journal of Psychiatry*, 141:900–901.

Sheldon, W. H. & Stevens, S. S. (1942). *The Varieties of Temperament*. New York: Harper & Brothers.

Sheppard, M. N., Polak, J. M., & Bloom, S. R. (1984). Neuropeptide tyrosine (NPY): A newly discovered peptide is present in the mammalian respiratory tract. *Thorax*, 39:326–330.

Sherrington, C. S. (1906). *The Integrative Activation of the Nervous System*. New Haven, Connecticut: Yale University Press.

Shershow, J. C., Kanarek, D. J., & Kazemi, H. (1976). Ventilatory response to carbon dioxide inhalation in depression. *Psychosomatic Medicine*, 38:282–287.

Shershow, J. S., King, A., & Robinson, S. (1973). Carbon dioxide sensitivity and personality. *Psychosomatic Medicine*, 35:155–160.

Shim, C. & Williams, M. N. (1986). Effect of odors in asthma. *The American Journal of Medicine*, 18–22.

Siesjo, B. K., Berntman, L., & Rehncrona, S. (1979). Effects of hypoxia on blood flow and metabolic flux in the brain. In Fahn, S. (ed.), *Advances in neurology* (vol. 26). New York: Raven Press.

Sietsema, K. E., Simon, J. I., & Wasserman, K. (1987). Pulmonary hypertension presenting as panic disorder. *Chest*, 91:910–912.

Sinclair, J. D. (1978). Exercise in pulmonary disease. In *Therapeutic Exercises*. See Basmajian (1978).

Singer, E. P. (1958). The hyperventilation syndrome in clinical medicine. *New York State Journal of Medicine*, 1:1494.

Singh, B. S. (1984a). Ventilatory response to CO_2: I. A psychologic marker of the respiratory system. *Psychosomatic Medicine*, 46:333–345.

Singh, B. S. (1984b). Ventilatory response to CO_2: II. Studies in neurotic psychiatric patients and practitioners of transcendental meditation. *Psychomatic Medicine*, 46:374–362.

Skarbek, A. (1970). A psychophysiological study of breathing behavior. *British Journal of Psychiatry*, 116:637.

Slaaf, D. W., Huub, H. E. O. V., Tangelder, G. J., & Reneman, R. S. (1988). Effective diameter as a determinant of local vascular resistance in presence of vasomotion. *American Journal of Physiology*, 255:H1240–1243.

Smith, A. T., Jukes, H. M., & Timmons, G. H. (1983). Data processing of respiratory activity from a vest pneumograph. *Biological Psychology*, 16:285–297.

Smyth, V. O. G. & Winter, A. L. (1964). The EEG in migraine. *EEG Clinical Neurophysiology*, 16:194–202.

Sobotta, J. & McMurrich, J. P. (1933). *Atlas of Human Anatomy*. New York: G. E. Stechert & Co.

Sodeman, W. A. & Sodeman, T. M. (1979). *Pathologic Physiology*. Philadelphia: W. B. Saunders.

Soderstrom, N. (1950). Clonic spasm of the diaphragm. Observations in three cases with special attention to the ECG findings. *Acta Medica Scandinavica*, 137:28–36.

Sokoloff, L. (1978). *Local Cerebral Energy Metabolism: Its Relationship to Local Functional Activity and Blood Flow*. See Purves.

Sokoloff, L., Mangold, R., Wechsler, R. L., Kennedy, S. S., & Kety, S. S. (1955). The effect of mental arithmetic on cerebral circulation and metabolism. *Journal of Clinical Investigation*, 34:1101–1108.

Soley, M. H. & Shock, N. W. (1938). The etiology of effort syndrome. *American Journal of Medical Science*, 196:840.

Sorenson, R. W. (1971). The chemical control of ventilation. *Acta Physiologica Scandinavia*, suppl. 361.

Spitzer, R. L. (ed.). (1981). DSM III—Casebook, 3d ed. Washington, D. C. American Psychological Association.

Sroufe, L. A. (1971). Effects of depth and rate of breathing on heart rate and heart rate variability. *Psychophysiology*, 8:648–655.

Stead, E. A. & Warren, J. V. (1943). The clinical significance of hyperventilation: The role of hyperventilation in the production, diagnosis, and treatment of certain anxiety symptoms. *American Journal of Medical Science*, 206:183–190.

Stefan, H., Bauer, J., Feistel, H., Schulemann, B., Neubauer, U., Wenzel, B., Wolf, F., Neundorfer, B., & Huk, W. J. (1990). Regional cerebral blood flow during total seizures of temporal and frontocentral onset. *Annals of Neurology*, 27:162–166.

Stein, J. H. (1983). *Internal Medicine*. Boston: Little Brown & Co.

Sterman, M. B. (1973). Neurophysiologic and clinical studies of sensorimotor biofeedback training: Some effects on epilepsy. In *Biofeedback: Behavioral Medicine*. See Birk (1973).

Sterman, M. B. (1977a). Effects of sensorimotor EEG feedback training on sleep and clinical manifestations of epilepsy. In Beatty, J. & Legewie, E. (eds.), *Biofeedback and Behavior*. New York: Plenum.

Sterman, M. B. (1977b). Clinical implications of EEG biofeedback training: A critical appraisal. In *Biofeedback Theory and Research*. See Schwartz & Beatty (1977).

Sterman, M. B. (1981a). EEG Biofeedback: Physiological behavior modification. *Neuroscience Biobehavior Review*, 5:405–412.

Sterman, M. B. (1981b). Power spectral analysis of EEG characteristics during sleep in epileptics. *Epilepsia*, 22:95–106.

Sterman, M. B. & Friar, L. (1972). Suppression of seizures in an epileptic following sensorimotor EEG feedback training. *EEG Clinical Neurophysiology*, 33:89–95.

Sterman, M. B., MacDonald, L. R., & Bernstein, I. (1977). Quantitative analysis of EEG sleep spindle activity in epileptic and non-epileptic subjects. *EEG Clinical Neurophysiology*, 42:724.

Stewart, R. S., Devous, M. D., & Rush, A. J. (1988). Cerebral blood flow changes during sodium-lactate-induced panic attacks. *American Journal of Psychiatry*, 145:442–449.

Stone, R. A. & DeLeo, J. (1976). Psychotherapeutic control of hypertension. *New England Journal of Medicine*, 294:80–84.

Strauss, H. & Selinsky, H. (1941). Electroencephalographic changes in patients with migrainous syndrome. *Transactions of the American Neurological Association*, 67:205–208.

Stroebel, C. F. (1982). *QR, The Quieting Reflex*. New York: Putnam.

Stroebel, C. F. & Glueck, B. (1977). Passive meditation: Subjective and clinical comparison with biofeedback. In Schwartz, G. & Shapiro, D. (eds.), *Consciousness and Self-Regulation*. New York: Plenum.

Suess, W. M., Alexander, A. B., Smith, D. D., Sweeney, H. W., & Marion, R. J. (1980). The effect of psychological stress on respiration: A preliminary study of anxiety on hyperventilation. *Psychophysiology*, 17:535–540.

Suler, J. R. (1985): Meditation and somatic arousal: A comment on Holmes' review. *American Psychologist*, 40:717.

Surwit, R. S. & Keefe, F. G. (1983). The blind leading the blind: Problems with "double-blind" design in clinical biofeedback research. *Biofeedback and Self-Regulation*, 8:1–2.

Surwit, R. S., Shapiro, D., & Feld, J. (1976). Digital temperature autoregulation and associated cardiovascular changes. *Psychophysiology*, 13:242–248.

Sutherland, G. F., Wolf, A., & Kennedy, F. (1938). The respiratory "fingerprints" of nervous states. *Medical Record*, 148:101–103.

Suthers, G. K., Henderson-Smart, D. J., & Read, D. J. C. (1977). Postnatal changes in the rate of high frequency bursts of inspiratory activity in cats and dogs. *Brain Research*, 132: 340–357.

Swanson, A. G., Stavney, L. S., & Plum, F. (1958). Effects of blood pH and carbon dioxide on cerebral electrical activity. *Neurology*, 8:787–792.

Szekely, G. (1965). Logical network for controlling limb movements in Urodela. *Acta Physiologica Hungarica*, 27:285–289.

Tachibana, S. (1966). Local temperature, blood flow, and electrical activity correlation in the posterior hypothalamus of the cat. *Experientia Neurologica*, 16:148–161.

Tachibana, S., Kuramoto, S., Inanaga, K., & Ikemi, Y. (1967). Local cerebrovascular responses in man. *Confina Neurologica*, 29:289–298.

Tamura, M., Itakura, K., Sayama, T., Murakami, T., & Suzuki, Y. (1983). Ventilatory response to CO_2 in bronchial asthma and chronic obstructive lung disease. *Japanese Journal of Medicine*, 22:190–194.

Tang, P. C. (1953). Localization of the pneumotaxic center in the cat. *American Journal of Physiology*, 172:645–652.

Tarlau, M. (1958). EEG changes in neurogenic chronic respiratory acidosis. *EEG Clinical Neurophysiology* 10:724–729.

Taub, E. & Emurian, C. S. (1976). Feedback-aided self-regulation of skin temperature with a single feedback locus. *Biofeedback and Self-Regulation*, 1:147–167.

Tharp, B. R., & Gersch, W. (1975). Spectral analysis of seizures in humans. *Computers and Biomedical Research*, 8:503–521.

Thayer, R. E. (1989). *The Biopsychology of Mood and Arousal*. New York: Oxford University Press.

Thompson, J. W. & Corwin, W. (1942). Correlation between patterns of breathing and personality manifestations. *Archives of Neurological Psychiatry*, 47:265–270.

Thompson, J. W., Corwin, W., & Aster-Salazar, J. H. (1937). Physiological patterns and mental disturbances. *Nature*, 140:1062–1063.

Thompson, W. P. (1943). The electrocardiogram in the hyperventilation syndrome. *American Heart Journal*, 25:372–390.

Tibbetts, V. & Peper, E. (1988). Incentive inspirometer feedback for desensitization with asthmatic provoking triggers: A clinical protocol. *Proceedings of the 19th Annual Meeting of the Biofeedback Society of America*. Wheat Ridge, Colorado, pp. 200–203.

Timmons, B. H. (1982). Breathing pattern measurements and monitoring: State of the art. *Journal of Medical Engineering and Technology*, 6:112–116.

Timmons, G., Salamy, J., Kamyia, J., & Girton, D. (1972). Abdominal-thoracic respiratory movements and level of arousal. *Psychonomic Science*, 27:173–175.

Tirala, L. G. (ca. 1935). *The Cure of High Blood Pressure by Respiratory Exercises*. New York: Westermann.

Tobin, M. J. (1990). Dyspnea: Pathophysiologic Basis, clinical presentation, and management. *Archives of Internal Medicine*, 150:1604–1613.

Tobin, M. J., Chadha, T. S., Jenouri, G., Birch, S. J., Hacik, B., Gazeroglu, H. B., & Sackner, M. A. (1983). Breathing patterns: 1. Normal subjects. *Chest*, 84:202–205.

Tohei, K. (1976). *Book of Ki: Co-ordinating Mind and Body*. Tokyo: Japan Publications.

Tortora, G. J. & Anagnostakos, H. P. (1984). *Principles of Anatomy and Physiology*, 4th ed. Cambridge: Harper & Row.

Toshikatsu, I. & Kazuya, A. (1980). Hyperventilation syndrome and beta receptor function— Clinical effects of beta blocker upon the syndrome. *Japan Journal of Psychosomatic Medicine*, 20:424–428.

Tower, D. B. (1960). *Neurochemistry of Epilepsy*. Springfield, Illinois: Charles C Thomas.

Towle, P. A. (1965). The electroencephalographic hyperventilation response in migraine. *EEG and Clinical Neurophysiology*, 19:390–393.

Townsend, H. R. A. (1966). The EEG in migraine. In Townsend, H. R. A. (ed.), *Background to Migraine*. New York: Springer-Verlag.

Townsend, R. E., House, J. F., & Addario, D. A. (1975). A comparison of biofeedback-mediated relaxation and group therapy in the treatment of chronic anxiety. *American Journal of Psychiatry*, 132:598–601.

Travis, T. A., Kondon, C. Y., & Knott, J. R. (1976). Heart rate, muscle tension, and alpha production of transcendental meditators and relaxation controls. *Biofeedback and Self-Regulation*, 1:287–294.

Triana, E., Frances, R. J., & Stokes, P. E. (1980). The relationship between endorphins and alcohol-induced subcortical activity. *American Journal of Psychiatry*, 137:491–493.

Tucker, G. J., Price, T. R. P., Johnson, V. B., & McCallister, T. (1986). Phenomenology of temporal lobe dysfunction: A link to atypical psychosis—A series of cases. *Journal of Nervous and Mental Diseases*, 174:348–356.

Upton, A. R. M. & Longmire, D. (1975). The effect of feedback on focal epileptic discharges in man. *Journal of Canadian Science of Neurology*, 3:153–168.

Vander, A. V., Sherman, J. H., & Luciano, D. S. (1975). *Human Physiology*, 2d ed. New York: McGraw-Hill.

van den Hout, M. & Griez, E. (1982). Cardiovascular and subjective responses to inhalation of carbon dioxide. *Psychotherapy and Psychosomatics*, 37:75–82.

van der Mollen, G. M. & van den Hout, M. A. (1988). Expectancy effects on respiration during lactate infusion. *Psychosomatic Medicine*, 50:439–443.

van Dixhoorn, J. & Duivenvoorden, H. J. (1985). Efficacy of Nijmegen questionnaire in recognition of the hyperventilation syndrome. *Journal of Psychosomatic Research*, 29: 199–206.

van Dixhoorn, J. & Duivenvoorden, H. J. (1986). Behavioral characteristics predisposing to hyperventilation complaints: "Emphasis on exhaling" and "time pressure." *Gedrag and Gesondheit*, 13:169–174.

van Doorn, P., Folgering, H., & Colla, P. (1982). Control of the end-tidal PCO_2 in the hyperventilation syndrome: Effects of biofeedback and breathing instructions compared. *Bulletin of European Physiopathology and Respiration*, 18:829–836.

Van Lysbeth, A. (1979). *Pranayama, the Yoga of Breathing*. London: Unwin.

Vasiliev, L. L. (1960). The physiological function of air ions. *American Journal of Physiological Medicine*, 39:124.

Vernon, H. M. (1909). The production of prolonged apnea in man. *Journal of Physiology*, 38: 18–20.

Vlannder-Van Der Giessen, C. J. M. & Janssen, R. H. C. (1983). Breathing instructions in the treatment of patients with hyperventilation. *Journal of Drug Resources*, 8:1888–1890.

Vogel, M. D. (1961). Conditioning and personality factors in alcoholics and normals. *Journal of Abnormal and Social Psychology*, 73:417–421.

Volkow, N. D., Harper, A., & Swann, A. C. (1986). Temporal lobe abnormalities and panick attacks. *American Journal of Psychiatry*, 143:1484–1485.

Volpicelli, J. R., Alterman, A. I., Hayashida, M., & O'Brien, C. P. (1992). Naltrexone in the treatment of alcohol dependence. *Archives of General Psychiatry*, 49:876–880.

Von Santha, K. & Cipriani, A. (1966). Focal alterations in subcortical circulation resulting from stimulation of the cerebral cortex. See Cobb, Frantz, Penfield, & Riley.

Waites, T. F. (1978). Hyperventilation, chronic and acute. *Archives of Internal Medicine*, 138:1700–1701.

Walker, H. E. (1984). Anxiety, panic, and the hyperventilation syndrome. Paper presented at the Annual Meeting of the American Psychiatric Association.

Walker, J. L. & Brown, A. M. (1970). Unified account of the variable effects of carbon dioxide on nerve cells. *Science*, 167:1502–1504.

Wallace, R. K. (1970a). Physiological Effect of Transcendental meditation. *Science*, 167:1751–1754.

Wallace, R. K. (1970b). *The Physiological Effect of Transcendental Meditation*. Los Angeles: Students International Meditation Society.

Wallace, R. K., Benson, H., & Wilson, A. F. (1971). A wakeful hypometabolic physiologic state. *American Journal of Physiology*, 221:795–799.

Waltz, A. G. & Ray, C. D. (1967). Inadequacy of "Rheoencephalography." *Archives of Neurology*, 16:94–102.

Wang, R. I. H. & Sonnenschein, R. E. (1955). pH of cerebral cortex during induced convulsions. *Journal of Neurophysiology*, 18:130–137.

Wang, S. C. & Ngai, S. H. (1964). Organization of central respiratory mechanisms. In *Handbook of Physiology*, Sec. 3: *Respiration*. See Fenn & Rahn.

Wang, S. C., Ngai, S. H., & Frumin, M. J. (1957). Organization of central respiratory mechanisms in the brain stem of the cat: Genesis of normal respiratory rhythmicity. *American Journal of Physiology*, 190:333–342.

Watanabe, T., Shapiro, D., & Schwartz, G. (1972). Meditation as an anoxic state: A critical review and theory. *Psychophysiology*, SPR abstr. 9:279.

Wehner, A. P. (1989). History of air ion research. In Charry, J. M. & Kavet, R. (eds.), *Air Ions: Physical and Biological Aspects*. Boca Raton: CRC Press.

Wei, L. Y. & Chow, P. (1985). Frequency distribution of human pulse spectra. *IEEE Transactions of Biomedical Engineering*, BME 32:245–256.

Weil, A. A. (1962). Observations on "dysrhythmic" migraine. *Journal of Nervous and Mental Diseases*, 134:277–281.

Weilburg, J. B., Bear, D. M., & Sachs, G. (1987). Three patients with concomitant panic attacks and seizure disorder: Possible clues to the neurology of anxiety. *American Journal of Psychiatry*, 144:1053–1056.

Weiner, H. (1977). *Psychobiology and Human Disease*. New York: Elsevier-North Holland.

Weissman, C., Askanazi, J., Milic-Emili, J., & Kinney, J. M. (1984). Effect of respiratory apparatus on respiration. *Journal of Applied Physiology: Respiration, Environment, and Exercise Physiology*, 475–480.

Welch, L. & Kubis, J. (1947a). The effect of anxiety on the conditioning rate and stability of the GSR. *Journal of Psychology*, 23:83–91.

Welch, L. & Kubis, J. (1947b). Conditioned PGR in states of pathological anxiety. *Journal of Nervous and Mental Disorders*, 105:372–381.

Werntz, D. A., Bickford, R. G., Bloom, F. E., & Shannahoff-Khalsa, D. S. (1983). Alternating cerebral hemispheric activity and the lateralization of autonomic nervous function. *Human Neurobiology*, 2:39–43.

Werntz, D. A., Bickford, R. G., & Shannahoff-Khalsa, D. S. (1987). Selective hemispheric stimulation by unilateral forced nostril breathing. *Human Neurobiology*, 6:165–171.

West, M. A. (1979). Physiological effects of meditation: A longitudinal study. *Journal of Social and Clinical Psychology*, 18:219–226.

West, M. A. (1985). Meditation and somatic arousal reduction. *American Psychologist*, 40: 717–719.

Whatmore, G. B. & Kohli, D. R. (1974). *The Physiopathology and Treatment of Functional Disorders*. New York: Grune & Stratton.

Whatmore, G. B. & Kohli, D. R. (1979). Dysponesis: A neurophysiological factor in functional disorders. In Peper, E., Ancoli, S., & Quinn, M. (eds.), *Mind–Body Integration*. New York: Plenum Press.

Wheatley, C. E. (1975). Hyperventilation syndrome: A frequent cause of angina. *Chest*, 68: 195–199.

Wheeler, E. O., White, P. D., Reed, E. W., & Cohen, M. E. (1950). Neurocirculatory asthenia (anxiety neurosis, effort syndrome, neurasthenia). *Journal of the American Medical Association*, 142:878–889.

White, P. D. (1942). The soldier's irritable heart. *Journal of the American Medical Association*, 196:270.

White, P. D. & Hahn, R. G. (1929). The symptom of sighing in cardiovascular diagnosis with spirometric observations. *American Journal of Medicine and Science*, 177:179–183.

Whittier, J. R. & Drymiotis, A. D. (1962). Age differences in the human electroencephalographic response to hyperventilation. *Journal of Gerontology*, 17:461.

Wickramasekera, I. (1973). Temperature feedback for the control of migraine. *Journal of Behavior Therapy and Experimental Psychiatry*, 4:343–345.

Wildenthal, K., Fuller, D. S., & Shapiro, W. (1968). Paroxysmal atrial arrhythmias by hyperventilation. *American Journal of Cardiology*, 21:436–441.

Wilder, J. (1959). The law of initial value in neurology and psychiatry: Facts and problems. *Journal of Nervous and Mental Disorders*, 125:73–86.

Wilkinson, I. M. S., Bull, J. W. D., Du Boulay, G. H., Marshall, J., Russell, R. W. R., & Symon, L. (1969). Regional blood flow in the normal cerebral hemisphere. *Journal of Neurology, Neurosurgery and Psychiatry*, 32:367–378.

Williams, R. B., Lane, J. D., Kuhn, C. M., Melosh, W., White, A. D., & Schanberg, S. M. (1982). Type A behavior and elevated physiological and neuroendocrine responses to cognitive tasks. *Science*, 218:483–485.

Williams, A. J., Tarn, A. C., De Belder, M. A., & Bailey, A. J. (1982). Nalaxone in acute respiratory failure. *Lancet*, 2:1470.

Winslow, R. M. & Monge, C. (1978). *Hypoxia, Polycythemia, and Chronic Mountain Sickness.* Baltimore: The Johns Hopkins University Press.

Wirz-Justice, A., Krauchel, K., Lichtsteiner, M., & Feer, H. (1978). Is it possible to modify serotonin receptor sensitivity? *Life Science,* 25:1249–1254.

Withrow, C. D. (1972). Systemic carbon dioxide derangements. In Purpura, D. P., Penry, J. K., Tower, D. B., Woodbury, D. M., & Walters, R. D. (eds.), *Experimental Models of Epilepsy.* New York: Raven Press.

Wittkower, E. (1935). Studies on the influence of emotions on the functions of the organs. *Journal of Mental Science,* 81:533–682.

Wolfe, L. S. & Elliott, K. A. C. (1962). Chemical studies in relation to convulsive conditions. In Elliott, K. A. C. Page, I. H., & Quastel, J. H. (eds.), *Neurochemistry,* 2nd ed. Springfield, Ill: Charles C Thomas.

Wolff, H. G. & Lennox, W. S. (1930). Cerebral circulation: XII. The effect on pial vessels of variations in the oxygen and carbon dioxide content of blood. *Archives of Neurology and Psychology,* 23:1097–1120.

Wolkove, N., Kreisman, H., Darragh, D., Cohen, C., & Frank, H. (1984). Effect of transcendental meditation on breathing and respiratory control. *Journal of Applied Physiology,* 56:607–612.

Wolpe, J. (1958). *Psychotherapy by Reciprocal Inhibition.* Stanford: Stanford University Press.

Wolpe, J. (1969). *The Practice of Behavior Therapy,* 2nd ed. Elmsford, New York: Pergamon Press.

Wolpe, J. & Lazarus, A. A. (1966). *Behavior Therapy Techniques.* Elmsford, New York: Pergamon Press.

Wood, P. (1941). Da Costa's (or effort) syndrome. *British Medical Journal,* 1:767.

Woodbury, D. M. & Kemp, J. W. (1970). Some possible mechanisms of action of antiepileptic drugs. *Pharmacopsychiatry and Neuropharmacology,* 3:201–226.

Woods, S. W., Charney, S. S., Loke, J., Goodman, W. K., Redmond, D. E., & Heninger, G. R. (1986). Carbon dioxide sensitivity in panic anxiety. *Archives of General Psychiatry,* 43:900–909.

Woodson, R. D. (1979). Physiological significance of oxygen dissociation curve shifts. *Critical Care in Medicine,* 7:368–373.

Woodson, R. D., Torrance, J. D., Shappell, S. D., & Lenfant, C. (1970). The effect of cardiac disease on hemoglobin-oxygen binding. *Journal of Clinical Investigation,* 49:1349–1356.

Woolfolk, R. L. (1975). Psychophysiological correlates of meditation. *Archives of General Psychiatry,* 32:1326–1333.

Wyrwicka, W. & Sterman, M. B. (1968). Instrumental conditioning of sensorimotor cortex spindles in the waking cat. *Physiology of Behavior,* 3:703–707.

Wyss, O. A. M. (1955–1956). Synchronization of inspiratory motor activity as compared between phrenic and vagus nerve. *Yale Journal of Biological Medicine,* 28:471–480.

Yasue, H. (1980). Pathophysiology and treatment of coronary arterial spasm. *Chest,* 78:216–233.

Yasue, H., Nagao, M., Omote, S., Takizawa, A., Miwa, K., & Tanaka, S. (1978). Coronary artery spasm and Prinzmetal's variant form of angina induced by hyperventilation and tri-buffer infusion. *Circulation,* 58:56–62.

Youmans, W. B. (1975). *Fundamentals of Human Physiology,* 2nd ed. Chicago: Year Book Medical Publishers.

Yu, P. N. & Yim, B. J. (1958). Electrocardiographic changes in hyperventilation syndrome: Possible mechanisms and clinical implications. *Transact Association of American Physicians,* 71:129–141.

Yu, P. N., Yim, B. J., & Stansfield, C. A. (1959). Hyperventilation syndrome. *Archives of Internal Medicine,* 103:902–913.

Zajonc, R. B., Murphy, S. T., & Inglehart, M. (1989). Feeling and facial efference: Implications of the vascular theory of emotion. *Psychological Review*, 96:395–416.

Ziegler, L. H. & Cash, P. T. (1938). A study of the influence of emotions and affect on the surface temperature of the body. *American Journal of Psychiatry*, 95:677–696.

Zyzanski, S. J., Jenkins, C. D., Ryan, T. J., Flessas, A., & Everist, M. (1976). Psychological correlates of coronary angiography findings. *Archives of Internal Medicine*, 136:1234–1237.

Index